Osteoarthritis

Guest Editor

DAVID J. HUNTER, MBBS, MSc, PhD

MEDICAL CLINICS OF NORTH AMERICA

www.medical.theclinics.com

January 2009 • Volume 93 • Number 1

SAUNDERS an imprint of ELSEVIER, Inc.

W.B. SAUNDERS COMPANY
A Division of Elsevier Inc.

1600 John F. Kennedy Boulevard • Suite 1800 • Philadelphia, Pennsylvania 19103-2899

http://www.theclinics.com

MEDICAL CLINICS OF NORTH AMERICA Volume 93, Number 1
January 2009 ISSN 0025-7125, ISBN-13: 978-1-4377-0499-0, ISBN-10: 1-4377-0499-9

Editor: Rachel Glover
Developmental Editor: Theresa Collier

Medical Clinics of North America (ISSN 0025-7125) is published bimonthly by W.B. Saunders, 360 Park Avenue South, New York, NY 10010-1710. Business and editorial offices: 1600 John F. Kennedy Boulevard, Suite 1800, Philadelphia, PA 19103-2899. Accounting and circulation offices: 6277 Sea Harbor Drive, Orlando, FL 32887-4800. Periodicals postage paid at New York, NY, and additional mailing offices. Subscription prices are USD 187 per year for US individuals, USD 334 per year for US institutions, USD 96 per year for US students, USD 238 per year for Canadian individuals, USD 434 per year for Canadian institutions, USD 151 per year for Canadian students, USD 288 per year for international individuals, USD 434 per year for international institutions and USD 151 per year for international students. To receive student/resident rate, orders must be accompanied by name of affiliated institution, date of term, and the *signature* of program/residency coordinator on institution letterhead. Orders will be billed at individual rate until proof of status is received. Foreign air speed delivery is included in all *Clinics* subscription prices. All prices are subject to change without notice. POSTMASTER: Send address changes to *Medical Clinics of North America*, Elsevier Periodicals Customer Service, 11830 Westline Industrial Drive, St. Louis, MO 63146. Customer Service (orders, claims, online, change of address): Elsevier Periodicals Customer Service, 11830 Westline Industrial Drive, St. Louis, MO 63146. Tel: 1-800-654-2452 (U.S. and Canada); 314-453-7041 (outside U.S. and Canada). Fax: 314-453-5170. E-mail: journalscustomerservice-usa@elsevier.com (for print support); journalsonlinesupport-usa@elsevier.com (for online support).

Reprints. For copies of 100 or more of articles in this publication, please contact the Commercial Reprints Department, Elsevier Inc., 360 Park Avenue South, New York, NY 10010-1710. Tel.: 212-633-3812; Fax: 212-462-1935; E-mail: reprints@elsevier.com.

Medical Clinics of North America is also published in Spanish by McGraw-Hill Interamericana Editores S. A., P.O. Box 5-237, 06500 Mexico, D.F., Mexico.

Medical Clinics of North America is covered in *MEDLINE/PubMed (Index Medicus), Current Contents, ASCA, Excerpta Medica, Science Citation Index,* and *ISI/BIOMED.*

Printed and bound in the United Kingdom

Transferred to Digital Print 2011

THE CLINICS ARE NOW AVAILABLE ONLINE!
Access your subscription at:
www.theclinics.com

Contributors

GUEST EDITOR

DAVID J. HUNTER, MBBS, MSc, PhD
Chief, Division of Research, New England Baptist Hospital, Boston, Massachusetts

AUTHORS

KIM L. BENNELL, PhD
Centre for Health, Exercise and Sports Medicine, School of Physiotherapy, The University of Melbourne, Carlton, Victoria, Australia

KENNETH D. BRANDT, MD
Clinical Professor of Medicine, Kansas University Medical Center, Kansas City, Kansas; Professor (Emeritus) of Medicine; Professor (Emeritus) of Orthopaedic Surgery, Indiana University School of Medicine, Indianapolis, Indiana

DEBORAH BURSTEIN, PhD
Associate Professor, Department of Radiology, Beth Israel Deaconess Medical Center, Harvard Medical School, Boston, Massachusetts

PHILIP G. CONAGHAN, MBBS, PhD, FRACP, FRCP
Professor of Musculoskeletal Medicine, Section of Musculoskeletal Disease, University of Leeds, Leeds, United Kingdom

PAUL DIEPPE, MD
Honorary Professor of Musculoskeletal Sciences, University of Oxford, Nuffield Department of Orthopaedic Surgery, Nuffield Orthopaedic Centre, Oxford, United Kingdom

FELIX ECKSTEIN, MD
Professor, Institute of Anatomy and Musculoskeletal Research, Paracelsus Medical University, Salzburg, Austria

MARTIN ENGLUND, MD, PhD
Epidemiologist, Musculoskeletal Sciences, Department of Orthopedics, Lund University, Lund, Sweden; Clinical Epidemiology Research and Training Unit, Boston University School of Medicine, Boston, Massachusetts

K. DOUGLAS GROSS, PT, ScD
Assistant Professor, MGH Institute of Health Professions, Graduate Programs in Physical Therapy, Charlestown Navy Yard, Boston, Massachusetts

STEVEN R. GOLDRING, MD
Chief Scientific Officer; St. Giles Chair, The Hospital for Special Surgery, Weill College of Medicine of Cornell University, New York, New York

ALI GUERMAZI, MD
Associate Professor; Section Chief, Musculoskeletal; Director, Quantitative Imaging Center, Department of Radiology, Boston University School of Medicine, Boston, Massachusetts

WILLIAM F. HARVEY, MD
Division of Rheumatology, Tufts Medical Center, Boston, Massachusetts

MARIE-PIERRE HELLIO LE GRAVERAND-GASTINEAU, MD, DSc, PhD
Senior Director, Pfizer Global Research and Development,
New London, Connecticut

HOWARD HILLSTROM, PhD
Director, Hospital for Special Surgery, Leon Root, M.D., Motion Analysis Lab, The Dana Center, New York, New York

RANA S. HINMAN, PhD
Centre for Health, Exercise and Sports Medicine, School of Physiotherapy, The University of Melbourne, Carlton, Victoria, Australia

MICHAEL A. HUNT, PhD
Centre for Health, Exercise and Sports Medicine, School of Physiotherapy,
The University of Melbourne, Carlton, Victoria, Australia

DAVID J. HUNTER, MBBS, MSc, PhD
Chief, Division of Research, New England Baptist Hospital, Boston, Massachusetts

JAMES D. JOHNSTON, MSc
PhD Student, Departments of Orthopaedics and Mechanical Engineering, University of British Columbia, Vancouver, British Columbia, Canada

FRANCIS J. KEEFE, PhD
Pain Prevention and Treatment Research Program, Department of Psychiatry and Behavioral Sciences, Duke University Medical Center, Durham, North Carolina

HELEN KEEN, MBBS, FRACP
Consultant Rheumatologist, Department of Medicine, School of Medicine and Pharmacology, University of Western Australia, Perth, Australia

BOON-WHATT LIM, MSc
School of Sport, Health and Leisure, Republic Polytechnic, Singapore

GRACE H. LO, MD, MSc
Tufts Medical Center, Division of Rheumatology, Boston, Massachusetts

JASON J. McDOUGALL, BSc, PhD
Department of Physiology and Biophysics, Faculty of Medicine, University of Calgary, Calgary, Alberta, Canada

EMILY J. McWALTER, MASc
PhD Student, Departments of Orthopaedics and Mechanical Engineering, University of British Columbia, Vancouver, British Columbia, Canada

STEPHEN P. MESSIER, PhD
J.B. Snow Biomechanics Laboratory, Department of Health and Exercise Science, Wake Forest University, Winston-Salem, North Carolina

ERIC RADIN, MD
Adjunct Professor of Orthopedic Surgery, Tufts University School of Medicine, Marion, Massachusetts

JOHN C. RICHMOND, MD
Chairman, Department of Orthopedic Surgery, New England Baptist Hospital, Boston, Massachusetts

FRANK W. ROEMER, MD
Associate Professor; Co-Director, Quantitative Imaging Center, Department of Radiology, Boston University School of Medicine, Boston, Massachusetts

TIMOTHY D. SPECTOR, MD, FRCP
Twin Research and Genetic Epidemiology Unit, St. Thomas Hospital Campus, Kings College, London School of Medicine, London, United Kingdom

ANA M. VALDES, PhD
Senior Lecturer, Twin Research and Genetic Epidemiology Unit, St. Thomas Hospital Campus, Kings College, London School of Medicine, London, United Kingdom

DAVID R. WILSON, DPhil
Associate Professor, Department of Orthopaedics, University of British Columbia, Vancouver, British Columbia, Canada

TIM V. WRIGLEY, MSc
Centre for Health, Exercise and Sports Medicine, School of Physiotherapy, The University of Melbourne, Carlton, Victoria, Australia

Contents

> Because of the implications for prevention and treatment, how a clinician views osteoarthritis (OA) matters. We view OA as an attempt to contain a mechanical problem in the joint and as failed repair of damage caused by excessive mechanical stress on the joint. OA is organ failure of the synovial joint. Because of insufficient focus on reduction of the habitually loaded contact area of the joint and on aberrant loading, we believe that therapeutic efforts aimed at pathogenetic mechanisms in OA have been misdirected: neither the large role that a reduction of excessive levels of mechanical stress plays in promoting the healing response in OA nor the evidence that relief of joint pain and improvement in function, rather than the appearance of the articular surface, are the most important outcomes of the healing process have been sufficiently emphasized. Various mechanical abnormalities can trigger the processes involved in repair and attempts by the joint to contain the mechanical insult, but without a return to mechanical normality, attempts at healing will fail. In our view, drugs may be helpful symptomatically, but cannot accomplish this. In our view, as long as the joint remains in the same adverse mechanical environment that got it into trouble in the first place, it is unlikely that a drug that inhibits a specific enzyme or cytokine in the pathways of cartilage breakdown, or further stimulates the already increased synthesis of cartilage matrix molecules will solve the problem of OA. Also, because the subchondral bone is critically important in containing the mechanical abnormalities that damage the cartilage, emphasis on cartilage repair alone is likely to be futile. On the other hand, if the abnormal stresses on the joint are corrected, intervention with a structure-modifying drug may be superfluous.

> Much of the attention in developing diagnostic tools and therapeutic interventions for the management of osteoarthritis (OA) has focused on the preservation or repair of articular cartilage. It is clear that all of the joint components, including the ligaments, tendons, capsule, synovial lining, and periarticular bone, undergo structural and functional alterations during the course of OA progression. This article focuses on the specific skeletal features of OA and the putative mechanisms involved in their pathogenesis.

The history of treating meniscal lesions has been characterized by firm belief in "radical" surgery, with serious long-term consequences for the individual and society. The menisci play a critical protective role for the knee joint through shock absorption and load distribution. Currently, the consensus in surgical treatment of meniscal tears is to preserve as much functional meniscal tissue as possible. Still, meniscal lesions are common, especially in the osteoarthritic knee. For health professionals, these lesions present a challenge in choosing the treatment that is best for the patient in both the short term and long term. A degenerative lesion, in the middleaged or older patient, could suggest early-stage knee osteoarthritis and should be treated accordingly. Surgical resection of nonobstructive degenerate lesions may only remove evidence of the disorder while the osteoarthritis degradation proceeds. Well-designed randomized, controlled clinical trials are needed.

Osteoarthritis (OA) is the most prevalent form of arthritis in the elderly. A large body of evidence, including familial aggregation and classic twin studies, indicates that primary OA has a strong hereditary component that is likely polygenic in nature. Traits related to OA, such as longitudinal changes in cartilage volume and progression of radiographic features, are also under genetic control. In recent years several linkage analyses and candidate gene studies have been performed and unveiled some of the specific genes involved in disease risk, such as *FRZB* and *GDF5*. This article discusses the impact that future genome-wide association scans can have on our understanding of the pathogenesis of OA and on identifying individuals at high risk for developing severe OA.

Mechanics play a role in the initiation, progression, and successful treatment of osteoarthritis. However, we don't yet know enough about which specific mechanical parameters are most important and what their impact is on the disease process to make comprehensive statements about how mechanics should be modified to prevent, slow, or arrest the disease process. The objectives of this review are (1) to summarize methods for assessing joint mechanics and their relative merits and limitations, (2) to describe current evidence for the role of mechanics in osteoarthritis initiation and progression, and (3) to describe some current treatment approaches that focus on modifying joint mechanics.

> This article delineates the characteristic symptoms and signs associated with OA and how they can be used to make the clinical diagnosis. The predominant symptom in most patients is pain. The remainder of the article focuses on what we know causes pain in OA and contributes to its severity. Much has been learned over recent years; however, for the budding researcher much of this puzzle remains unexplored or inadequately understood.

> Osteoarthritis (OA) is the most prevalent joint disease; it is increasingly common in the aging population of Western society and has a major health economic impact. Despite surgery and symptom-oriented approaches there is no efficient treatment. Conventional radiography has played a role in the past in confirming diagnosis and demonstrating late bony changes and joint space narrowing. MRI has become the method of choice in large research endeavors and may become important for individualized treatment planning. This article focuses on radiography and MRI, with insight into other modalities, such as ultrasound, scintigraphy, and CT. Their role in OA diagnosis, follow-up, and research is discussed.

> This article presents a general outline for the management of the patient with osteoarthritis in the form of a narrative review considering diagnosis, investigation, and treatment. It is not a comprehensive discussion (subsequent articles on imaging, weight management, exercise, braces and orthotics, pharmacologic intervention, and surgery provide more detail); rather, it provides the clinician with an overview of what is available. Inevitably, there is much the interested clinician can do rather than practice nihilistic waiting. The authors encourage active clinician involvement and instilling self-management strategies in patients to further promote effective long-term treatment of this pervasive disease.

> The mechanisms by which obesity affects osteoarthritis (OA) are of great concern to osteoarthritis researchers and clinicians who manage this disease. Inflammation and joint loads are pathways commonly believed to cause or to exacerbate the disease process. This article reviews the physiologic and mechanical consequences of obesity in older adults who have knee OA, the effects of long-term exercise and weight-loss interventions,

the most effective nonpharmacologic treatments for obesity, and the use-fulness and feasibility of translating these results to clinical practice.

This article outlines the influence of muscle activity on knee-joint loading, describes the deficits in muscle function observed in people with knee osteoarthritis, and summarizes available evidence pertaining to the role of muscle in the development and progression of knee osteoarthritis. The article focuses on whether muscle deficits can be modified in knee osteoarthritis and whether improvements in muscle function lead to improved symptoms and joint structure. This article concludes with a discussion of exercise prescription for muscle rehabilitation in knee osteoarthritis.

Osteoarthritis (OA) is an epidemic for which there is no known cure. There is enormous popular demand for noninvasive and nonpharmacologic ther-apies for OA, and there is a pressing need for primary care physicians to respond by updating their pattern of practice. Despite increasing concern about the capacity of our health care system to meet rising demands, rou-tine primary care for knee OA has changed little over several decades. This article introduces physicians to many of the most important noninvasive devices used in the conservative management of symptomatic knee OA.

The most important goals of therapy in patients with osteoarthritis are pain management, improvement in function and disability, and, ultimately, dis-ease modification. This review discusses the current pharmacologic regi-men available to address these goals. Specific attention is paid to current trends and controversies related to pharmacologic management, includ-ing the use of oral, topical, and injectable agents.

The role of surgical treatment in osteoarthritis of the knee continues to evolve. The indications for arthroscopy have narrowed. Orthopedic sur-geons continue to explore options less invasive than total knee replace-ment for isolated unicompartmental arthritis of the knee joint. In addition to arthroscopy, this article discusses the merits and drawbacks of and in-dications for osteotomy, interpositional arthroscopy, patellofemoral re-placements, and emerging technologies for total knee replacements.

This review describes the potential of disease-modifying osteoarthritis drugs (DMOADs), distinguishing between preventing, retarding, stopping, and reversing disease and what might be clinically meaningful. The authors also describe whether there is any evidence to suggest that one can modify disease, and whether the current tissue that is predominantly focused on, namely, cartilage, is an appropriate target. The methodologic approaches and other obstacles to demonstrating efficacy of these agents in clinical trials are considered. This discussion is a narrative review in a field that is rapidly evolving. It is hoped the reader appreciates the complexity of the field and the likely road ahead to DMOAD development.

Preface

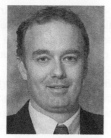

David J. Hunter, MBBS, MSc, PhD
Guest Editor

The evolution of our society has been accompanied by increasing obesity and aging, and, with this, increasing prevalence of osteoarthritis (OA). With these societal trends, new insights are developing into the pervasive disease we know as OA. Critically, the disease is no longer viewed as a passive, degenerative disorder, but rather an active disease process driven primarily by mechanical factors. Many define OA as a condition that primarily affects hyaline articular cartilage, including William Hunter, who in 1743 stated soberly "From Hippocrates to the present age it is universally allowed that ulcerated cartilage is a troublesome thing and that once destroyed, is not repaired."[1] We now conceptualize OA as a disease of the whole joint organ.

Drs. Brandt, Dieppe, and Radin have coauthored a provocative review critiquing the current definition and understanding of OA and providing important insights into the etiopathogenesis of the pathologic changes associated with disease, the tissue changes important for symptoms, and how this should inform disease management. Hopefully the diminishing remnants of our scientific community who hold so firmly to the centrality of cartilage and terms such as "degenerative and passive" will be better informed after reading this sagely work by founding members of our field.

With the centrality of cartilage now cast aside, and a more thoughtful focus on the whole joint organ, two tissues that are worthy of more extensive investigation include the bone and meniscus. Dr Goldring provides a stimulating review of the specific skeletal features of OA and the putative mechanisms involved in their pathogenesis. In addition, the relationship of these boney changes to the alterations in other tissues comprising the diarthrodial joint are appraised. Dr Englund has provided a thorough review of the critical role of meniscus in joint function, the role they play in the incipient development of OA, and the overwhelming need to preserve their integrity rather than the penchant to attribute knee symptoms to them and remove them.

OA has a strong hereditary component that is likely polygenic in nature. In recent years several linkage analysis and candidate gene studies have been carried out and unveiled some of the specific genes involved in disease risk. Much of this work

---

A version of this article originally appeared in the 34:3 issue of the *Rheumatic Disease Clinics of North America*.

Med Clin N Am 93 (2009) xv–xviii
doi:10.1016/j.mcna.2008.09.010
0025-7125/08/$ – see front matter © 2008 Elsevier Inc. All rights reserved.

has been led by Drs. Valdes and Spector, and in their considered review they appraise what we know and what impact future genome wide scans will have on providing further insights.

Mechanics plays a critical role in the initiation, progression, and successful treatment of OA. Dr. Wilson, a true pioneer in this field, and colleagues summarize the methods for assessing joint mechanics, describes the current evidence for the role of mechanics in OA initiation and progression, and further describes some current treatment approaches that focus on modifying joint mechanics.

OA causes substantial physical and psychosocial disability. I had the privilege of coauthoring a review with Drs. McDougall and Keefe that delineates the characteristic symptoms and signs associated with OA and how they can be used to make the clinical diagnosis. We also describe what we know causes pain in OA and what contributes to its severity.

Conventional radiography has played an important role in confirming the diagnosis of OA demonstrating late bony changes and joint space narrowing and has been applied as an endpoint for disease progression in clinical trials. However, OA is a disease of the whole joint, including cartilage, bone, and intra- and peri-articular soft tissues. Thus, the importance to image and assess all joint structures has been recognized in recent years largely using magnetic resonance imaging. Leaders in this field, Drs. Guermazi, Burstein, Conaghan, Eckstein, Hellio Le Graverand-Gastineau, Keen, and Roemer review radiography and MRI in OA and also give insight into other modalities (such as ultrasound, scintigraphy and computed tomography (CT), and CT-arthrography), discussing their role in the diagnosis, follow-up, and research in OA.

Sir William Osler, considered to be the "Father of Modern Medicine," once said "osteoarthritis is an easy disease to take care of—when the patient walks in the front door, I walk out the back door."[2] No one denies that the management of OA is a challenge, however modern clinicians are armed with a plethora of effective treatment options. We are also charged with discerning what agents are less effective yet still receive generous publicity rigorously eulogizing their benefits. The review of the management of OA provides an overview of what is available to the clinician managing OA. It is not comprehensive relying on subsequent articles (on imaging, weight management, exercise, braces and orthotics, pharmacologic intervention, and surgery) to provide more detail, but rather provides the clinician an opportunity to put the multitude of therapeutic options in perspective. I and Dr. Lo encourage active clinician involvement, to instill much of what are self-management strategies in patients, to further promote more effective long-term treatment of this pervasive disease.

For practicing clinicians, arming themselves with evidence for disease management is critical, and the ensuing articles—particularly those on obesity, muscle, and device use—are critical, as these are far too frequently overlooked in clinical practice. It is important that symptomatic improvement serve the purpose of increasing tolerance for functional activity. Ultimately, an efficacious treatment for any progressive disorder should also control the factors and forces that drive disease progression. These sections highlight this need.

The impact of and mechanisms by which obesity affects osteoarthritis are of great concern. Dr. Messier, a master in this field, reviews the physiologic and mechanical consequences of obesity on older adults with knee OA; the effects of long-term exercise and weight-loss interventions; the most effective nonpharmacological treatments for obesity; and the utility and feasibility of translating these results to clinical practice.

Drs. Bennell, Hunt, Wrigley, Lim, and Hinman provide a thorough review of the influence of muscle activity on knee joint loading, describe the deficits in muscle function observed in people with knee OA, and summarize available evidence pertaining to the role of muscle in the development and progression of knee OA. They focus on whether muscle deficits can be modified in knee OA and whether improvements in muscle function lead to improved symptoms and joint structure, then conclude with a discussion of exercise prescription for muscle rehabilitation in knee OA.

The goal of many noninvasive devices for knee OA is to alter joint biomechanics in such a way as to limit regional exposure to potentially damaging and provocative mechanical stresses. Because of their targeted intention, optimal prescription of most noninvasive devices requires that we first specify which mechanical stresses we wish to reduce, and in which knee region. Drs. Gross and Hillstrom lend their expertise and review several of the most important devices currently used in the treatment of knee OA.

Ultimately, many patients seek assistance for pain relief in the form of pharmacologic intervention. Dr. Harvey and I review the current trends and controversies related to pharmacologic management, including the use of oral, topical, and injectable agents.

Failing prior interventions for knee OA, surgery may become necessary. While the indications for arthroscopy have narrowed, joint replacement continues to play a pivotal role in disease management. Dr. Richmond reviews the plethora of surgical options and the evidence to support their efficacy. Orthopedic surgeons continue to explore options less invasive than total knee replacement for isolated unicompartmental arthritis of the knee joint.

The Holy Grail for many in this field is to modify the underlying structural changes. Dr. Hellio Le Graverand-Gastineau and I review the evidence to suggest we can modify the disease, and if the current tissue we are predominantly focused upon, namely cartilage, is an appropriate target. We will also consider the methodologic approaches and other obstacles to demonstrating efficacy of these agents in clinical trials.

Looking forward, we are reminded by the late Sir Henry Tizard that "the secret of science is to ask the right question, and it is the choice of problem more than anything else that marks the man of genius in the scientific world." We have been afforded an opportunity to study a much maligned disease that is rapidly evolving. Let's learn from the insights our research is providing to focus even more on important modifiable risk factors, such as mechanics and obesity, as we develop the therapeutic armamentarium of the 21st century. Assuming we maintain a meaningful motivation with the patient at the forefront of our mind, we have an opportunity to make a difference in millions of people's lives. I look forward to the evolution ahead.

I would sincerely like to thank my friends and colleagues for their valuable contributions to this issue of *Medical Clinics of North America*. They were a pleasure to work with, and I am sure you will see that the contents here reflect wonderful insight and appraisal of a complex and developing field.

David J. Hunter, MBBS, MSc, PhD
Division of Research
New England Baptist Hospital
125 Parker Hill Avenue
Boston, MA 02120, USA

E-mail address:
djhunter@caregroup.harvard.edu (D.J. Hunter)

REFERENCES

1. Buchanan WW. William Hunter (1718–1783). Rheumatology 2003;42(10):1260–1.
2. Balint G, Rooney PJ, Buchanan WW. A legacy for rheumatology from Sir William Osler. Clinical Rheumatology 1987;6(3):423–35.

Etiopathogenesis of Osteoarthritis

Kenneth D. Brandt, MD[a,b,*], Paul Dieppe, MD[c], Eric Radin, MD[d]

KEYWORDS

- Osteoarthritis • Joint failure
- Mechanical stress • Microklutz • Joint pain

CURRENT DEFINITIONS OF OSTEOARTHRITIS

In 1995, at a workshop of experts in osteoarthritis (OA) sponsored by the American Academy of Orthopaedic Surgeons; the National Institute of Arthritis, Musculoskeletal, and Skin Diseases; the National Institute on Aging; the Arthritis Foundation; and the Orthopaedic Research and Education Foundation, OA was defined as follows:

> Osteoarthritis is a group of overlapping distinct diseases which may have different etiologies, but with similar biologic, morphologic, and clinical outcomes. The disease processes not only affect the articular cartilage, but involve the entire joint, including the subchondral bone, ligaments, capsule, synovial membrane, and periarticular muscles. Ultimately, the articular cartilage degenerates with fibrillation, fissures, ulceration, and full thickness loss of the joint surface. OA diseases are a result of both mechanical and biologic events that destabilize the normal coupling of degradation and synthesis of articular cartilage of chondrocytes and extracellular matrix, and subchondral bone. Although they may be initiated by multiple factors, including genetic, developmental, metabolic, and traumatic, OA changes involve all of the tissues of the diarthrodial joint. Ultimately, OA diseases are manifested by morphologic, biochemical, molecular, and biomechanical changes of both cells and matrix which lead to a softening, fibrillation, ulceration, loss of articular cartilage, sclerosis and eburnation of subchondral bone, osteophytes, and subchondral cysts. When clinically evident, OA diseases

---

A version of this article originally appeared in the 34:3 issue of the *Rheumatic Disease Clinics of North America*.

Some of the thoughts expressed herein are contained in a chapter, "Neuromuscular Aspects of Osteoarthritis" written by Kenneth D. Brandt, that is to be published by Wiley-Blackwell in the book *Osteoarthritis Pain*, edited by D.T. Felson and H-G Schaible.

[a] Kansas University Medical Center, 5755 Windsor Drive, Fairway, Kansas City, KS 66205, USA
[b] Indiana University School of Medicine, Indianapolis, IN, USA
[c] University of Oxford, Nuffield Department of Orthopaedic Surgery, Nuffield Orthopaedic Centre, Windmill Road, Headington, Oxford, OX3 7LD, UK
[d] Tufts University School of Medicine, PO Box 561, Marion, MA 02738, USA
* Corresponding author.
E-mail address: kenbrandt@yahoo.com (K.D. Brandt).

Med Clin N Am 93 (2009) 1–24
doi:10.1016/j.mcna.2008.08.009
0025-7125/08/$ – see front matter © 2008 Elsevier Inc. All rights reserved.

are characterized by joint pain, tenderness, limitation of movement, crepitus, occasional effusion, and variable degrees of inflammation without systemic effects.[1]

Nine years earlier, the definition that emerged from a multidisciplinary workshop on the etiopathogenesis of OA sponsored by the National Institute of Arthritis, Diabetes, Digestive, and Kidney Diseases; the National Institute on Aging; the American Academy of Orthopaedic Surgeons; the National Arthritis Advisory Board; and the Arthritis Foundation was similarly comprehensive.[2]

Such inclusive definitions offer something for everyone but are not helpful in understanding the etiopathogenesis of OA. They emphasize joint damage, in general, and loss of articular cartilage, in particular, but fail to recognize an important point that is misunderstood by many clinicians: OA reflects a process within the joint that is attempting to contain damage caused by a local mechanical problem.

Furthermore, the current definitions do not distinguish between "garden-variety" OA (ie, the common clinical picture of the condition that is familiar to clinicians) and various similar joint diseases that are often labeled OA. For example, rare systemic diseases (eg, ochronosis, chondroepiphyseal dysplasia that results from a point mutation in a gene that codes for type II procollagen,[3] other collagen gene abnormalities, and Gaucher's disease) can all cause an arthritis that has radiographic features similar to those in garden-variety OA. They have phenotypes that differentiate them from the latter, however, and in our view should not be thought of as OA. Garden-variety OA itself is heterogeneous; it can arise from many different congenital, developmental, or acquired abnormalities that result in abnormal stress on the joint, such as an abnormal joint shape, obesity, trauma, instability, or micro-incoordination. The long-held distinction between primary and secondary OA is not meaningful: OA is always secondary to *something*, and usually to a combination of factors.

The definitions mentioned earlier say nothing about abnormal mechanics of the joint. The more recent definition considers OA to be the "...result of both mechanical and biologic events that destabilize..."[1] the normal metabolic equilibrium of cartilage and subchondral bone but, like its predecessor, does not mention joint biomechanics. **Box 1** lists several facts about OA that are not apparent in the current definitions.

Box 1
Key points that are not recognized by the current definitions of osteoarthritis

The clinical presentation of OA

There are multiple causes of OA

The most common clinical presentation (ie, garden-variety OA) can result from a wide variety of insults to the joint

Etiopathogenesis

OA is initiated by a mechanical insult to the joint

OA is a manifestation of attempts to heal the joint and ameliorate the abnormal biomechanics

The OA process may cause joint pain but is often successful in leading to a stable, painless joint

Radiology of OA

Radiographic changes of OA are extremely common in the population

Many people who have severe radiographic changes of OA are asymptomatic

Radiographic progression of OA is usually slow and may cease completely for many years

A CURRENT VIEW OF THE ETIOPATHOGENESIS OF OSTEOARTHRITIS

We view OA as a process that is attempting to contain a mechanical problem in the joint. We believe OA is best defined as failed repair of damage that has been caused by excessive mechanical stress (defined as force/unit area) on joint tissues. Because the body's innate mechanisms for repairing the damaged tissues cannot be effective in the face of the underlying mechanical abnormality, they cannot solve the problem of OA; for example, remodeling of subchondral bone may reduce the excessive stress and contain the mechanical abnormality, but may result in joint pain (see later discussion).

Because OA represents the failure of an organ (the synovial joint), any of the tissues of that organ may be the first to fail. It is to be expected, therefore, that there are many causes of OA, and there are. For this reason, OA has no common pathophysiologic pathway, but only a final common end stage.[4] The inflammatory changes in OA are secondary and are caused by particulate and soluble breakdown products of cartilage and bone. OA should not be considered to be a degenerative joint disease insofar as the cells of the cartilage and bone are normal and, if the high levels of intra-articular stress are reduced, can restore the damaged tissue to normal.[5] Furthermore, apart from the inaccuracy, consider the pessimism, sense of futility, and nihilism that are engendered in a patient who has painful OA when her physician tells her she has "degenerative joint disease."

The common mechanical factor underlying OA is a pathologic increase in intra-articular stress, which can result either from a decrease in the load-bearing area on the joint surface or a quantitative increase or qualitative aberration in joint loading (ie, repetitive impulsive loading).[6] Excessive loading of a joint, in and of itself, causes bone to fracture, rather than fracturing the cartilage.[7] In contrast, subfracture impulsive loads cause micro-injury of the subchondral bone and articular cartilage that may exceed the ability of the joint to repair the damage.

The capacity for intrinsic repair of damaged articular cartilage is limited, but if the local environment permits, cells that are extrinsic to the cartilage can provide a mechanism for repair.[5] Although the new cartilage they produce, fibrocartilage, is not histologically, biochemically, or biomechanically comparable to normal hyaline articular cartilage, in the presence of physiologic loading it nonetheless permits normal joint function, prevents further deterioration, and, most important, permits the patient to function asymptomatically.[5] Data indicate that joint healing in OA depends not only on a source of cells but also on normalization of intra-articular stress and movement of the joint.[8] Neither the large role that reduction of the excessive levels of mechanical stress plays in promoting the healing response in OA, nor evidence that relief of joint pain and improvement of function, rather than the histologic appearance of the articular surface, are the most important outcomes of the healing process, is sufficiently recognized.

The essential importance of abnormal joint mechanics in the etiopathogenesis of OA cannot be overemphasized. For example, in the classic experimental canine model of knee OA that is induced by transection of the anterior cruciate ligament, if loading of the unstable limb is markedly restricted by immobilization immediately after instability is created, OA does not develop.[9] Immobilization effectively reduces the instability and loss of the load-bearing surface and the stresses on joint tissues that exceed physiologic limits.

On the other hand, when stresses on joint tissues exceed physiologic limits (eg, because of obesity, varus-valgus malalignment, meniscus damage, or developmental or genetic factors) and overwhelm the protective mechanisms, OA ensues. In cases of OA such as those mentioned above, even though loads on the joint may be physiologic, the accumulation of abnormal biomaterials in joint tissues (eg, polymers of homogentisic acid oxidase in ochronosis) results in abnormal tissue mechanics and, eventually, breakdown of the joint.

The cells in cartilage and bone in an OA joint are essentially normal but in highly loaded areas of the joint they seem abnormal because they are literally being crushed. If the abnormal joint mechanics can be restored to a physiologic range, joints can heal.[5] Although the process is slow, the fibrocartilage and woven bone that have been mistakenly characterized as a failed attempt at healing are clinically functional and may be associated with symptomatic relief. If normal joint mechanics can be sustained, these transitional tissues may eventually remodel into normal hyaline cartilage and trabecular bone.[5]

Eventually, all of the tissues of the joint are involved in OA, including synovium, periarticular muscle, nerves, ligaments, and, if present, meniscus, along with the articular cartilage and subchondral bone. It follows that the focus of clinical management and OA research should be on limiting and treating the increased intra-articular stress that is causing joint damage rather than, almost exclusively, as is currently the case, on the loss of articular cartilage.

Because OA is more than a cartilage problem,[10] it is notable in the above context that although the impression is widespread that Heberden nodes, which are generally interpreted as a manifestation of OA of the distal interphalangeal joints (DIPJs) and have been reported to be a risk factor for incident knee OA[11] and for the progression of established knee OA,[12] can be associated with various DIPJ pathologies.[13] One of the slides that was included in the section on degenerative joint disease in the 1972 Arthritis Foundation Clinical Teaching Collection, depicting a histologic section through a Heberden node (**Fig. 1**),[14] illustrates this point.

The slide shows a prominent osteophyte at the articular margin of the distal phalanx that is unaccompanied by changes in either the surface integrity or the thickness of the load-bearing articular cartilage or by thickening of the subchondral bone which, in combination, are pathognomonic for OA. We believe that the slide does not show an OA joint but is consistent with observations that osteophytes are not

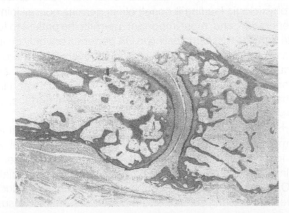

Fig. 1. Histologic section through a distal interphalangeal joint of a patient who had nodal "OA." A prominent dorsal osteophyte is present but there is no thinning of the articular cartilage or loss of surface integrity and no thickening of the subchondral bone (pathognomonic features of OA). (*From* The American College of Rheumatology Clinical Slide Collection. Atlanta (GA): American College of Rheumatology; © 1972–2004 American College of Rheumatology Slide Collection. Used with permission.)

pathognomonic for OA. Hernborg and Nilsson[15] concluded in 1973 that, in the absence of other bony changes (ie, subchondral sclerosis or cysts), knee osteophytes may be a manifestation of aging, rather than of OA.

We suggest that our long-standing inability to effectively manage patients who have OA pharmacologically is the result of a persistent overemphasis on articular cartilage as the major focus of OA damage and on cartilage in the progression of joint failure. Excessive emphasis has been placed also on the inflammatory phase of OA. It has been insufficiently appreciated that the synovial joint is an organ, that OA is organ failure, and that it can be initiated by abnormalities arising in any of its tissues. In our view, our failure to focus on the reduction in the contact area in the joint and on aberrant joint loading has misdirected our therapeutic efforts in OA.

We believe that effecting cures that aim at the causes of OA requires the understanding that OA can be the result of traumatic joint damage or inherited predilections. Many of the cases of OA that do not follow significant (macro) joint injury may be related to abnormalities in genes that create or promote the development of structurally abnormal joints that result in aberrant loads or increased intra-articular stress, leading to cumulative tissue microdamage and remodeling that are detrimental to joint function.[16]

Not all abnormal joints develop OA, however. Among subjects who had hip dysplasia, slipped capital femoral epiphysis, or Legg-Calve-Perthes disease in childhood, the frequency of OA at a 30-year follow-up evaluation was 60% to 70%, not 100%.[17] Although all had hips that were at increased risk for developing OA, the likelihood that a predisposed individual developed OA was presumably affected by the severity of the structural abnormality, the amount of repetitive unprotected loading, and the adequacy of the mechanisms that normally protect joints from excessive mechanical stress (see later discussion).

ARTICULAR CARTILAGE HEALING AND REMODELING: MECHANOBIOLOGY OF THE CHONDROCYTE

The remodeling of connective tissues requires removal of damaged matrix to allow for its replacement. Inflammation and alterations of cell metabolism are an essential part of this healing process. In a normal joint, articular cartilage chondrocytes are subjected to physiologic dynamic and static compressive and deep shear stresses. This physical perturbation of the chondrocytes is associated with changes in expression of genes for aggrecan, collagen, matrix metalloproteinases, growth factors, and cytokines that are transduced into metabolic responses.[18]

The rate of loading may be more injurious to cartilage than the magnitude of the load. When normal rabbits were subjected to repeated acute (50 milliseconds, onset to peak) impulsive loading of the knee (ie, square wave loading), the articular cartilage and subchondral bone were damaged. Loads of greater magnitude, when applied more gradually (500 milliseconds, onset to peak, [ie, sine wave loading]) had no adverse effect.[19] Rapid delivery of load does not permit sufficient time for periarticular muscle, the major shock absorber protecting the joint (see later discussion), to prepare for and absorb the load.[20]

In vitro, a single injurious compression of a cartilage explant resulted in a 250-fold increase in expression of the gene for matrix metalloproteinase-3 (stromelysin), 40-fold increase in gene expression for ADAMTS-5 (aggrecanase), and 12-fold increase in gene expression for tissue inhibitor of matrix metalloproteinases (TIMP).[21] Changes of this proportion in the quantities of the relevant proteins that are expressed could lead to breakdown of the articular cartilage matrix. We consider the metabolic responses of articular cartilage to mechanical injury as evidence of an attempt by the chondrocytes to repair damage to the extracellular matrix. The criteria for identifying cartilage injury, however, may not be sufficiently sensitive to detect microdamage.[21]

The effect on joint cartilage of loading forces and of cytokines (eg, tumor necrosis factor, interleukin-1) that are involved in the healing of subfracture levels of damage may be additive.[22] Observations suggest that beyond the direct effects of the mechanical insult to the cartilage itself, the capsule/synovium of the OA joint may contribute to degradation of the damaged cartilage in an attempt to heal the joint.

Although dose-response curves that are relevant to loading of joint cartilage in vivo are not well defined, the data suggest that the breakdown of OA cartilage is mediated by matrix metalloproteinases whose production is stimulated by interleukin-1 and tumor necrosis factor, and that these cytokines could be produced by the chondrocytes themselves in response to mechanical loads. It is reasonable to consider that the process may be driven by abnormal mechanical stresses on the joint that arise, eg, as a result of muscle weakness or neuropathy that interfere with protective muscular reflexes,[23] or ligamentous instability.

Changes seen in organ culture in vitro are not identical to what happens in an OA joint in vivo. Excessive loading of a joint leads to fracture of the bone before it produces obvious damage to the articular cartilage.[7] Although metalloproteinases can weaken the mechanical integrity of articular cartilage in OA, mechanical factors would seem to play the major role; pharmacologic inhibition of metalloproteinases has by no means been uniformly successful in halting the progression of OA.[24,25] Based on the readily apparent shards of articular cartilage embedded in OA synovium[26] and the duplication and advance of the tidemark,[27,28] much of the loss of articular cartilage in OA seems to be attributable to the breaking off, like icebergs from a glacier, of enzymatically weakened segments of the joint surface. Although vertical splits (fibrillation) in the proteoglycan-depleted cartilage can persist without fragmentation of the joint surface, the thinned cartilage is subject also to deep horizontal splits (**Fig. 2**).[29] When these join with the common vertical splits, the result is the breaking off of cartilage shards that may be detected in the synovial fluid before they become incorporated into the synovial membrane, where they incite inflammation. In addition, endochondral ossification, due to reactivation of the secondary center of ossification, moves toward the joint surface with duplication and advance of the tidemark, gradually thinning the cartilage from below.[27] Most of the loss of articular cartilage in OA seems to be attributable to these two processes.

WHY DOES ANY OF THIS MATTER? LACK OF RELEVANCE OF CHONDROPROTECTIVE DRUGS TO THE UNDERLYING PROCESS

How a clinician views OA matters, in particular, because of the implications for treatment of patients. Because synovial inflammation in OA is secondary to mechanical damage to the cartilage and bone (see later discussion), it stands to reason that nonsteroidal anti-inflammatory drugs (NSAIDs), although they may be symptomatically effective, cannot arrest the process. Efforts to develop disease-modifying OA drugs that can interrupt or reverse the pathogenetic processes underlying OA have not been unambiguously effective.[24,25] We believe the reason for this lack of success is our failure to appreciate sufficiently that OA, from its earliest stages and in whichever joint it occurs, is mechanically induced.[10,25]

Various mechanical abnormalities can trigger the many processes involved in joint repair and attempts to contain the mechanical insult. Without a return to mechanical normality, however, attempts at healing fail. Drugs cannot accomplish this. As long as the joint remains in the same adverse mechanical environment that got it into

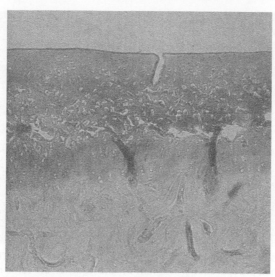

Fig. 2. Histologic section of articular cartilage from a rabbit whose hind limb has been subjected to repetitive impulsive loading (see Ref.[19]). In addition to vertical splits (fibrillation) at the surface, horizontal tears are apparent running near the base of the cartilage. In OA, when horizontal tears join with the vertical fissures they result in fragmentation of the joint surface and are responsible for the presence of particulate cartilage debris in the synovial space, which may then become incorporated into the synovial membrane and cause synovitis, as may soluble breakdown products of cartilage matrix molecules (safranin O–fast green, original magnification ×25). (*Courtesy of* D.B. Burr, PhD, Department of Anatomy, Indiana University School of Medicine, Indianapolis, IN.)

trouble in the first place, we consider it highly unlikely that a drug that, for example, inhibits a specific enzyme or cytokine in the pathways of cartilage breakdown or further stimulates the already increased synthesis of cartilage matrix molecules by the chondrocytes will solve the problem of OA. Indeed, if the increased joint stresses are normalized, such drugs may be superfluous. In addition, because the subchondral bone is critical for containment of the mechanical abnormalities that damage the articular cartilage, emphasis on cartilage repair alone is likely to be futile.

In our view, the genes whose identification will be required to allow us to get at the root problems in OA are not the genes that regulate chondrocyte metabolism. Rather, it will be those genes that control developmental and congenital deformities that lead to a reduction in the habitually loaded area of the joint surface and result in the concentration of peak dynamic loads, or the genes that create microincoordination ("microklutziness") during physical activity.[6]

Lowering the stress on a joint can result in healing of OA.[5] Notably, healing can be brought about only by mechanical means; drugs have not been shown to accomplish this. Although arthroplasty (essentially, an amputation of the joint and replacement with a prosthesis) is the popular current treatment of OA, with a carefully executed osteotomy the load-bearing surface can be increased (**Fig. 3**) or the force of a selected muscle acting across a joint reduced by increasing its leverage or weakening the muscle by lengthening.[30,31]

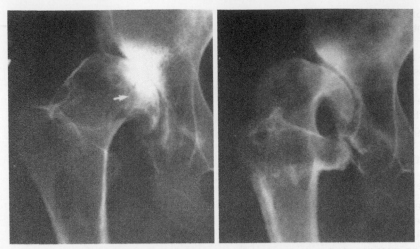

Fig. 3. Radiographs of a patient who had hip dysplasia that led to OA. The radiograph on the left was obtained preoperatively. The film on the right, of the same hip, was obtained 7 years after a successful osteotomy. At surgery, the alignment of the femur was altered so that the large, inferomedial beak osteophyte was shifted to the load-bearing region of the joint. Note the marked decrease in subchondral sclerosis and the widening of the joint space after surgery. (*From* Maquet P. Biomechanics of the hip as applied to osteoarthritis and related conditions. Berlin: Springer; 1985. p. 114. With the kind permission of Springer Science and Business Media, and of Dr. Maquet.)

WHY DON'T WE ALL DEVELOP PROGRESSIVE OSTEOARTHRITIS? MECHANISMS PROTECTING THE JOINT FROM MICRODAMAGE

In normal walking, 3 to 4 times the weight of the body is transmitted through the knee; during a deep knee bend, the patellofemoral joint is subjected to a load 9 to10 times body weight. Adaptive mechanisms must protect the joint from these physiologic loads. Although the bulk properties of articular cartilage would make it an excellent shock absorber, at most sites it is too thin to serve as much of a shock-absorbing structure in a joint.

Periarticular Muscle as a Shock Absorber for the Joint

The body's most active shock-absorbing mechanisms for joints are the use of muscles and joint motion. Although contraction of muscles can move a joint, muscles can also act as large rubber bands. When a slightly stretched muscle is subjected to greater stretch as a result of movement of a joint, it can absorb a large amount of energy. Most of the muscle activity generated during activity is not used to propel the body forward but to absorb energy to decelerate the body.[32]

For example, when we jump off a ledge or table we normally land on our toes, come down on our heels, and straighten our flexed knees and hips. During this smooth action our muscles perform negative work (ie, they absorb energy). As we dorsiflex our ankles, we stretch our calf muscles; as we straighten our knees and hips we stretch our hamstrings. The amount of energy absorbed as a result of this is enormous.[33] The energy produced by normal walking is sufficient to tear all the ligaments of the knee; that this does not occur routinely attests to the importance and effectiveness of this active energy absorption mechanism in the muscles that surround our joints and cushion them from mechanical stress.

Small, unexpected loads for which we are unprepared are much more damaging to joints than large ones that we have anticipated. Consider what happens when we come down stairs, misjudge a step, and abruptly skip a step. Because our muscles are not prepared to accommodate the load, we feel a sharp jolt. To prepare a neuro-muscular reflex to handle an impact load requires approximately 75 milliseconds. A fall of brief duration (e.g, of only about 1 in) does not afford sufficient time to bring protec-tive muscular reflexes into play.[20] Under such conditions, the load is transmitted to the cartilage and bone. In contrast, during an unexpected fall from a slightly greater height, sufficient time is available for activation of the appropriate reflexes so that the lengthening of the muscles that cross the joint results in protection of its articular cartilage by absorbing the energy of impact.[33]

The Quadriceps Muscle: Implications for Knee Osteoarthritis

Quadriceps weakness (see later discussion) or an increase in the latent period of the reflex, which may occur with peripheral neuropathy because of aging or other causes, reduces the effectiveness of the above shock-absorbing mechanism.

The quadriceps muscle protects the knee from mechanical damage because it is the major antigravity muscle of the lower extremity and serves as a brake on the pendular action of the lower limb during ambulation, thereby minimizing the forces generated with heelstrike. In addition, it is important in stabilizing the knee. Quadri-ceps weakness may thus generate abnormal mechanical stresses on the joint.

After a femoral nerve block (to temporarily paralyze the quadriceps), the load rate in normal subjects who had no force-transient profile during gait increased more than twofold—to approximately 150 times body weight/sec[34] The data suggest that a force transient can be caused by failure to decelerate the lower extremity before heelstrike. In normal individuals, minor incoordination in muscle recruitment, resulting in failure to decelerate the leg before heelstrike, may generate rapidly applied impulsive forces at the knee that are as high as 65 times body weight/sec.[6] Whether the microincoordina-tion of muscular control in some normal humans that results in generation of a heel-strike transient at the knee with walking is a risk factor for knee pain or for structural changes of knee OA remains to be established in prospective longitudinal studies.

Although the periarticular muscles serve a primary motor function, Hurley[35] has emphasized the importance of the sensory function of muscle and of the propriocep-tive impulses that originate in muscle and are transmitted to the central nervous system. Data suggest that muscle weakness due to reflex inhibition of muscle contraction because of intra-articular pathology may result in joint degeneration.

Quadriceps weakness is common in patients who have knee OA, in whom it has generally been considered to arise as a consequence of the pain that occurs with load-ing of the arthritic joint, which leads the patient to minimize load bearing, thereby lead-ing to atrophy. It may exist also in subjects who have knee OA who have no history of joint pain, however, and in whom quadriceps muscle mass is not diminished but is normal or even increased (as a result of obesity).[36] Longitudinal studies suggest that quadriceps weakness may not only result from painful knee OA but may itself be a risk factor for structural damage.[36–38] Among women who had no radiographic evidence of knee OA at the initial examination but who had developed OA changes some 30 months later, baseline knee extensor strength was significantly lower than that in women who did not develop radiographic changes of OA.[36] When the presence of knee OA (based on radiographic changes, with or without knee pain) as a function of sex, body weight, age, and lower extremity strength was modeled, it was found that each 10 lb/ft increase in knee extensor strength was associated with a 20% reduction in the odds of developing radiographic OA and 29% reduction in the odds of developing symptomatic knee OA. A relatively small increase in strength (approximately 20% of the mean for men and 25% for women) was predicted to result in a 20% to 30% decrease in the odds of having knee OA.[36]

Although the question has not been examined, the shock-absorbing function of periarticular muscle in protecting joints other than the knee is likely to be important also. The expression of OA with respect to, for example, the frequency and severity of joint pain and the rate of progression of joint damage, may vary at different joint sites and some of this variability may be because of the adequacy of the physiologic shock-absorbing mechanisms that protect the joint.

As we get older our nervous systems, like our muscles, age, leaving us not only with less strength but also with less coordination and poorer proprioception, all of which may result in microincoordination. This change may help explain the strong association between OA and age.

Subchondral Bone as a Passive Shock Absorber for the Joint

The normal joint

Normally, in the unloaded state, the opposing surfaces of a joint are incongruent. Under load, the cartilage and bone on both sides of the joint space deform, maximizing the contact area and thereby minimizing the stress within the cartilage.[39] This normal deformation of the articular cartilage when it is subjected to a compressive load provides the self-pressurized hydrostatic weeping lubrication needed for effortless motion. With increasing load, however, cartilage deformation alone is insufficient; deformation of the underlying bone must also occur and, under high loads, is more important than deformation of cartilage in reducing stress.

Joint damage due to excessive loading is related to the rate, and not only the magnitude, of loading because the chondroprotective effect of the shock-absorbing capacity of subchondral bone becomes limited as the bone becomes thicker and sclerotic.[40] In brief, normal subchondral bone is viscoelastic (ie, it deforms less, or becomes limited as the bone becomes stiffer, when load is applied rapidly than when it is loaded more gradually). Rapid loading of the joint does not allow time for the viscoelastic flow of interstitial fluid out of the bone, which would absorb the energy transmitted and protect the cartilage matrix and chondrocytes. If deformation under an impulsive load is restricted, therefore, the cartilage does not conform completely to the load, the size of the contact area is restricted, and high stresses are generated in the cartilage matrix. This process is exacerbated by thinning of the cartilage and is the reason that rapid impulsive loading is eventually detrimental to the integrity of the articular cartilage.

The cancellous subchondral bone, although 10 times stiffer than the cartilage, is much softer than cortical bone and serves as a major shock absorber. Because the cartilage is too thin to function effectively as a shock absorber, the subchondral bone, by providing a pliable bed that absorbs energy, protects it from damage caused by repetitive impulse loads,[39] which are capable of fracturing the subchondral trabeculae.

Theoretically, the transfer of load from the articular surface to the diaphyseal cortex should create large shear stresses in the subchondral bone, particularly under the edges of the contact area.[41] Because of the undulations of the tidemark and the osteochondral junction, however, the interposed zone of calcified cartilage, whose stiffness is intermediate between that of the overlying hyaline cartilage and underlying subchondral bone,[42] tends to transform these shear stresses into compressive and tensile stresses,[43] which the articular cartilage is better able to withstand.

Joint lubrication is so effective that shear forces along the surface of the cartilage are unlikely.[44] Furthermore, by constraining radial deformation of the cartilage under load,[45] the existence of subchondral bone raises the threshold for cartilage damage. Grasping with the hand, for example, or walking (in most normal individuals) does not generate impulsive loads on contact of the joint surfaces.[6] The joint can withstand up to five times the peak deformation that occurs with walking, suggesting that normal subchondral bone can protect it from all but impulsive loads. The reason for this is that bone, like cartilage, is viscoelastic (ie, the fluid in the tissue acts to dampen the effects of loading).

With rapidly applied impulsive loads, however, the viscoelasticity of the tissue becomes problematic. Viscoelastic damping requires time to have an effect: fluid must flow. About one third of normal adults have been shown to exhibit microklutziness.[6] In these individuals, the important muscle-based protective mechanisms needed to dampen the forces of joint loading are not fully coordinated. They, therefore, subject their knees to impulsive loading during walking. The consequence of impulsive loading is that the subchondral bone takes the brunt of the blow and, along with the calcified cartilage, sustains microdamage. If this is repetitive, it causes reactivation of the secondary center of ossification and remodeling of the subchondral bone, with advance of the tidemark leading to thinning of the articular cartilage.[27]

The osteoarthritic joint

Normal subchondral bone attenuates loads through the joint more than either the articular cartilage or surrounding soft tissues.[46] In a normal joint, it absorbs up to 50% of the load and the cartilage only 1% to 3%.[46,47] In an OA joint, however, the sclerotic subchondral bone is less able to absorb and dissipate the energy of an impulsive load, increasing the force transmitted through the joint. The OA knee therefore absorbs only about half as much load as a normal knee.[47] As noted by Burr,[48] the total volume of subchondral trabecular bone in OA increases by an average of 10% to 15%, chiefly because of thickening of the trabeculae and some increase in the number of trabeculae and reduction in trabecular separation. This process is reflected by the subchondral sclerosis that is a cardinal radiographic feature of OA and by an increase in the apparent density (bone volume/total volume of the tissue) of OA bone, in comparison with normal bone. Because the subchondral bone in OA is actively remodeling in response to the increased mechanical stress, however, much of the newly formed bone does not have sufficient time to fully mineralize. From a material standpoint, however, it is less highly mineralized, and less stiff, than bone from age-matched nonarthritic controls.[49,50] To retain a normal degree of tissue stiffness, or even that seen in osteoporosis, the volume of subchondral bone in an OA joint must increase markedly, to at least twice that in a normal joint.[48]

An earlier hypothesis that stiffened subchondral bone, present in the OA joint as a consequence of the healing of cumulative microfractures, drives the destruction of the overlying articular cartilage was not supported by finite element models, which have shown that even a marked increase in the density of subchondral bone would cause only a modest increase in mechanical stress in the overlying cartilage.[51] The amount of stiffening of the bone required to significantly increase stresses in the cartilage is far beyond that which is likely to occur in vivo. Although stiffening of subchondral bone may be an important feature of OA, these data suggest that, on a mechanical basis, it alone is not sufficient to account for destruction of the articular cartilage.[28] It is the thinning of the cartilage as the subchondral bone thickens and advances toward the joint space that eventually causes the cartilage to fragment.

Microcracks in the subchondral bone or calcified cartilage stimulate focal remodeling and account for increased vascularity in OA joints. They are found routinely in calcified cartilage from femoral heads of middle-aged nonarthritic humans and are associated with foci of remodeling in OA cartilage.[48] Single or repetitive high-impact loads have been shown to cause microcracks,[52] which are followed by remodeling of the subchondral bone and degeneration of the overlying cartilage. Microdamage in the calcified cartilage caused by mechanical stress, and the ensuing endochondral ossification, may thus play a vital role in the pathogenesis of OA.

With remodeling and disruption of the articular plate by microfractures, bone necrosis, as reflected by empty lacunae devoid of osteocytes, is seen in association with extensive resorption, repair, and apposition of new bone on the existing subchondral trabeculae. Scintigraphy may show a generalized subarticular zone of increased uptake, whose presence correlates with pain on loading of the joint, subchondral sclerosis, and progression of the structural damage of OA.[53] The appearance is different from that of primary osteonecrosis, however, in which a sequestrum of subchondral bone underlies viable articular cartilage. The contribution of this secondary osteonecrosis to collapse of the articular surface in OA is unclear, but it has been considered to be related to occlusion of small intramedullary arteries and has been reported to occur in nearly one of every six femoral heads resected surgically for advanced OA.[54]

Whether changes in the subchondral bone precede or follow those in the overlying cartilage in OA is unclear. It is likely that both sequences occur.[55–58] Even in circumstances in which bony changes are not involved in the initiation of cartilage damage, however, they are critically important in the progression of cartilage breakdown in OA.

ETIOPATHOGENESIS OF OSTEOARTHRITIS PAIN

For the patient and clinician, the essential problem associated with OA is joint pain. If OA were not painful, it would receive little attention. Liang[59] succinctly captured the issue: "...x-rays don't weep." Patients weep.

Among people who have OA, those who have more severe radiographic changes are somewhat more likely to have difficulty with mobility, but the radiographic progression of OA is usually slow and the course is unpredictable.[60] Symptoms wax and wane independent of radiographic progression.[61] Among people who have far advanced radiographic changes of hip OA, nearly half may not have hip pain.[62,63] On the other hand, the overall prevalence of radiographic OA is high: the Framingham study suggested it occurs in one third of all people aged 63 years and older.[64] Even if joint pain occurs in only a minority of these individuals, the absolute numbers are so large as to present a major public health problem with huge medicoeconomic and socioeconomic costs.

At different joint sites, the balance of risk factors for OA, symptomatic presentation, relationship between radiographic changes and symptoms, and rate of progression vary. For example, radiographic OA of the elbow is seldom symptomatic and hip OA tends to progress much more rapidly than knee OA.

In view of the poor correlation between symptoms and radiographic changes of OA, it is notable that criteria for case definition have traditionally relied on the presence of radiographic features of OA. Use of radiographic criteria to define cases of OA for clinical studies or as the sole criterion for surgical intervention has serious limitations, however. The association between radiographic changes of OA and reported pain in the hip or knee may be statistically significant in groups of people but in an individual patient the correlation between the severity of radiographic changes (ie, structural damage) and the severity of symptoms is often poor. At the community level many people who have an advanced grade of radiographic OA have no symptoms.

Given that the real problem is, in fact, not radiographic OA, but painful OA, it is also notable that although current reports of OA research often contain a statement to the effect that OA is not merely a disease of cartilage, but of the entire joint, the large amounts of time, money, and brainpower that are invested in efforts to develop a chondroprotective drug, image miniscule (and clinically meaningless) changes in articular cartilage, and identify markers of cartilage damage in body fluids suggest that this proposition is not really accepted. Current textbooks discuss in detail the biochemical changes associated with the breakdown of articular cartilage in OA.[65–67] Biochemists and molecular biologists studying cartilage or bone from OA joints, investigators imaging OA joints, and those assaying biologic fluids for molecules derived from the tissues of OA joints have yet to explain why some OA joints are painful and others are not. Anxiety, depression, and quadriceps weakness may be better predictors of pain in subjects who have knee OA than the severity of radiographic changes.[68] Understanding the etiopathogenesis of OA pain may be much more relevant than understanding the mechanisms of articular cartilage breakdown in this disease.

The pathogenesis and the tissue origins of OA pain may vary from patient to patient and, within the same patient, from visit to visit. A variety of evidence points to the synovium and subchondral bone as the major sources of joint pain in patients who have OA, but ligaments, menisci, periarticular muscles, entheses, and joint capsules can all be painful.

Synovitis

The synovial membrane from patients who have advanced OA commonly exhibits hyperplasia of the lining cell layer and focal infiltration of lymphocytes and monocytes. In advanced OA the intensity of the synovitis may resemble that in rheumatoid arthritis. Synovitis in OA may be due to phagocytosis of wear particles of cartilage and bone from the abraded joint surface[26,69,70], release from the cartilage of soluble matrix macromolecules[71] (eg, proteoglycans, collagen, fibronectin fragments), or the presence of crystals of calcium pyrophosphate dihydrate or calcium hydroxyapatite.[72] In some cases, immune complexes containing antigens derived from the cartilage matrix may be sequestered in collagenous tissue of the joint, such as meniscus, leading to chronic low-grade inflammation.[73]

Earlier in the course of OA, however, the synovium—even from symptomatic patients who have full-thickness ulceration of their articular cartilage—may be histologically normal, suggesting that the early pain in those cases is not attributable to synovitis.[74] Conversely, in patients who have knee OA who have no joint pain, the severity of articular cartilage damage and of synovitis may be as great as in those who have knee pain.

Synovitis is an important cause of pain in patients who have OA, however. In cross-sectional MRI analyses of subjects who had knee OA, synovial thickening was much more common in those who had pain than in those who were asymptomatic and, among those who had knee pain, was associated with more severe pain.[75] Furthermore, in a 30- month longitudinal study of patients who had symptomatic knee OA,[76] changes in synovitis, as graded by MRI, correlated only modestly with changes in knee pain. The relatively weak correlation suggests that synovitis was not the only, or even the major, cause of the joint pain. Furthermore, pain was not correlated with the loss of articular cartilage in either the tibiofemoral or patellofemoral compartment and changes in synovial effusion were not correlated with changes in pain. In contrast, in a sample of symptomatic subjects from the Osteoarthritis Initiative (OAI), Lo and colleagues[77] found that maximal joint effusion scores on MRI were highly associated with knee pain even after adjustment for bone marrow lesion (BML) scores, suggesting that effusion (a manifestation of underlying synovitis) was independently associated with knee pain.

We expressed previously our reservations about the success of pharmacologic modification of joint damage in OA unless a more favorable local mechanical environment is established. Among these reservations is that it is by no means established that a chondroprotective drug would ameliorate symptoms. If such an agent stabilized the cartilage surface, some have suggested that it might reduce that component of joint pain caused by synovitis attributable to the breakdown of cartilage and bone. There is no reason to believe it would reduce pain due to the reaction to phlogistic breakdown products that had already been incorporated by the synovium. In addition, in the face of increased intra-articular stress, the assumption that pharmacologic chondroprotection is feasible is questionable.

Subchondral Bone

In the 1930s the French found that drilling a hole in the femoral head (fomage), which is performed today for some patients who have osteonecrosis of the femoral head, relieved pain in some patients who had early hip OA, at least temporarily.[78] The procedure was adopted for a time by the Mayo Clinic.[79]

In the early 1970s, Arnoldi and colleagues[80,81] demonstrated the importance of increased intraosseous pressure as a cause of pain in OA. These investigators demonstrated marked increases in intramedullary pressure and stasis of medullary blood flow in patients who had hip OA, presumably because of the distortion of blood flow through subchondral trabeculae that had been thickened as a result of remodeling in response to abnormal stress. Normalization of the hemodynamic changes by an osteotomy (ie, an operation that, without entering the joint, cuts the bone and fixes it into an alignment that relieves mechanical stress across the joint by decreasing the resultant force on the joint or increasing the surface area available to carry that force) or by any procedure that transects the metaphyseal bone, can promptly alleviate joint pain.

In 1980, Arnoldi and colleagues[82] described 25 patients who had rest pain in the hip or knee due to OA or to intraosseous engorgement-pain syndrome, who exhibited venous stasis on intraosseous phlebography, increased intraosseous pressure in the intramedullary space near the painful joint, and high uptake of technetium-99m polyphosphate on bone scintigraphy. In patients who had other types of pain these correlations did not exist. The authors suggested that the similarity of the three findings in patients who had intraosseous engorgement-pain syndrome and those who had OA reflected a common pathogenetic mechanism for the patients' pain.

Notably, McAlindon and colleagues,[83] in a 1991 study that correlated findings on MRI, scintigraphy, and radiography in 12 patients who had knee OA, found that nine OA knees exhibited diffuse loss of the medial or lateral tibiofemoral subchondral marrow signal on the proton density image, with corresponding hyperintensity on the STIR sequence and reported that this MRI abnormality was very strongly associated with an extended pattern of isotope on bone scintigraphy.

In a cross-sectional scintigraphic study of 100 patients who had knee OA recruited from a rheumatology clinic, McCrea and colleagues[53] found a very strong correlation between a pattern of generalized uptake of the isotope around the joint on the delayed (bone phase) scan and knee pain. Similarly, a very strong correlation was observed between isotope retention in the subchondral bone in late phase scans and subchondral sclerosis on the radiograph. Furthermore, Dieppe and colleagues[84] documented the predictive value of the bone scan for radiographic progression of knee OA, as reflected by joint space narrowing (JSN). Among scans that did not show focal areas of isotope retention, no progression was noted over a 5-year follow-up period. In contrast, among patients who had OA who had a "hot" knee scan at baseline, progression of JSN was seen in approximately 50%.

Since the reports by Arnoldi and colleagues, however, osteotomy has been largely superceded by arthroplasty as a surgical treatment of symptomatic OA. In the hands of most surgeons it is a more reliable procedure and, for the patient, is associated with a much more rapid return to weight-bearing activity. Nonsurgical treatment of OA pain continues to be based chiefly on systemic pharmacologic therapy with analgesics and nonselective or selective NSAIDs that fail to take into account the altered vascular physiology of the joint.

A recent preliminary report by Hunter and colleagues[85] confirms a link between elevated intraosseous pressures and BMLs, which are commonly seen on MRI of OA knees as focal areas of increased signal in the subchondral marrow in fat-suppressed T2-weighted images. The lesions that are now called BMLs are consistent with the marrow lesions that McAlindon and colleagues[83] described in 1991 and showed to be strongly associated with isotope retention on bone scintigraphy. Histologic examination of these lesions, which have erroneously been called bone marrow "edema," has shown them to be foci of fibrosis and of osteonecrosis and bone remodeling.[86] BMLs are not specific for OA, but may be seen with insufficiency fractures, osteonecrosis, and various other conditions. In subjects who have knee OA, they have been associated with varus-valgus malalignment[87] and the progression of structural damage,[83,87] and, in some studies, with joint pain.[53,88] Using a dynamic contrast-enhanced MRI sequence, Hunter and colleagues[85] found that BMLs in patients who had advanced knee OA were sites of venous hypertension that showed reduced runoff of contrast material, in comparison with the surrounding tissue. Results were consistent with reduced perfusion, intraosseous venous hypertension, and increased permeability at sites of BMLs.

Whether pharmacologic agents that act directly on vascular flow would be efficacious in treatment of OA pain is unknown. In a recent uncontrolled trial in 104 patients who had painful BMLs attributable to various causes, including OA, Meizer and colleagues[89] found that parenteral administration of iloprost, a stable analog of prostacyclin, significantly improved pain and decreased the size of the BMLs. Aigner and colleagues[90] compared results over 11 months in patients who had bone marrow edema syndrome (with BMLs on MRI but not necessarily with OA) who were treated with iloprost with those in a control group who was treated with core decompression of the femoral head. Clinical improvement and improvement in the MRI changes were marked in both groups and as good, or better, with iloprost as with core decompression. It would be of interest to know whether iloprost or other vasoactive agents are of symptomatic benefit in patients who have OA and, if so, whether improvement can be predicted by the presence of a BML on MRI. It would also be important to know how long such changes persist.

In a cross-sectional study, Lo and colleagues[77] found that the maximal BML score was highly associated with knee pain even after adjustment for synovial effusion score, suggesting that each is independently associated with joint pain. In a 15-month longitudinal study of the relationship between BML and knee pain in older subjects who had knee OA or were at high risk for developing knee OA, Felson and colleagues[91] reported that among those who had no knee pain at baseline, but developed knee pain during the study, an increase in the BML volume score at 15 months, relative to the baseline score, was much more common than in subjects who did not develop knee pain.

In a preliminary report of a cross-sectional study of subjects who have symptomatic OA who are enrolled in the OAI, a multicenter study of the natural history of knee OA, Lo and colleagues[92] found a strong association between maceration of the meniscus and BMLs. Large BMLs in the medial tibiofemoral compartment were observed only if there was evidence of maceration of the medial meniscus. The authors suggested that meniscus maceration was a prerequisite for a large BML and that BMLs may be a consequence of impact forces in a knee with aberrant load distribution or instability due to meniscus damage, but a longitudinal study will be needed to establish causality. As further indication of the strong association between BMLs and mechanical stress, BMLs are much more prevalent in the medial tibiofemoral compartment of varus knees than in knees with neutral or valgus alignment (~74% versus 16%). In valgus knees, BMLs tend to localize to the lateral compartment.[87]

The recent interest in BMLs as a source of pain in patients who have OA is reminiscent of the work of Ahlbäck and colleagues[93] in the 1960s, in which the investigators described periarticular osteonecrotic lesions in the bone marrow of patients who had spontaneous knee pain.

In addition to the question of the tissue of origin of pain in an OA joint, the clinician is faced with the problem that other sources of pain may be confused with OA pain. For example, pain in the knee is often referred from the hip or is due to lumbar radiculopathy or a periarticular problem, such as anserine bursitis. The presence of radiographic knee OA is no assurance that the patient's knee pain is attributable to knee OA. The implications of an accurate diagnosis of the patient's pain are obvious. Misinterpretation of the signs and symptoms, of the radiograph and of laboratory tests may all lead to a misdiagnosis. Bálint and Szebenyi[94] published a useful analysis of the clinical problems that underlie the diagnosis of OA and the factors that may confound the clinician.

RELIEF OF OSTEOARTHRITIS PAIN BY PHYSIOLOGIC INTERVENTIONS: FURTHER REASON TO CONSIDER A MECHANICAL ETIOPATHOGENESIS OF OSTEOARTHRITIS

In considering risk factors for OA from an epidemiologic perspective, Felson[95] suggested that elimination of obesity, prevention of knee injury, and elimination of jobs requiring knee bending and carrying heavy loads, each of which can cause increased stress on the joints under consideration, would significantly decrease the incidence of OA of the hip and knee. We contend that such considerations may be important not only in the prevention of incident OA but also in treatment of established symptomatic disease. Several examples of the relief of OA pain by a mechanical (ie, physiologic) rather than pharmacologic intervention can be cited.

Patients who have knee OA who undergo valgus osteotomy to alter the mechanical stresses across the hip joint report relief of knee pain on follow-up examination. Notably, improvement at 2 years was unrelated to whether the hyaline articular cartilage remains unchanged from baseline, shows worsening of OA pathology, or is replaced with fibrocartilage.[96] Langlais and colleagues[97] reported that 83% of patients who had severe hip OA were pain-free 3 to 10 years (average, 6 years) after having undergone valgus osteotomy.

Reduction of the abnormally high stresses in an OA joint by osteotomy has been shown to result in gradual loss of the subchondral sclerosis in the radiograph (**Fig. 3**) and an increase in the formerly narrowed joint space.[30,31] Whether the latter represents growth of new hyaline cartilage or fibrocartilage may be immaterial to the clinical outcome.

A recent systematic review and meta-analysis of patellar taping for patellofemoral OA by Warden and colleagues[98] focuses on another example of successful treatment of painful OA mechanically. Taping to exert a medially directed force on the patella of patients who had symptomatic radiographic patellofemoral OA significantly decreased chronic knee pain in comparison with no taping or sham taping. The results are consistent with evidence that anterior knee pain in patients who have patellofemoral OA is due to lateral displacement of the patella, with increased loading of the lateral facet.[99] Surgical advancement of the tibial tubercle, to weaken the quadriceps muscle by increasing its leverage, can also be symptomatically beneficial on a long-term basis in patients who have patellofemoral OA.[100]

Recent preliminary reports of the results of joint distraction in treatment of severe symptomatic OA provide further evidence.

Among nine patients who had severe tibiofemoral OA who were candidates for joint arthroplasty, distraction of the knee joint for 2 months by way of an external fixation frame that was fitted with springs that bridged the knee and hinges to maintain intermittent synovial fluid pressure resulted in striking reductions in joint pain and improvement in function and clinical status, with almost complete normalization by 6 months.[101] In 5 patients who have been followed for 2 years after undergoing knee distraction, the improvement has been sustained. Longitudinal MRI examinations suggest articular cartilage repair, with a 30% increase in total cartilage volume and 25% increase in mean cartilage thickness, relative to baseline. Urinary biomarker analyses were consistent with high levels of turnover of articular cartilage and bone during distraction, which subsequently normalized. These results are consistent with demonstrations of the prolonged clinical efficacy of distraction in treatment of severe hip and ankle OA[102–104] and reports of clinical improvement in the latter persisting for at least 7 years.[105]

We noted earlier the inverse relationship between knee extensor strength and the risk for developing knee OA.[36] Several randomized controlled trials have shown that quadriceps exercise regimens that were diverse in content, intensity, and frequency improved quadriceps strength, reduced joint pain, improved function, and reduced reflex inhibition of the quadriceps in patients who had knee OA.[106] As reviewed by Minor,[107] longer trials tended to be more effective than shorter ones; the higher the dose of exercise, the more effective the intervention; and only weight-bearing exercise seemed to improve function.

Considerable interest has focused on the importance in knee OA of the peak adduction moment, which is considered to be a proxy for the dynamic load on the medial tibiofemoral compartment of the knee.[108] In cross-sectional studies the peak adductor moment was significantly greater in patients who had medial compartment knee OA than in controls and in patients who had more severe OA than in those who had less severe disease.[109,110] It has been shown to strongly predict radiographic progression in patients who have medial compartment OA[111] and development of knee pain in asymptomatic older subjects.[112] Chang and colleagues[113] recently reported that a greater degree of toe-out during gait, which shifts the ground reaction force vector closer to the center of the knee, thereby reducing the adductor moment, decreased the risk for radiographic progression of knee OA over 18 months.

In subjects who had relatively mild structural changes of knee OA, Thorp and colleagues[114] found that those who had knee pain had significantly higher medial compartment loads than those who were asymptomatic, whereas loads in those who were asymptomatic were no different from those in normal controls. The results suggest that at this stage of structural damage, individuals who have symptomatic OA differ biomechanically from those who have asymptomatic disease. The possibility that the two groups differed with respect to the prominence of repetitive impulsive loading warrants consideration.

In gait analyses performed on subjects who had knee OA while they were wearing their everyday walking shoes and also while walking barefoot, peak loads at the hips and knees decreased significantly with barefoot walking, with nearly 12% reduction in the knee adduction moment.[115] In a recent preliminary report,[116] the same researchers found that a shoe that was designed to incorporate essential features of natural foot motion reduced dynamic loading of the medial compartment of the knee during gait.

Finally, Schnitzer and colleagues,[117] in a 4-week study of 18 patients who had symptomatic knee OA and varus deformity, found that treatment with the NSAID piroxicam reduced the level of joint pain but significantly increased the adductor moment (ie, it increased loading of the already damaged medial tibiofemoral compartment). Whether this would have resulted in acceleration of structural damage if treatment had been maintained for longer periods, possibly because of a faster gait and greater impulsive loading because of relief of joint pain, is not known, but the question has potential clinical importance insofar as many patients who have OA pain are treated with NSAIDs for years.

REFERENCES

1. Kuettner K, Goldberg VM. Introduction. In: Kuettner K, Goldberg VM, editors. Osteoarthritic disorders. Rosemont (IL): American Academy of Orthopaedic Surgeons; 1995. p. xxi–v.
2. Brandt KD, Mankin HJ, Shulman LE. Workshop on etiopathogenesis of osteoarthritis. J Rheumatol 1986;13:1126–60.
3. Knowlton RG, Katzenstein PL, Moskowitz RW, et al. Genetic linkage of a polymorphism in the type II procollagen gene (COL 2A1) to primary osteoarthritis associated with mild chondrodysplasia. N Engl J Med 1990;322:526–30.
4. Radin EL, Burr DB, Caterson B, et al. Mechanical determinants of osteoarthrosis. Semin Arthritis Rheum 1991;21(Suppl 2):12–21.
5. Radin EL, Burr DB. Hypothesis: joints can heal. Semin Arthritis Rheum 1984;13:293–302.
6. Radin EL, Yang KH, Riegger C, et al. Relationship between lower limb dynamics and knee joint pain. J Orthop Res 1991;9:398–405.
7. Radin EL, Paul IL, Pollock D. Animal joint behavior under excessive loading. Nature 1970;226:554–5.
8. Convery FR, Akeson WH, Keown GH. The repair of large osteochondral defects. An experimental study in horses. Clin Orthop Relat Res 1972;82:253–62.
9. Palmoski M, Brandt KD. Immobilization of the knee prevents osteoarthritis after anterior cruciate ligament transaction. Arthritis Rheum 1982;25:1201–8.
10. Brandt KD, Radin EL, Dieppe PA, et al. Yet more evidence that OA is not a cartilage disease. Ann Rheum Dis 2006;65:1261–4.
11. Doherty M, Watt I, Dieppe P. Influence of primary generalized osteoarthritis on development of secondary osteoarthritis. Lancet 1983;2:8–11.
12. Schouten JSAG, van den Ouweland FA, Valkenburg HA. A twelve-year follow-up study in the general population on prognostic factors of cartilage loss in osteoarthritis of the knee. Ann Rheum Dis 1992;51:932–7.
13. Smythe HA. The mechanical pathogenesis of generalized steoarthritis. J Rheumatol 1983;10(Suppl 9):10–2.

14. American college of rheumatology. Clinical slide collection. Atlanta, GA: American College of Rheumatology; 1972–2004.

15. Hernborg J, Nilsson BE. The relationship between osteophytes in the knee joints, osteoarthritis and aging. Acta Orthop Scand 1973;44:69–74.

16. Radin EL. Osteoarthrosis: a perspective. Acta Orthop Scand 1995;66(Suppl 266):6–9.

17. Weinstein SL. Long-term follow-up of pediatric orthopaedic conditions. Natural history and outcomes of treatment. J Bone Joint Surg 2000;82A:980–90.

18. Fitzgerald JB, Jin M, Dean D, et al. Mechanical compression of cartilage explants induces multiple time-dependent gene expression patterns and involves intracellular calcium and cyclic AMP. J Biol Chem 2004;279:19502–11.

19. Radin EL, Boyd RD, Martin RB, et al. Mechanical factors influencing cartilage damage. In: Peyron JG, editor. Osteoarthritis: current clinical and fundamental problems. Paris: Geigy; 1985. p. 90–9.

20. Jones CM, Watt DG. Muscular control of landing from unexpected falls in man. J Physiol 1971;219:729–37.

21. Lee JH, Fitzgerald JB, Dimmico MA, et al. Mechanical injury of cartilage explants causes specific time-dependant changes in chondrocyte gene expression. Arthritis Rheum 2005;52:2386–95.

22. Lee JH, Bai Y, Flannery CR, et al. Cartilage mechanical injury and co-culture with joint capsule tissue increase abundance of ADAMTS-5 protein and aggrecan-G1-NITEGE product. Trans Orthop Res Soc 2006;31.

23. Stokes M, Young A. The contribution of reflex inhibition to arthrogenous muscle weakness. Clin Sci 1984;67:7–14.

24. Felson DT, Kim Y. The futility of current approaches to chondroprotection. Arthritis Rheum 2007;56:1378–83.

25. Brandt KD, Radin EL, Dieppe PA, et al. Letter. The futility of current approaches to chondroprotection—a different perspective: comment on the special article by Felson and Kim. Arthritis Rheum 2007;56:3873–4.

26. Myers SL, Flusser D, Brandt KD, et al. Prevalence of cartilage shards in synovium and their association with synovitis in patients with early and end stage osteoarthritis. J Rheumatol 1992;19:1247–51.

27. Burr DR, Schaffler MB. The involvement of subchondral mineralized tissues in osteoarthrosis: quantitative microscopic evidence. Microsc Res Tech 1997;37:353–7.

28. Burr DB, Radin EL. Microfractures and microcracks in subchondral bone: are they relevant to osteoarthrosis. Rheum Dis Clin North Am 2003;29:675–85.

29. Meachim G, Bentley G. Horizontal splitting in patellar articular cartilage. Arthritis Rheum 1978;21:669–74.

30. Pauwels F. Biomechanics of the normal and diseased hip: theoretical foundation, technique and results of treatment. Berlin: Springer-Verlag; 1976. p. 129–268.

31. Maquet P, Radin EL. Osteotomy as an alternative to total hip replacement in young adults. Clin Orthop Relat Res 1977;123:138–42.

32. Hill AV. Production and absorption of work by muscle. Science 1960;131:897–903.

33. Radin EL. Role of muscles in protecting athletes from injury. In: Astrand PO, Grimby G. editors. Physical activity in health and disease. Acta Med Scand Series No. 2 (Suppl 711): 1986. p. 143–7.

34. Radin EL, Yang KH, Whittle MW, et al. The generation and transmission of heel-strike transient and the effect of quadriceps paralysis. In: Harris D, editor. Gait analysis and medical photogrammetry. Oxford: Oxford Orthopaedic Engineering Centre; 1987. p. 34–45.

35. Hurley MV. The role of muscle weakness in the pathogenesis of osteoarthritis. Rheum Dis Clin North Am 1999;25:299–314.
36. Slemenda C, Brandt KD, Heilman D, et al. Quadriceps weakness and osteoarthritis of the knee. Ann Intern Med 1997;127:97–104.
37. Slemenda C, Heilman D, Brandt KD, et al. Reduced quadriceps strength relative to body weight: a risk factor for knee osteoarthritis in women? Arthritis Rheum 1998;41:1951–9.
38. Brandt KD, Heilman DK, Slemenda C, et al. Quadriceps strength in women with radiographically progressive osteoarthritis of the knee and those with stable radiographic changes. J Rheumatol 1999;26:2431–7.
39. Radin EL, Paul IL. Does cartilage compliance reduce skeletal impact loads? The relative force-attenuating properties of articular cartilage, synovial fluid, periarticular soft tissues and bone. Arthritis Rheum 1970;13:139–44.
40. Burr DB. Subchondral bone in the pathogenesis of osteoarthritis. Mechanical aspects. In: Brandt KD, Doherty M, Lohmander LS, editors. Osteoarthritis. 2nd edition. Oxford: Oxford University Press; 2003. p. 125–33.
41. Hayes WC, Swenson LW Jr, Schurman DJ. Axisymmetric finite element analysis of the lateral tibial plateau. J Biomech 1978;11:21–33.
42. Mente P, Lewis JL. The elastic modulus of calcified cartilage is an order of magnitude less than that of subchondral bone. J Orthop Res 1994;12:637–47.
43. Redler I, Mow VC, Zimny ML, et al. The ultrastructure and biomechanical significance of the tidemark of articular cartilage. Clin Orthop Relat Res 1975;112:357–62.
44. Radin EL, Paul IL. A consolidated concept of joint lubrication. J Bone Joint Surg 1972;54A:607–16.
45. Finlay JB, Repo RU. Cartilage impact in vitro: effect of bone and cement. J Biomech 1978;11:379–88.
46. Radin EL, Paul IL, Lowy M. A comparison of the dynamic force transmitting properties of subchondral bone and articular cartilage. J Bone Joint Surg 1970;52(A):444–56.
47. Hoshino A, Wallace WA. Impact-absorbing properties of the human knee. 1987. J Bone Joint Surg 1987;69(B):807–11.
48. Burr DB. The importance of subchondral bone in the progression of osteoarthritis. J Rheumatol 2004;31(Suppl 70):77–80.
49. Li B, Aspden RM. Mechanical and material properties of the subchondral bone plate from the femoral head of patients with osteoarthritis or osteoporosis. Ann Rheum Dis 1997;56:247–54.
50. Grynpas MD, Alpert B, Katz I, et al. Subchondral bone in osteoarthritis. Calcif Tissue Int 1991;49:20–6.
51. Brown TD, Radin EL, Martin RB, et al. Finite element studies of some juxtarticular stress changes due to localized subchondral stiffening. J Biomech 1984;17:11–24.
52. Vener MJ, Thompson RC Jr, Lewis JL, Oegema TR Jr. Subchondral damage after acute transarticular loading: an in vitro model of joint injury. J Orthop Res 1992;10:759–65.
53. McCrae F, Shouls J, Dieppe P, et al. Scintigraphic assessment of osteoarthritis of the knee joint. Ann Rheum Dis 1992;51:938–42.
54. Franchi A, Bullough PG. Secondary avascular necrosis in coxarthrosis: a morphologic study. J Rheumatol 1992;19:1263–8.
55. Newberry WN, Zukosky OK, Haut RC. Subfracture insult to a knee joint causes alterations in the bone and in the functional stiffness of overlying cartilage. J Orthop Res 1997;15:450–5.

56. Dedrick OK, Goulet R, Huston L, et al. Early bone changes in experimental osteoarthritis using microscopic computer tomography. J Rheumatol 1991; 18(Suppl 27):44–5.

57. Dedrick OK, Goldstein SA, Brandt KD, et al. A longitudinal study of subchondral plate and trabecular bone in cruciate-deficient dogs with osteoarthritis followed for up to 54 months. Arthritis Rheum 1993;36:1460–7.

58. Myers SL. Effects of a bisphosphonate on bone histomorphometry and dynamics in the canine cruciate-deflciency model of osteoarthritis. J Rheumatol 1999; 26:2546–53.

59. Liang MH. Pushing the limits of patient-oriented outcome measurements in the search for disease modifying treatments for osteoarthritis. J Rheumatol 2004;31:61–5.

60. Hadler NM. Knee pain is the malady—not osteoarthritis. Ann Intern Med 1992; 116:598–9.

61. Massardo L, Watt I, Cushnaghan J, et al. Osteoarthritis of the knee joint: an eight year prospective study. Ann Rheum Dis 1989;48:893–7.

62. Lawrence JS, Bremmer JM, Bier F. Osteo-arthrosis. Prevalence in the population and relationship between symptoms and x-ray changes. Ann Rheum Dis 1966;25:1–24.

63. Lawrence JS. Osteoarthrosis. In: Lawrence JS, editor. Rheumatism in populations. London: Heinemann Medical Books, Ltd; 1977. p. 98–155.

64. Felson DT, Naimark A, Anderson J, et al. The prevalence of knee osteoarthritis in the elderly. Arthritis Rheum 1987;30:914–8.

65. Sandell LS, Heinegard D, Hering TM. Cell biology, biochemistry, and molecular biology of articular cartilage in osteoarthritis. In: Moskowitz RW, Altman RD, Hochberg MC, Buckwalter JA, Goldberg VM, et al, editors. Osteoarthritis. 4th edition. Philadelphia: Lippincott Willams and Wilkins; 2007. p. 73–106.

66. Poole AR, Guilak F, Abramson SB. Etiopathogenesis of osteoarthritis. In: Sandell LS, Heinegard D, Hering TM. Cell biology, biochemistry, and molecular biology of articular cartilage in osteoarthritis. In: Osteoarthritis. edited by: Moskowitz RW, Altman RD, Hochberg MC, et al. Lippincott Willams and Wilkins; 4th edition. Philadelphia: 2007. p. 27–49.

67. Sandy J. Proteolytic degradation of normal and osteoarthritic cartilage matrix. In: Brandt KD, Doherty M, Lohmander LS, editors. Osteoarthritis. 2nd edition. Oxford: Oxford University Press; 2003. p. 82–92.

68. O'Reilly SC, Muir KR, Doherty M. Knee pain and disability in the Nottingham Community: association with poor health status and psychological distress. Br J Rheumatol 1998;57:588–94.

69. Evans CH, Mears DC, McKnight JL. A preliminary ferrographic survey of the wear particles in human synovial fluid. Arthritis Rheum 1981;24:912–8.

70. Evans CH. Cellular mechanisms of hydrolytic enzyme release in osteoarthritis. Semin Arthritis Rheum 1981;11(Suppl 1):93–5.

71. Boniface RJ, Cain PR, Evans CH. Articular responses to purified cartilage proteoglycans. Arthritis Rheum 1998;31:258–66.

72. Schumacher HR, Gordon G, Paul H, et al. Osteoarthritis, crystal deposition and inflammation. Semin Arthritis Rheum 1981;11:116–9.

73. Jasin HE. Immune mechanisms in osteoarthritis. Semin Arthritis Rheum 1989; 18(Suppl 2):86–90.

74. Myers SL, Brandt KD, Ehlich JW, et al. Synovial inflammation in patients with early osteoarthritis of the knee. J Rheumatol 1990;17:1662–9.

75. Hill CL, Gale DG, Chaisson CE, et al. Knee effusions, popliteal cysts and synovial thickening. Association with knee pain in those with and without osteoarthritis. J Rheumatol 2001;28:1330–7.

76. Hill CL, Hunter DJ, Niu J, et al. Synovitis detected on magnetic resonance imaging and its relation to pain and cartilage loss in knee osteoarthritis. Ann Rheum Dis 2007;66:1599–603.
77. Lo G, McAlindon T, Niu J, et al. Strong association of bone marrow lesions and effusion with pain in osteoarthritis. Arthritis Rheum 2007;56(Suppl):S790.
78. Graber-Duvernay J. Un traitement nouveau de l'arthrite chronique de la hanche: le forage de l'epiphyse femorale. J Med Lyon 1932;XIII:531–4 [in French].
79. Ghormley RK, Coventry MB. Surgical treatment of painful hips of adults. J Bone Joint Surg 1942;24:424–8.
80. Arnoldi CC, Linderholm H, Mussbichler H. Venous engorgement and intraosseous hypertension in osteoarthritis of the hip. J Bone Joint Surg Br 1972;54:409–21.
81. Arnoldi CC, Lempberg RK, Linderholm H. Immediate effect of osteotomy on the intramedullary pressure of the femoral head and neck in patients with degenerative osteoarthritis. Acta Orthop Scand 1971;42:357–65.
82. Arnoldi CC, Djurhuus JC, Heerfordt J, et al. Intraosseous phlebography, intraosseous pressure measurements and 99m Tc-polyphosphate scintigraphy in patients with various painful conditions in the hip and knee. Acta Orthop Scand 1980;51:19–28.
83. McAlindon TEM, Watt I, McCrae F, et al. Magnetic resonance imaging in osteoarthritis of the knee: correlation with radiographic and scintigraphic findings. Ann Rheum Dis 1991;50:14–9.
84. Dieppe P, Cushnaghan J, Young P, et al. Prediction of the progression of joint space narrowing in osteoarthritis of the knee with bone scintigraphy. Ann Rheum Dis 1993;52:557–63.
85. Hunter DJ, Niu J, Zhang Y, et al. Altered perfusion and venous hypertension is present in regions of bone affected by BMLs in knee OA. Osteoarthritis Cartilage 2007;15(Suppl C):C171.
86. Zanetti M, Bruder E, Romero J, et al. Bone marrow edema pattern in osteoarthritic knees: correlation between MR imaging and histologic findings. Radiology 2000;215:835–40.
87. Felson DT, McLaughlin S, Goggins J, et al. Bone marrow edema and its relation to progression of knee osteoarthritis. Ann Intern Med 2003;139:330–6.
88. Felson DT, Chaisson CE, Hill CL, et al. The association of bone marrow lesions with pain in knee osteoarthritis. Ann Intern Med 2001;134:541–9.
89. Meizer R, Radda C, Stolz G, et al. MRI-controlled analysis of 104 patients with painful bone marrow edema in different joint locations treated with the prostacyclin analogue iloprost. Wien Klin Wochenschr 2005;8:278–86.
90. Aigner N, Petje G, Schneider W, et al. Bone marrow edema syndrome of the femoral head: treatment with the prostacyclin analogue iloprost vs. core decompression: an MRI-controlled study. Wien Klin Wochenschr 2005;117:130–5.
91. Felson DT, Niu J, Guermazi A, et al. Correlation of the development of knee pain with enlarging bone marrow lesions on magnetic resonance imaging. Arthritis Rheum 2007;56:2986–92.
92. Lo G, Hunter D, Nevitt M, et al. Strong association of meniscal maceration and bone marrow lesions in osteoarthritis. Arthritis Rheum 2007;56(Suppl):S125.
93. Ahlbäck S, Bauer GC, Bohne WH. Spontaneous osteonecrosis of the knee. Arthritis Rheum 1968;11:705–33.
94. Bálint G, Szebenyi B. Diagnosis of osteoarthritis. Guidelines and current pitfalls. Drugs 1996;52(Suppl 3):1–13.
95. Felson DT. Preventing knee and hip osteoarthritis. Bull Rheum Dis 1998;47:1–4.

96. Bergennud H, Johnell O, Redlund-Johnell I, et al. The articular cartilage after osteotomy for gonarthrosis: biopsies after 2 years in 19 cases. Acta Orthop Scand 1992;63:413–6.
97. Langlais F, Roure JL, Maquet P. Valgus osteotomy in severe osteoarthritis of the hip. J Bone Joint Surg 1979;61:424–31.
98. Warden SJ, Hinman RS, Watson MA Jr, et al. Patellar taping and bracing for the treatment of chronic knee pain: a systematic review and meta-analysis. Arthritis Rheum 2008;59:73 83.
99. Niu J, Zhang YQ, Nevitt M, et al. Patellar malalignment is associated with prevalent patellofemoral osteoarthritis: the Beijing osteoarthritis study. Arthritis Rheum 2005;52(Suppl 9):S456–7.
100. Maquet P. Biomechanics of the knee. With application to the pathogenesis and the surgical treatment of osteoarthritis. Berlin: Springer; 1984. p. 144–56; 279–82.
101. Intema F, van Roermund PM, Castelein RM, et al. Joint distraction in the treatment of knee osteoarthritis; the first clinical results. Osteoarthritis Cartilage 2007;15(Suppl C):C234.
102. Aldegheri R, Trivella G, Saleh M. Articulated distraction of the hip: conservative surgery for arthritis in young patients. Clin Orthop Relat Res 1994;301: 94–101.
103. Marijnissen AC, Van Roermund PM, van Melkebeek J, et al. Clinical benefit of joint distraction in the treatment of severe osteoarthritis of the ankle. Arthritis Rheum 2002;46:2893–902.
104. Paley D, Lamm BM. Ankle joint distraction. Foot Ankle Clin 2005;10:685–98.
105. Ploegmakers JJ, van Roermund PM, van Melkebeek J, et al. Prolonged clinical benefit from joint distraction in the treatment of ankle osteoarthritis. Osteoarthritis Cartilage 2005;13:582–8.
106. Minor MA. Exercise for the patient with osteoarthritis. In: Brandt KD, Doherty M, Lohmander LS, editors. Osteoarthritis. 2nd edition. Oxford: Oxford University Press; 2003. p. 299–310.
107. Minor MA. Impact of exercise on osteoarthritis outcomes. J Rheumatol 2004; 31(Suppl 70):81–6.
108. Birmingham TB, Hunt MA, Jones IC, et al. Test-retest reliability of the peak knee adduction moment during walking in patients with medial compartment knee osteoarthritis. Arthritis Rheum 2007;57:1012–7.
109. Baliunas AJ, Hurwitz DE, Ryals AB, et al. Increased knee joint loads during walking are present in subjects with knee osteoarthritis. Osteoarthritis Cartilage 2002;10:573–9.
110. Mundermann A, Dyrby CO, Hurwitz DE, et al. Potential strategies to reduce medial compartment loading in patients with knee osteoarthritis of varying severity: reduced walking speed. Arthritis Rheum 2004;50:1172–8.
111. Miyazaki T, Wada M, Kawahara H, et al. Dynamic load at baseline can predict radiographic disease progression in medial compartment knee osteoarthritis. Ann Rheum Dis 2002;61:617–22.
112. Amin S, Luepongsak N, McGibbon CA, et al. Knee adduction moment and development of chronic knee pain in elders. Arthritis Rheum 2004;51:371–6.
113. Chang A, Hurwitz D, Dunlop D, et al. The relationship between toe-out angle during gait and progression of medial tibiofemoral osteoarthritis. Ann Rheum Dis 2007;66:1271–5.
114. Thorp LE, Sumner DR, Wimmer MA, et al. Relationship between pain and medial knee joint loading in mild radiographic knee osteoarthritis. Arthritis Rheum 2007; 57:1254–60.

115. Shakoor N, Block JA. Walking barefoot decreases loading on the lower extremity joints in knee osteoarthritis. Arthritis Rheum 2006;54:2923–7.
116. Shakoor N, Lidtke RH, Sengupta M, et al. Mobility footwear reduces dynamic loads in subjects with osteoarthritis of the knee. Osteoarthritis Cartilage 2007; 15:C219.
117. Schnitzer TJ, Popovich JM, Andersson GB, et al. Effect of piroxicam on gait in patients with osteoarthritis of the knee. Arthritis Rheum 1993;36:1207–13.

Role of Bone in Osteoarthritis Pathogenesis

Steven R. Goldring, MD

KEYWORDS

- Osteoarthritis • Bone • Cartilage • Biomechanics
- Remodeling

PERIARTICULAR BONE STRUCTURE AND MECHANISMS OF ADAPTATION IN OSTEOARTHRITIS

Much of the attention in developing diagnostic tools and therapeutic interventions for the management of osteoarthritis (OA) has focused on the preservation or repair of articular cartilage. It is clear that all of the joint components, including the ligaments, tendons, capsule, synovial lining, and periarticular bone, undergo structural and functional alterations during the course of OA progression. This article focuses on the specific skeletal features of OA and the putative mechanisms involved in their pathogenesis.

In considering the skeletal alterations that occur during the course of OA, it is important to appreciate that the organization and functional properties of the periarticular bone are not uniform. The specific skeletal sites can be separated into distinct anatomic entities that include the subchondral cortical bone plate, the subchondral trabecular bone, and the bone at the joint margins. The subchondral bone plate consists of cortical bone, which is relatively nonporous and poorly vascularized. It is separated from the overlying articular cartilage by a zone of calcified cartilage. The so-called "tide-mark," which can be distinguished based on its enhanced metachromatic staining pattern, provides a line of demarcation between the hyaline articular cartilage and calcified cartilage (**Fig. 1**). Because the local environmental influences at each of the skeletal sites differ, the structural reorganization and adaptation during the course of OA progression assume different and distinct patterns.[1–3] The capacity of bone to adapt its structural organization in response to mechanical forces is embodied in the Wolff hypothesis that states that the distribution and material properties of bone are determined by the magnitude and direction of applied load.[4]

A version of this article originally appeared in the 34:3 issue of the *Rheumatic Disease Clinics of North America*.

The Hospital for Special Surgery, Weill College of Medicine of Cornell University, 535 East 70th Street, New York, NY 10021, USA

E-mail address: goldrings@hss.edu

Med Clin N Am 93 (2009) 25–35
doi:10.1016/j.mcna.2008.09.006
0025-7125/08/$ – see front matter © 2008 Elsevier Inc. All rights reserved.

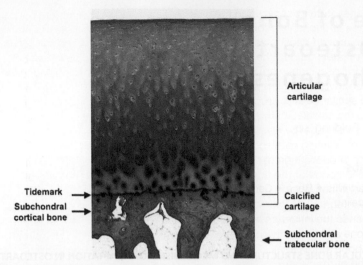

Fig. 1. Histologic features of a normal joint. The articular cartilage is separated from the underlying subchondral bone by a region of calcified cartilage. The tidemark denotes the interface between the calcified cartilage and adjacent hyaline articular cartilage. The subchondral bone is organized into a region of subchondral cortical bone overlying the adjacent trabecular bone and bone marrow space. (*Courtesy of* Edward DiCarlo, MD, Hospital for Special Surgery, New York, NY.)

The architecture and properties of the periarticular cortical and trabecular bone are modified during the course of OA through the cellular processes of remodeling and modeling. In addition, mechanical factors may directly alter the structural and functional features of the bone tissue by generation of discontinuities (microcracks) in the absence of direct cellular activity.[2–5] The remodeling process is initiated by the preparation of quiescent bone surfaces and the activation of a phase of bone resorption mediated by osteoclasts, which are highly specialized monocyte-macrophage lineage cells that are uniquely adapted to the removal of the mineralized bone matrix.[6,7] The phase of bone resorption is followed by a phase of bone formation mediated by osteoblasts. In physiologic conditions the quantities of bone removed during the resorption and formation phases are exquisitely balanced such that bone mass is maintained, although the shape and architecture of the bone may be modified. This equilibrium is related to so-called "coupling" of the activities of the osteoclasts and osteoblasts and is an intrinsic feature of the remodeling unit. This cellular system permits adaptation of the skeleton to changing mechanical influences and, importantly, provides a mechanism for repairing damage that occurs to the skeleton during mechanical loading.[3,8]

Modeling represents an additional mechanism for changing the architecture and volume of bone. In contrast to the remodeling process, the events of resorption and formation are not coupled, and bone may be formed or lost without compensatory balancing of the two events. In general, modeling represents a mechanism for local addition of bone tissue by direct apposition to existing bone surfaces.

Remodeling and modeling are processes that modify the structural and functional properties of subchondral cortical and trabecular bone architecture during the course of OA. An additional mechanism affecting periarticular bone involves the process of endochondral ossification in which new bone is formed by replacement of a cartilaginous matrix.[2,5,9–11] During the period of growth and development this complex multicellular system is localized to the growth plates and to the centers of ossification and provides a mechanism for skeletal growth and enlargement. At skeletal maturity, longitudinal growth ceases associated with discontinuation of cellular activity within the growth plates. During the course of OA, the cellular processes associated with endochondral ossification are reactivated at the joint margins, giving rise to the formation of osteophytes, which represent one of the radiographic hallmarks of OA.[11,12] In addition, a similar cellular process is activated at the site of the tidemark, immediately adjacent to the calcified cartilage. The initial event involves the penetration of the zone of calcified cartilage by vascular elements followed by chondrocyte hypertrophy, deposition of calcified cartilage, and eventual replacement with bone.[2,3,13–15] This process results in duplication of the tidemark and advancement of the calcified cartilage into the deep zones of the articular cartilage (**Fig. 2**). The replacement of the hyaline cartilage contributes to thinning of the articular cartilage zone and likely adversely affects the integrity and biomechanical properties of the articular surface.

In addition to the influence of bone architecture and structure, the mechanical properties of bone also are influenced by an additional factor, namely the material properties of the bone matrix itself. These properties are determined by the organization and composition of the organic phase of bone and the chemistry and content of the mineral phase. Inherited disorders of bone matrix molecules or genetic defects that affect mineralization may have profound effects on the material properties of bone. Many of these conditions affect the skeleton during the period of development and growth and are manifest in growth retardation and skeletal deformities that are often accompanied by the premature development of OA. In a vast majority of individuals the skeletal changes associated with OA occur in the absence of overt heritable underlying metabolic or genetic abnormalities, and the skeletal alterations are a reflection of adaptation of the bone tissue that are mediated though the same cellular and biochemical processes that are operative during physiologic bone remodeling.

The state of mineralization is one of the major determinants of the material properties of the bone matrix.[16–18] The degree of mineralization is highly dependent on rate of bone formation and turnover. In the remodeling cycle, the initial deposition of the organic phase (osteoid) of bone by osteoblasts lasts for several weeks and is associated with rapid mineralization. The process of mineralization, however, continues for an extended time, and this late phase of mineral accretion markedly affects the material properties of the bone matrix. In high bone turnover states, the late phase of mineral deposition is attenuated leading to a state of relative hypomineralization, which produces bone with a lowered modulus of elasticity that is more easily deformed under

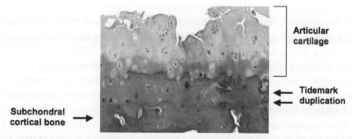

Fig. 2. Histologic features associated with advanced osteoarthritis. There is fragmentation and fissuring the articular cartilage. There is duplication of the tidemark with advancement of the calcified cartilage into the lower zones of the articular cartilage further contributing to thinning of the cartilage lining. (*Courtesy of* Edward DiCarlo, MD, Hospital for Special Surgery, New York, NY.)

load.[3,16,19] In contrast, in low bone turnover states, the continued deposition of mineral may lead to a state of hypermineralization, resulting in bone that has an increased modulus and is therefore more resistant to deformation and more brittle. During the course of OA progression marked changes occur in the rate and extent of remodeling in the subchondral cortical plate and the underlying trabecular bone. These alterations, especially when accompanied by changes in the shape and contour of the subchondral plate, may adversely affect the capacity of the adjacent articular cartilage to adapt to mechanical loads.[1,16,20] In addition, the altered loading environment may impact adversely on the remodeling and repair capacity of the resident chondrocytes.

PERIARTICULAR BONE CHANGES ASSOCIATED WITH OSTEOARTHRITIS

Periarticular bone changes associated with OA can be segregated into distinct patterns based on the anatomic location and pathogenic mechanisms. These alterations include progressive increase in subchondral plate thickness, alterations in the architecture of subchondral trabecular bone, formation of new bone at the joint margins (osteophytes), development of subchondral bone cysts, and advancement of the tidemark associated with vascular invasion of the calcified cartilage. These skeletal changes also may be associated with marked alteration in the contour of the adjacent articulating surfaces resulting in modification in joint congruity that further contributes to an adverse biomechanical environment.[1,2,5,21,22]

Numerous approaches have been used to establish that the changes in periarticular bone occur early in the development of OA, and these studies support the concept that the skeletal adaptations antedate detectable alterations in the structural integrity of the articular cartilage. In part, this may be related to the marked differential capacity of cartilage and bone to adapt to mechanical loads and damage. Cortical and trabecular bone rapidly alter skeletal architecture and shape in response to load by way of cell-mediated remodeling and modeling. Recent studies have shown that chondrocytes also modulate their functional state in response to loading.[23–29] The capacity of these cells to repair and modify their surrounding extracellular matrix is relatively limited in comparison to skeletal tissues, however. This differential adaptive capacity likely underlies the more rapid appearance of detectable skeletal changes in OA, especially after injuries that acutely alter joint mechanics. The imbalance in the adaptation of the cartilage and bone disrupts the physiologic relationship between these tissues that is essential for maintenance of normal joint structure and function and in this way further contributes to the development of OA pathology.

Evidence that skeletal changes occur early in the course of OA have been provided by studies using isotope-labeled bone-seeking agents and radiographic techniques.[30–33] Bone scans reveal that the increased retention of the radiolabel conforms to regions of enhanced bone remodeling. Results indicate that the changes in bone turnover precede the evidence of detectable radiographic bony changes, and the scintigraphic changes are predictive of the subsequent development of osteophytes and subchondral bone sclerosis.[34,35] These studies also demonstrate that the development of osteophytes and subchondral sclerosis precede detectable changes in articular cartilage thickness and joint space narrowing.[1]

Insights into sequential skeletal changes associated with OA onset have been provided by the study of individuals who have posttraumatic OA in which the onset of the pathologic process can be linked to the date of a specific injury. Particularly informative have been the observations of Buckland-Wright and colleagues[36] who used quantitative macroradiography in a cross-sectional study of patients who had anterior cruciate ligament rupture to rigorously define the sequence of periarticular bone changes. They observed that ligament rupture was associated with thickening of the subchondral horizontal trabeculae reaching significance by 3 to 4 years. Osteophytes were present in approximately 50% of the injured knees by the third year. Within these time intervals, no changes were detected in joint space width or cortical plate thickness. Of interest, the findings in patients who had OA of the knee not associated with a discrete injury differed in that the cortical plate thickness in these individuals antedated the trabecular alterations, suggesting the existence of differential biomechanical and adaptive influences in these two populations.[37,38] In studies of the periarticular changes in hand and wrist OA, similar increases in cortical plate thickness were detected. In approximately one third of the subjects, there was a decrease in thickness. The authors speculated that the reduced thickness might be related to the effects of local inflammation on bone remodeling.[39]

SUBCHONDRAL CORTICAL AND TRABECULAR BONE CHANGES IN OSTEOARTHRITIS

There has been considerable controversy regarding the effects of the subchondral bone changes on the biomechanical properties of the bone tissue and the influences of these changes on the overlying articular cartilage. It was originally proposed by Radin and Rose[22] that the increased thickness and volume in the subchondral bone in OA was associated with increased stiffness in the bone tissue and that these changes adversely affected the biomechanical environment of the overlying cartilage. Numerous analytic and imaging techniques have confirmed that OA is associated with an increase in subchondral bone volume and these changes account for the pattern of subchondral sclerosis detected with standard radiographic techniques.[3] Bone volume, however, is only one of the factors that determine the mechanical properties of bone. Additional factors include the architecture and material properties of the tissue. Particularly informative have been the studies of Day and colleagues[16] who used finite element models constructed from micro-CT scans of subchondral trabecular bone obtained from the proximal tibiae from cadaver specimens from subjects who had early OA cartilage damage. Direct mechanical testing was combined with finite element analysis to determine the effective tissue modulus. Although the volume fraction of trabecular bone was increased, they observed that the bone tissue modulus was reduced by 60% in the medial condyles of the samples with cartilage damage compared to the control specimens. They related this reduction in modulus to an overall decrease in mineral density attributable to incomplete mineralization due to the increased rate of remodeling and bone turnover. Similar observations have been made by other investigators.[3,19] Importantly, these findings indicate that the adverse mechanical environment in the overlying calcified and hyaline cartilage associated with the changes in the properties of the subchondral bone in OA may be associated with a decrease rather than an increase in the bone tissue modulus (ie, stiffness). These conclusions, if correct, have significant implications with respect to the OA treatment approaches that target subchondral and periarticular bone remodeling. Therapies that are designed to inhibit bone resorption and reduce remodeling (eg, bisphosphonates) would be expected to initially increase bone volume by filling in of the remodeling space and increasing bone mineral content by reducing bone turnover. This process would eventually lead to subchondral bone with increased stiffness. It would also interfere with the adaptation of the periarticular bone to changing biomechanical environment influences, the effects of which may be beneficial or adverse depending on the stage of OA progression. The lack of efficacy of a recent trial with risedronate in the treatment of OA despite compelling preclinical and early human study data highlights the complexity of the issues surrounding the influences of bone adaptation and its effects on the natural history of OA.[40,41]

In considering the alterations in bone volume and mineral composition of the subchondral bone, it also is important to identify the specific anatomic site, because the adaptive changes in the cortical and underlying trabecular bone, although intimately related, may differ. In human studies, analysis of the bone mineral density of the subchondral trabecular bone reveal reduced levels deep to the thickened cortical bone.[42] Recently Messent and colleagues[43–45] used a computerized method of textural image analysis (Fractal Signature Analysis) to assess the architecture of subchondral trabecular bone. They showed that OA progression was associated with an increase in vertical trabeculae, which tended to be thinner and fenestrated, resulting in the development of relatively osteoporotic bone consistent with the decrease in mineral density detected in this region observed using dual energy x-ray absorptiometry.[42] Horizontal trabeculae increased throughout the course of OA but the size varied depending on stage of early or late OA. The authors speculated that the thickened cortical plate and retention of the horizontal trabeculae was associated with enhanced absorption of load-bearing stress, resulting in reduced transmission to the underlying trabecular bone and the development of progressive osteoporotic change.

TIDEMARK ADVANCEMENT

An additional finding in analysis of hand OA has been the presence of advancement of the zone of calcified cartilage.[14] Similar changes have been detected in large joints, such as the hip, shoulder, and knee (**Fig. 2**).[2] The precise mechanisms involved in this process have not been definitively established and could include the release of proangiogenic factors from chondrocytes in the deep zones of the articular cartilage that have undergone hypertrophy or the influences of microcracks that have initiated focal remodeling in the calcified cartilage in an attempt to repair the microdamage through a process of targeted remodeling.[5,8,27,28,46,47] The advancement and duplication of the tidemark contributes to overall thinning of the articular cartilage. In addition, this process markedly increases the mechanical stresses in the deep zones of the cartilage matrix, which likely contributes to the acceleration in OA cartilage deterioration.[5]

BONE MARROW EDEMA AND BONE CYSTS

The introduction of MRI has provided a powerful diagnostic tool for quantitating changes in the tissues that make up the diarthrodial joint in patients who have OA. The term "bone marrow edema" was introduced in 1988 by Wilson and colleagues[48] who identified regions of increased signal intensity using fluid-sensitive magnetic resonance sequences and decreased signal intensity in the T1-weighted sequences. Subsequently, several groups have demonstrated that the presence of bone marrow edema detected by MRI correlates with the severity of pain and with the progression of OA cartilage and bone lesions.[49–54] Taljanovic and colleagues[54] recently analyzed the histopathologic findings associated with bone marrow edema in a series of patients who had advanced hip OA. They observed that 70% of the patients had pseudocysts in the regions of bone marrow edema and these changes corresponded to regions of the most severe damage in the overlying cartilage. Observations by other investigators support the speculation that the bone cysts associated with OA develop in the focal areas of bone damage and necrosis.[55,56] In the studies of Taljanovic and colleagues[54] microfractures of the trabecular bone at various stages of healing were present in the regions of bone marrow edema and the findings correlated with the areas of most severe cartilage loss. All of the femoral heads had regions of fat necrosis and localized marrow fibrosis. Hoffman and colleagues[57] examined bone specimens from core decompression in a series of patients who had nontraumatic bone marrow edema and also noted the presence of focal necrosis, marrow fibrosis, and evidence of microdamage and bone repair. Similar histologic findings were reported by Zanetti and colleagues.[58] Actual edema in the marrow was not a major feature in any of the studies, supporting the more recent generic description of these changes as "bone marrow lesions." The correspondence of the sites of bone marrow edema with regions of skeletal and cartilage damage strongly supports a primary role for a mechanical and traumatic cause for the marrow alterations. Supporting this conclusion are the histologic features, which are most consistent with localized activation of bone repair processes that accompany targeted bone remodeling.[3,5]

OSTEOPHYTES

Osteophytes represent fibrocartilaginous and skeletal outgrowths that are localized to the joint margins and are a radiographic hallmark of OA. Animal models of OA have been particularly useful in defining the sequence of events associated with osteophyte development.[11] These studies have shown that the initiation of the osteophyte is associated with proliferation of periosteal cells at the joint margin. These cells undergo differentiation into chondrocytes, which hypertrophy, and through the process of endochondral ossification create an enlarging skeletal outgrowth at the joint margin.[11] Local production of growth factors has been strongly implicated in the formation of osteophytes based on their presence within the developing osteochondral outgrowth.[59,60] These conclusions are supported by experimental approaches in which investigators have directly injected transforming factor β or bone morphogenic protein-2 (growth factors implicated in endochondral bone formation) into joints of experimental animals or selectively inactivated these growth factors or their signal pathways and shown inhibition of osteophyte formation.[9,10,61–63]

There remains uncertainty regarding the pathogenic role of osteophytes in OA. In human and animal models of OA, osteophytes may form in the absence of cartilage damage and cartilage damage associated with OA is not invariably associated with

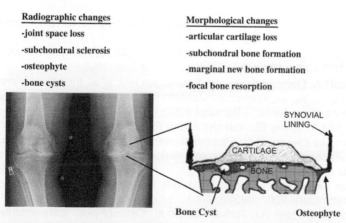

Correlation of radiographic and structural changes in OA

Radiographic changes
-joint space loss
-subchondral sclerosis
-osteophyte
-bone cysts

Morphological changes
-articular cartilage loss
-subchondral bone formation
-marginal new bone formation
-focal bone resorption

SYNOVIAL LINING

CARTILAGE

BONE

Bone Cyst   Osteophyte

Fig. 3. Periarticular bone changes associated with OA and the associated radiographic changes that are the diagnostic hallmarks of OA.

osteophyte formation. Nevertheless, there is an association between the presence of cartilage changes of OA and osteophyte formation, and the localization of osteophytes to sites of joint loading strongly implicates local mechanical factors in their formation. Several lines of evidence support the concept that osteophytes represent a skeletal adaptation to local mechanical factors that in fact contribute to maintenance of joint function and stability.[11,12,64]

SUMMARY

Fig. 3 is a depiction of the periarticular bone changes associated with OA and the relationship of these structural alterations to the radiographic findings that are used clinically to diagnose and monitor OA progression. The skeletal adaptations reflect responses of bone cells that remodel the bone tissue to alterations in the mechanical and biologic influences that are present at these sites. An understanding of the factors responsible for these changes and their relationship and effects on the other tissues that make up the joint are essential for the development of rational and effective therapies to improve the outcomes in patients who have OA.

REFERENCES

1. Buckland-Wright C. Subchondral bone changes in hand and knee osteoarthritis detected by radiography. Osteoarthr Cartil 2004;12(Suppl A):S10–9.
2. Bullough PG. The role of joint architecture in the etiology of arthritis. Osteoarthr Cartil 2004;12(Suppl A):S2–9.
3. Burr DB. Anatomy and physiology of the mineralized tissues: role in the pathogenesis of osteoarthrosis. Osteoarthr Cartil 2004;12(Suppl A):S20–30.
4. Frost HM. Perspective: genetic and hormonal roles in bone disorders: insights of an updated bone physiology. J Musculoskelet Neuronal Interact 2003;3(2):118–35.
5. Burr DB, Schaffler MB. The involvement of subchondral mineralized tissues in osteoarthrosis: quantitative microscopic evidence. Microsc Res Tech 1997;37(4):343–57.
6. Teitelbaum SL. Osteoclasts: what do they do and how do they do it? Am J Pathol 2007;170(2):427–35.
7. Teitelbaum SL, Ross FP. Genetic regulation of osteoclast development and function. Nat Rev Genet 2003;4(8):638–49.
8. Martin RB. Targeted bone remodeling involves BMU steering as well as activation. Bone 2007;40(6):1574–80.
9. Scharstuhl A, Glansbeek HL, van Beuningen HM, et al. Inhibition of endogenous TGF-beta during experimental osteoarthritis prevents osteophyte formation and impairs cartilage repair. J Immunol 2002;169(1):507–14.
10. Scharstuhl A, Vitters EL, van der Kraan PM. Reduction of osteophyte formation and synovial thickening by adenoviral overexpression of transforming growth factor beta/bone morphogenetic protein inhibitors during experimental osteoarthritis. Arthritis Rheum 2003;48(12):3442–51.
11. van der Kraan PM, van den Berg WB. Osteophytes: relevance and biology. Osteoarthr Cartil 2007;15(3):237–44.
12. Messent EA, Ward RJ, Tonkin CJ, et al. Osteophytes, juxta-articular radiolucencies and cancellous bone changes in the proximal tibia of patients with knee osteoarthritis. Osteoarthr Cartil 2007;15(2):179–86.

13. Muir P, McCarthy J, Radtke CL, et al. Role of endochondral ossification of articular cartilage and functional adaptation of the subchondral plate in the development of fatigue microcracking of joints. Bone 2006;38(3):342–9.
14. Patel N, Buckland-Wright C. Advancement in the zone of calcified cartilage in osteoarthritic hands of patients detected by high definition macroradiography. Osteoarthr Cartil 1999;7(6):520–5.
15. Lane LB, Villacin A, Bullough PG. The vascularity and remodelling of subchondrial bone and calcified cartilage in adult human femoral and humeral heads. An age- and stress-related phenomenon. J Bone Joint Surg Br 1977; 59(3):272–8.
16. Day JS, Ding M, van der Linden JC, et al. A decreased subchondral trabecular bone tissue elastic modulus is associated with pre-arthritic cartilage damage. J Orthop Res 2001;19(5):914–8.
17. Faibish D, Ott SM, Boskey AL. Mineral changes in osteoporosis: a review. Clin Orthop Relat Res 2006;443:28–38.
18. Meunier PJ, Boivin G. Bonse mineral density reflects bone mass but also the degree of mineralization of bone: therapeutic implications. Bone 1997;21(5): 373–7.
19. Li B, Aspden RM. Mechanical and material properties of the subchondral bone plate from the femoral head of patients with osteoarthritis or osteoporosis. Ann Rheum Dis 1997;56(4):247–54.
20. Day JS, Van Der Linden JC, Bank RA, et al. Adaptation of subchondral bone in osteoarthritis. Biorheology 2004;41(3–4):359–68.
21. Messent EA, Ward RJ, Tonkin CJ, et al. Differences in trabecular structure between knees with and without osteoarthritis quantified by macro and standard radiography, respectively. Osteoarthr Cartil 2006;14(12):1302–5.
22. Radin EL, Rose RM. Role of subchondral bone in the initiation and progression of cartilage damage. Clin Orthop Relat Res 1986;213:34–40.
23. Goldring SR, Goldring MB. The role of cytokines in cartilage matrix degeneration in osteoarthritis. Clin Orthop 2004;427(Suppl):S27–36.
24. Hunziker EB. Articular cartilage repair: basic science and clinical progress. A review of the current status and prospects. Osteoarthr Cartil 2002;10(6): 432–63.
25. Maroudas A, Bayliss MT, Uchitel-Kaushansky N, et al. Aggrecan turnover in human articular cartilage: use of aspartic acid racemization as a marker of molecular age. Arch Biochem Biophys 1998;350(1):61–71.
26. Plaas A, Osborn B, Yoshihara Y, et al. Aggrecanolysis in human osteoarthritis: confocal localization and biochemical characterization of ADAMTS5-hyaluronan complexes in articular cartilages. Osteoarthr Cartil 2007;15(7):719–34.
27. Sandell LJ, Aigner T. Articular cartilage and changes in arthritis. An introduction: cell biology of osteoarthritis. Arthritis Res 2001;3(2):107–13.
28. Goldring MB, Goldring SR. Osteoarthritis. J Cell Physiol 2007;213(3):626–34.
29. Goodwin JL, Farley ML, Swaim B, et al. Dual proline labeling protocol for individual "baseline" and "response" biosynthesis measurements in human articular cartilage. Osteoarthr Cartil 2008;16:1263–6.
30. Buckland-Wright JC, Macfarlane DG, Fogelman I, et al. Technetium 99m methylene diphosphonate bone scanning in osteoarthritic hands. Eur J Nucl Med 1991;18(1):12–6.
31. Hutton CW, Higgs ER, Jackson PC, et al. 99mTc HMDP bone scanning in generalised nodal osteoarthritis. I. Comparison of the standard radiograph and four hour bone scan image of the hand. Ann Rheum Dis 1986;45(8):617–21.

32. Hutton CW, Higgs ER, Jackson PC, et al. 99mTc HMDP bone scanning in generalised nodal osteoarthritis. II. The four hour bone scan image predicts radiographic change. Ann Rheum Dis 1986;45(8):622–6.
33. Macfarlane DG, Buckland-Wright JC, Emery P, et al. Comparison of clinical, radionuclide, and radiographic features of osteoarthritis of the hands. Ann Rheum Dis 1991;50(9):623–6.
34. Dieppe P, Cushnaghan J, Young P, et al. Prediction of the progression of joint space narrowing in osteoarthritis of the knee by bone scintigraphy. Ann Rheum Dis 1993;52(8):557–63.
35. McCrae F, Shouls J, Dieppe P, et al. Scintigraphic assessment of osteoarthritis of the knee joint. Ann Rheum Dis 1992;51(8):938–42.
36. Buckland-Wright JC, Lynch JA, Dave B. Early radiographic features in patients with anterior cruciate ligament rupture. Ann Rheum Dis 2000;59(8):641–6.
37. Buckland-Wright JC, Lynch JA, Macfarlane DG. Fractal signature analysis measures cancellous bone organisation in macroradiographs of patients with knee osteoarthritis. Ann Rheum Dis 1996;55(10):749–55.
38. Buckland-Wright JC, Macfarlane DG, Jasani MK, et al. Quantitative microfocal radiographic assessment of osteoarthritis of the knee from weight bearing tunnel and semiflexed standing views. J Rheumatol 1994;21(9):1734–41.
39. Buckland-Wright JC, MacFarlane DG, Lynch JA. Relationship between joint space width and subchondral sclerosis in the osteoarthritic hand: a quantitative microfocal radiographic study. J Rheumatol 1992;19(5):788–95.
40. Bingham CO 3rd, Buckland-Wright JC, Garnero P, et al. Risedronate decreases biochemical markers of cartilage degradation but does not decrease symptoms or slow radiographic progression in patients with medial compartment osteoarthritis of the knee: results of the two-year multinational knee osteoarthritis structural arthritis study. Arthritis Rheum 2006;54(11): 3494–507.
41. Buckland-Wright JC, Messent EA, Bingham CO 3rd, et al. A 2 yr longitudinal radiographic study examining the effect of a bisphosphonate (risedronate) upon subchondral bone loss in osteoarthritic knee patients. Rheumatology (Oxford) 2007;46(2):257–64.
42. Karvonen RL, Miller PR, Nelson DA, et al. Periarticular osteoporosis in osteoarthritis of the knee. J Rheumatol 1998;25(11):2187–94.
43. Messent EA, Buckland-Wright JC, Blake GM. Fractal analysis of trabecular bone in knee osteoarthritis (OA) is a more sensitive marker of disease status than bone mineral density (BMD). Calcif Tissue Int 2005;76(6):419–25.
44. Messent EA, Ward RJ, Tonkin CJ, et al. Cancellous bone differences between knees with early, definite and advanced joint space loss; a comparative quantitative macroradiographic study. Osteoarthr Cartil 2005;13(1):39–47.
45. Messent EA, Ward RJ, Tonkin CJ, et al. Tibial cancellous bone changes in patients with knee osteoarthritis. A short-term longitudinal study using Fractal Signature Analysis. Osteoarthr Cartil 2005;13(6):463–70.
46. Aigner T, Bartnik E, Sohler F, et al. Functional genomics of osteoarthritis: on the way to evaluate disease hypotheses. Clin Orthop Relat Res 2004;427(Suppl): S138–43.
47. Aigner T, Fundel K, Saas J, et al. Large-scale gene expression profiling reveals major pathogenetic pathways of cartilage degeneration in osteoarthritis. Arthritis Rheum 2006;54(11):3533–44.
48. Wilson AJ, Murphy WA, Hardy DC, et al. Transient osteoporosis: transient bone marrow edema? Radiology 1988;167(3):757–60.

49. Felson DT, Niu J, Guermazi A, et al. Correlation of the development of knee pain with enlarging bone marrow lesions on magnetic resonance imaging. Arthritis Rheum 2007;56(9):2986–92.
50. Hernandez-Molina G, Guermazi A, Niu J, et al. Central bone marrow lesions in symptomatic knee osteoarthritis and their relationship to anterior cruciate ligament tears and cartilage loss. Arthritis Rheum 2008;58(1):130–6.
51. Hunter DJ, Zhang Y, Niu J, et al. Increase in bone marrow lesions associated with cartilage loss: a longitudinal magnetic resonance imaging study of knee osteoarthritis. Arthritis Rheum 2006;54(5):1529–35.
52. Lo GH, Hunter DJ, Zhang Y, et al. Bone marrow lesions in the knee are associated with increased local bone density. Arthritis Rheum 2005;52(9):2814–21.
53. Reichenbach S, Guermazi A, Niu J, et al. Prevalence of bone attrition on knee radiographs and MRI in a community-based cohort. Osteoarthr Cartil 2008;16: 1005–10.
54. Taljanovic MS, Graham AR, Benjamin JB, et al. Bone marrow edema pattern in advanced hip osteoarthritis: quantitative assessment with magnetic resonance imaging and correlation with clinical examination, radiographic findings, and histopathology. Skeletal Radiol 2008;37(5):423–31.
55. Bancroft LW, Peterson JJ, Kransdorf MJ. Cysts, geodes, and erosions. Radiol Clin North Am 2004;42(1):73–87.
56. Carrino JA, Blum J, Parellada JA, et al. MRI of bone marrow edema-like signal in the pathogenesis of subchondral cysts. Osteoarthr Cartil 2006;14(10):1081–5.
57. Hofmann S, Engel A, Neuhold A, et al. Bone-marrow oedema syndrome and transient osteoporosis of the hip. An MRI-controlled study of treatment by core decompression. J Bone Joint Surg Br 1993;75(2):210–6.
58. Zanetti M, Bruder E, Romero J, et al. Bone marrow edema pattern in osteoarthritic knees: correlation between MR imaging and histologic findings. Radiology 2000; 215(3):835–40.
59. Zoricic S, Maric I, Bobinac D, et al. Expression of bone morphogenetic proteins and cartilage-derived morphogenetic proteins during osteophyte formation in humans. J Anat 2003;202(Pt 3):269–77.
60. Blaney Davidson EN, van der Kraan PM, van den Berg WB. TGF-beta and osteoarthritis. Osteoarthr Cartil 2007;15(6):597–604.
61. van Beuningen HM, Glansbeek HL, van der Kraan PM, et al. Differential effects of local application of BMP-2 or TGF-beta 1 on both articular cartilage composition and osteophyte formation. Osteoarthr Cartil 1998;6(5):306–17.
62. van Beuningen HM, Glansbeek HL, van der Kraan PM, et al. Osteoarthritis-like changes in the murine knee joint resulting from intra-articular transforming growth factor-beta injections. Osteoarthr Cartil 2000;8(1):25–33.
63. van Beuningen HM, van der Kraan PM, Arntz OJ, et al. Transforming growth factor-beta 1 stimulates articular chondrocyte proteoglycan synthesis and induces osteophyte formation in the murine knee joint. Lab Invest 1994;71(2):279–90.
64. Pottenger LA, Phillips FM, Draganich LF. The effect of marginal osteophytes on reduction of varus-valgus instability in osteoarthritic knees. Arthritis Rheum 1990;33(6):853–8.

The Role of the Meniscus in Osteoarthritis Genesis

Martin Englund, MD, PhD[a,b],*

KEYWORDS

• Osteoarthritis • Meniscus • Knee • Epidemiology • Treatment

The menisci are two semicircular fibrocartilage structures located between the articular surfaces of the femur and tibia in the medial and lateral joint compartments. Each covers approximately two thirds of the corresponding articular surface of the tibia. In cross section, both menisci are wedge-shaped with a thick peripheral base infiltrated by capillaries and nerves that penetrate 10% to 30% of the meniscus width.[1,2]

The sparse meniscal population of fibrochondrocytes produces and maintains the meniscal matrix. The main functions of the menisci are shock absorption and load transmission during knee-joint movement and loading.[3–5] The menisci distribute stress over a large area of the articular cartilage. When the knee is loaded, the tensile strength of the meniscal matrix (hoop tension) counteracts extrusion of the meniscus. Therefore, the healthy meniscus mainly responds to load with compression. The meniscus may also be important in joint stability, proprioception, and joint lubrication.[6–8]

DIFFERENT TYPES OF MENISCAL LESIONS

Normally configured menisci are rare in knees with osteoarthritis. Instead, menisci in osteoarthritic knees are often torn, macerated, or even destroyed, suggesting a strong association between the disorder and the meniscus.[9,10] There are two major categories of meniscal injuries: traumatic lesions and gradual degeneration with aging or other degenerative processes.[11–14] Traumatic lesions, which usually occur in younger active individuals, stem from distinct knee trauma where the meniscus often splits vertically and parallel to the circumferentially oriented collagen fibers.

A version of this article originally appeared in the 34:3 issue of the *Rheumatic Disease Clinics of North America.*
[a] Musculoskeletal Sciences, Department of Orthopedics, Lund University, Hs 32, Box 117, SE-221 00 Lund, Sweden
[b] Clinical Epidemiology Research and Training Unit, Boston University School of Medicine, Boston, MA, USA
* Musculoskeletal Sciences, Department of Orthopaedics, Lund University, Hs 32, Box 117, SE-221 00 Lund, Sweden.
E-mail address: martin.englund@med.lu.se

Med Clin N Am 93 (2009) 37–43
doi:10.1016/j.mcna.2008.08.005
0025-7125/08/$ – see front matter © 2008 Elsevier Inc. All rights reserved.

Degenerative lesions, described as horizontal cleavages, flaps (oblique), complex tears, or meniscal maceration or destruction, are associated with older age and osteoarthritic disease.[11–14] These tears are common. In asymptomatic subjects with a mean age of 65 years, a tear was found in 67% using MRI, whereas in patients with symptomatic knee osteoarthritis, a meniscal tear was found in 91%.[9] Similar findings have been made in necropsy cases, where 60% of the subjects had a horizontal cleavage lesion.[12] Recent figures using a sample randomly drawn irrespective of the presence of osteoarthritis from the general population in Framingham, Massachusetts, revealed a prevalence of meniscal tear in about every third knee, and most lesions were found in knees with no pain.[15] Other studies support these findings.[16]

Meniscal lesions may be associated with knee-joint symptoms, but most lesions are actually not, and degenerative meniscal lesions are particularly poorly associated with knee pain.[9,15] This is in particular true for the latter category of degenerative meniscal lesions. Still, some meniscal tears may cause severe knee discomfort or even locking of the knee because of a dislocated tear fragment. In such cases, surgical treatment often becomes necessary.

PAST, PRESENT, AND FUTURE TREATMENT STRATEGIES OF A TORN MENISCUS

The first report of meniscal surgery that we know of described a meniscal repair procedure. In 1883, a British surgeon successfully sutured a torn medial meniscus.[17] However, 4 years later, in another report, he justified total removal of the meniscus rather than repair, and that view prevailed for over 80 years.[18] In the late 1940s, Fairbank[19] speculated that frequent radiographic changes found after total meniscectomy were due to the loss of the load-protective function of the menisci, resulting in remodeling of the joint. However, total removal of the menisci was considered a mostly benign procedure for at least another 20 years. From the late 1960s to the 1980s an increasing number of follow-up reports of meniscectomy were published, all indicating a high frequency of radiographic osteoarthritis and reduced knee function.[20–28] However, lack of standardized radiographic assessment and outcome measures precluded consistent quantification of the osteoarthritis risk. In 1998, a study showed a sixfold increase in the risk of radiographic osteoarthritis 21 years after total meniscectomy, compared with controls matched for age and sex.[29]

Not until the 1970s, when arthroscopic techniques were introduced, did interest increase in excising only the damaged portion of the meniscus rather than performing the previously popular complete resection with an open procedure. During that same period, several biomechanical studies reported on the load-bearing and shock-absorbing functions of the menisci.[3–5,30,31] The arthroscopic technique of surgery and partial meniscal resection offers several short-term benefits in terms of length of hospital stay, rehabilitation, and other measures.[32–34] Furthermore, with a substantial portion of the circumferentially oriented matrix fibers intact in the residual meniscus, hoop tension may still develop to counteract meniscal extrusion when the knee is loaded. Substantial shock-absorption and load-transmission function may thus remain in the residual meniscus, yielding a lower risk of radiographic changes related to osteoarthritis than that following a total meniscectomy.[35] However, the frequency of symptomatic knee osteoarthritis was not substantially lowered, which suggested that partial removal of the meniscus was not the final answer.

In consequence, for younger individuals with traumatic injury to the meniscus, meniscal repair is presently advocated when the lesion is located in the vicinity of the vascularized zone (with the potential to heal). Interestingly, we are back to where it all started in 1883. However, rehabilitation after repair is much more demanding than after meniscal resection, and the long-term outcome of meniscal repair compared with partial meniscectomy with respect to osteoarthritis is still unknown.[36,37] Thus, in practice, meniscal resection remains the most frequently performed procedure by orthopedic surgeons in the United States.[38]

Meniscal replacement using allogenic, xenogenic, or artificial materials is being tested in younger individuals who have undergone total meniscectomy. However, transplant survival is variable and long-term results using standardized outcomes are lacking.[39,40] Even so, as there is evidence that meniscal damage *without* surgery would otherwise lead to radiographic osteoarthritis, it is conceivable that treatments aimed at restoring meniscal function may lower this risk.[41] The treatment modality may be particularly suitable for younger individuals who have a severely torn meniscus, but surgery is hardly the answer for the one third of middle-aged and older adults in the general population who have meniscal damage.[9,15]

So, for many patients, the preferred goal of treatment is to preserve or restore the meniscus. But preservation or restoration is not feasible or practical in all patients, including the overwhelming majority of patients with osteoarthritis and degenerative tears. This leads to the question: In the middle-aged or older adult, what does a meniscal lesion not caused by knee trauma indicate?

MENISCAL TEAR—A CAUSE OR RESULT OF OSTEOARTHRITIS?

Although preserving meniscal tissue during meniscal surgery may provide some benefits, preservation, compared with total resection, appears to offer only modest reductions in frequency of knee osteoarthritis.[35] The reason this reduction is so modest could be because many of the middle-aged and older patients operated on already have early-stage knee osteoarthritis at the time of "meniscal" symptoms. It is plausible that they just happen to be referred to an orthopedic surgeon, perhaps after a meniscal tear was found during a routine MRI examination to investigate unclear knee-joint symptoms. In this age category, knee symptoms are weakly associated with meniscal tears, but may be strongly associated with other features of osteoarthritis.[15,42]

The menisci and articular cartilage share many similar components and properties, and are exposed to similar stresses. The pathologic processes active in the early-stage osteoarthritis joint that eventually lead to the cartilage destruction characteristic of osteoarthritis are not limited to the joint cartilage only, but would be expected to affect meniscus and ligament integrity as well. A tear in a meniscus with degenerative changes is often associated with pre-existing structural changes in the articular cartilage that may represent early-stage osteoarthritis.[12] Shear stress and early degradation of the collagenous meniscal matrix may result in decreased tensile strength. A meniscal tear could be the result of decreased ability of the compromised meniscus to withstand loads and force transmissions during normal knee-joint loads. A lesion may develop spontaneously (eg, when squatting) or in conjunction with minor knee trauma. Patients with "meniscal" symptoms due to a degenerative tear may thus constitute a subpopulation enriched in individuals with incipient osteoarthritis. For these patients, a tear and surgical resection may result in loss of some meniscus function, leading to increased biomechanical loading of the joint cartilage, further driving the development of the osteoarthritis that has already been established.

Meniscal displacement is common, particularly in osteoarthritic knees.[43,44] It is often another sign of a degraded or torn meniscus and a possible osteoarthritis disease process. Meniscal displacement may also contribute to increased joint space narrowing seen on radiographs, and meniscal tear and displacement are strong determinants of the rate of cartilage loss in knee osteoarthritis.[45–47] In middle-aged or elderly people, knees with meniscal damage but without cartilage lesions are at much higher risk of knee osteoarthritis than knees with intact menisci, suggesting that, in many instances, the meniscal damage comes before visible cartilage changes.[41]

GENE-ENVIRONMENT INTERACTION

A degenerative meniscal lesion was more frequently found in patients with radiographic hand osteoarthritis, and subjects with bilateral knee osteoarthritis had radiographic hand osteoarthritis more frequently than did subjects with unilateral knee osteoarthritis.[48] These findings provide additional support for an interaction between genetic and environmental risk factors in osteoarthritis, although metabolic effects cannot be excluded. Worse outcome after lateral meniscectomy compared with medial has been shown in several studies. The lateral meniscus carries higher loads in the knee compared with the medial meniscus. Consequently, if removed, the slightly convex lateral tibial plateau is exposed to relatively more cartilage contact stress,[3,4] which may further facilitate the osteoarthritis process. By comparison, the removal of the medial meniscus exposes the more concave medial tibial plateau.[22,27,28,35,49,50] This may provide yet another example of the interaction of local environmental factors with the inherent risk for the individual.

ONGOING CHALLENGES AND UNMET NEEDS

The middle-aged and older patients with "meniscal" pain and meniscal lesions represent a challenge for the health professional. It is difficult to discriminate between symptoms caused by a meniscal tear and symptoms of early-stage knee osteoarthritis. The weak evidence base for many of the current treatments suggests that this therapeutic area is in great need of well-designed randomized controlled clinical trials to assess the true effects of arthroscopic meniscal resection, meniscal repair or transplant, or nonsurgical treatments, compared with placebo or sham treatment.[51–53] Stratification with regard to lesion type, age, activity level, and other variables will provide a challenge in trial design, but there is no shortage of patients. Blinding of patient and assessor, and ethical issues represent additional challenges.

REFERENCES

1. Day B, Mackenzie WG, Shim SS, et al. The vascular and nerve supply of the human meniscus. Arthroscopy 1985;1(1):58–62.
2. Arnoczky SP, Warren RF. Microvasculature of the human meniscus. Am J Sports Med 1982;10(2):90–5.
3. Seedhom BB, Hargreaves DJ. Transmission of the load in the knee joint with special reference to the role of the meniscus. Part I+II. Eng Med 1979;4:207–28.
4. Walker PS, Erkman MJ. The role of the menisci in force transmission across the knee. Clin Orthop 1975;109:184–92.
5. Kurosawa H, Fukubayashi T, Nakajima H. Load-bearing mode of the knee joint: physical behavior of the knee joint with or without menisci. Clin Orthop 1980; 149:283–90.
6. Levy IM, Torzilli PA, Warren RF. The effect of medial meniscectomy on anterior-posterior motion of the knee. J Bone Joint Surg Am 1982;64(6):883–8.
7. Levy IM, Torzilli PA, Gould JD, et al. The effect of lateral meniscectomy on motion of the knee. J Bone Joint Surg Am 1989;71(3):401–6.
8. Assimakopoulos AP, Katonis PG, Agapitos MV, et al. The innervation of the human meniscus. Clin Orthop 1992;(275):232–6.

9. Bhattacharyya T, Gale D, Dewire P, et al. The clinical importance of meniscal tears demonstrated by magnetic resonance imaging in osteoarthritis of the knee. J Bone Joint Surg Am 2003;85(1):4–9.
10. Hunter DJ, Zhang YQ, Niu JB, et al. The association of meniscal pathologic changes with cartilage loss in symptomatic knee osteoarthritis. Arthritis Rheum 2006;54(3):795–801.
11. Poehling GG, Ruch DS, Chabon SJ. The landscape of meniscal injuries. Clin Sports Med 1990;9(3):539–49.
12. Noble J, Hamblen DL. The pathology of the degenerate meniscus lesion. J Bone Joint Surg Br 1975;57(2):180–6.
13. Noble J. Lesions of the menisci. Autopsy incidence in adults less than fifty-five years old. J Bone Joint Surg Am 1977;59(4):480–3.
14. Smillie IS. Surgical pathology of the menisci. Injuries of the knee joint. 3rd edition. Baltimore (MD): The Williams and Wilkins Co.; 1962. p. 51–90.
15. Englund M, Guermazi A, Gale D, et al. Incidental meniscal findings on knee MRI in middle-aged and elderly persons. N Engl J Med 2008;359:1108–15.
16. Ding C, Martel-Pelletier J, Pelletier JP, et al. Meniscal tear as an osteoarthritis risk factor in a largely non-osteoarthritic cohort: a cross-sectional study. J Rheumatol 2007;34(4):776–84.
17. Annandale T. An operation for displaced semilunar cartilage. Br Med J 1885;1: 779.
18. Annandale T. Excision of the internal semilunar cartilage, resulting in perfect restoration of the joint-movements. Br Med J 1889;1:291–2.
19. Fairbank TJ. Knee joint changes after meniscectomy. J Bone Joint Surg Br 1948; 30:164–70.
20. Gear MW. The late results of meniscectomy. Br J Surg 1967;54(4):270–2.
21. Tapper EM, Hoover NW. Late results after meniscectomy. J Bone Joint Surg Am 1969;51(3):517–26.
22. Johnson RJ, Kettelkamp DB, Clark W, et al. Factors affecting late results after meniscectomy. J Bone Joint Surg Am 1974;56(4):719–29.
23. Noble J. Clinical features of the degenerate meniscus with the results of meniscectomy. Br J Surg 1975;62(12):977–81.
24. Noble J, Erat K. In defence of the meniscus. A prospective study of 200 meniscectomy patients. J Bone Joint Surg Br 1980;62-B(1):7–11.
25. Sonne-Holm S, Fledelius I, Ahn NC. Results after meniscectomy in 147 athletes. Acta Orthop Scand 1980;51(2):303–9.
26. Doherty M, Watt I, Dieppe P. Influence of primary generalised osteoarthritis on development of secondary osteoarthritis. Lancet 1983;2(8340):8–11.
27. Allen PR, Denham RA, Swan AV. Late degenerative changes after meniscectomy. Factors affecting the knee after operation. J Bone Joint Surg Br 1984;66(5): 666–71.
28. Jørgensen U, Sonne-Holm S, Lauridsen F, et al. Long-term follow-up of meniscectomy in athletes. A prospective longitudinal study. J Bone Joint Surg Br 1987;69(1):80–3.
29. Roos H, Lauren M, Adalberth T, et al. Knee osteoarthritis after meniscectomy: prevalence of radiographic changes after twenty-one years, compared with matched controls. Arthritis Rheum 1998;41(4):687–93.
30. Shrive NG, O'Connor JJ, Goodfellow JW. Load-bearing in the knee joint. Clin Orthop 1978;131:279–87.
31. Fukubayashi T, Kurosawa H. The contact area and pressure distribution pattern of the knee. A study of normal and osteoarthrotic knee joints. Acta Orthop Scand 1980;51(6):871–9.

32. Dandy DJ. Early results of closed partial menisectomy. Br Med J 1978;1(6120): 1099–100.

33. Oretorp N, Gillquist J. Transcutaneous meniscectomy under arthroscopic control. Int Orthop 1979;3(1):19–25.

34. Northmore-Ball MD, Dandy DJ, Jackson RW. Arthroscopic, open partial, and total meniscectomy. A comparative study. J Bone Joint Surg Br 1983;65(4):400–4.

35. Englund M, Lohmander LS. Risk factors for symptomatic knee osteoarthritis fifteen to twenty-two years after meniscectomy. Arthritis Rheum 2004;50(9): 2811–9.

36. Steenbrugge F, Verdonk R, Verstraete K, et al. Long-term assessment of arthroscopic meniscus repair: a 13-year follow-up study. Knee 2002;9(3):181–7.

37. Rockborn P, Messner K. Long-term results of meniscus repair and meniscectomy: a 13-year functional and radiographic follow-up study. Knee Surg Sports Traumatol Arthrosc 2000;8(1):2–10.

38. Hall MJ, Lawrence L. Ambulatory surgery in the United States, 1996. Adv Data 1998;300:1–16.

39. Noyes FR, Barber-Westin SD, Rankin M. Meniscal transplantation in symptomatic patients less than fifty years old. J Bone Joint Surg Am 2005;87(Suppl 1(Pt 2)): 149–65.

40. Lohmander LS, Englund PM, Dahl LL, et al. The long-term consequence of anterior cruciate ligament and meniscus injuries: osteoarthritis. Am J Sports Med 2007;35(10):1756–69.

41. Englund M, Guermazi A, Roemer FW, et al. The effect of meniscal damage on incident radiographic knee osteoarthritis. [abstract]. Arthritis Rheum 2007; 56(9):S316.

42. Englund M, Niu J, Guermazi A, et al. Effect of meniscal damage on the development of frequent knee pain, aching, or stiffness. Arthritis Rheum 2007;56(12): 4048–54.

43. Adams JG, McAlindon T, Dimasi M, et al. Contribution of meniscal extrusion and cartilage loss to joint space narrowing in osteoarthritis. Clin Radiol 1999;54(8): 502–6.

44. Gale DR, Chaisson CE, Totterman SM, et al. Meniscal subluxation: association with osteoarthritis and joint space narrowing. Osteoarthr Cartil 1999;7(6): 526–32.

45. Berthiaume MJ, Raynauld JP, Martel-Pelletier J, et al. Meniscal tear and extrusion are strongly associated with progression of symptomatic knee osteoarthritis as assessed by quantitative magnetic resonance imaging. Ann Rheum Dis 2005; 64(4):556–63.

46. Hunter DJ, Zhang YQ, Niu JB, et al. The association of meniscal pathologic changes with cartilage loss in symptomatic knee osteoarthritis. Arthritis Rheum 2006;54:795–801.

47. Ding C, Martel-Pelletier J, Pelletier JP, et al. Knee meniscal extrusion in a largely non-osteoarthritic cohort: association with greater loss of cartilage volume. Arthritis Res Ther 2007;9(2):R21.

48. Englund M, Paradowski PT, Lohmander LS. Association of radiographic hand osteoarthritis with radiographic knee osteoarthritis after meniscectomy. Arthritis Rheum 2004;50(2):469–75.

49. Chatain F, Adeleine P, Chambat P, et al. A comparative study of medial versus lateral arthroscopic partial meniscectomy on stable knees: 10-year minimum follow-up. Arthroscopy 2003;19(8):842–9.

50. Hede A, Larsen E, Sandberg H. The long term outcome of open total and partial meniscectomy related to the quantity and site of the meniscus removed. Int Orthop 1992;16(2):122–5.
51. Moseley JB, O'Malley K, Petersen NJ, et al. Arthroscopic lavage or debridement did not reduce pain more than placebo did in patients with osteoarthritis. J Bone Joint Surg Am 2003;85-A(2):387.
52. Herrlin S, Hallander M, Wange P, et al. Arthroscopic or conservative treatment of degenerative medial meniscal tears: a prospective randomised trial. Knee Surg Sports Traumatol Arthrosc 2007;15:393–401.
53. Kirkley A, Birmingham TB, Litchfield RB, et al. A randomized trial of arthroscopic surgery for osteoarthritis of the knee. N Engl J Med 2008;359:1097–107.

The Contribution of Genes to Osteoarthritis

Ana M. Valdes, PhD*, Timothy D. Spector, MD, FRCP

KEYWORDS

• Osteoarthritis • Genetic association • Polymorphism

Osteoarthritis (OA) is the most prevalent form of arthritis in the elderly. Primary osteoarthritis is an idiopathic phenomenon, occurring in previously intact joints, with no apparent initiating factor, such as joint injury or developmental abnormalities. The disease is characterized by softening, splitting, and fragmentation (fibrillation) of articular cartilage. This process is usually accompanied by sclerosis of the bone providing support for the cartilage of the articular surface (subchondral bone), bone cysts, and bony outgrowths at the joint margins (osteophytes).[1] In the United States alone the prevalence of clinical OA has grown to nearly 27 million, up from an estimate of 21 million for 1995,[2] and it is the third most prevalent condition causing work disability.[3] OA may be local (ie, confined to one joint) or generalized.[4] Generalized OA refers to the involvement in disease of at least three joints or a group of joints (eg, the interphalangeal joints). Two types of generalized disease have been described: nodal and non-nodal. The nodal type features Heberden nodes (hard or bony swellings) of the distal interphalangeal joints and predominates in women. The hereditary nature of Heberden nodes was noted as early as the nineteenth century[5] and by the 1940s it was concluded that the phenotype was inherited as a dominant trait.[6] Further studies established that nodal OA often occurred in the context of OA at multiple sites and even suggested polygenic inheritance of the disease.[7]

Understanding the genetic contribution to OA has two important clinical implications. First, by finding genes involved in disease risk or involved in progression we will better understand the molecular pathogenesis of OA and this may open areas for therapeutic intervention. Second, by identifying sets of genetic variants associated with risk for disease or with progression of OA it will be possible to detect individuals at high risk and to better monitor disease progression. This article reviews the current

A version of this article originally appeared in the 34:3 issue of the *Rheumatic Disease Clinics of North America*.

This work was supported by EC framework 7 programme grant 200800 TREAT-OA and by Arthritis and Research Campaign project grant 17716.

Twin Research and Genetic Epidemiology Unit, St. Thomas Hospital Campus, Kings College, London School of Medicine, London SE1 7EH, UK

* Corresponding author.

E-mail address: ana.valdes@kcl.ac.uk (A.M. Valdes).

knowledge relating to evidence for the genetic contribution to OA, focusing mostly on the hip and the knee, and on the specific genetic regions and genes involved.

Several strategies can be used to investigate the role of genetics in OA, including familial aggregation studies, twin studies, linkage analyses, and candidate gene association studies (**Fig. 1**).[5,8,9] Some of these methods have also been applied to risk factors or components of disease, such as cartilage volume, and to some longitudinal traits relating to OA incidence and progression. Nevertheless, the strategies geared toward the identification of the genes and variants actually involved in disease have to date only been applied to radiographic or clinical OA status.

FAMILIAL AGGREGATION

The risk ratio for a relative of an affected individual compared with the population prevalence is a measure for familial aggregation of complex diseases.[10] It has been extensively applied in genetic epidemiology to derive the statistical power available for a given condition to detect genetic linkage to a complex genetic disorder.[11] For affected sib pairs this sib recurrence risk is termed the lambda sib (λ_s). **Table 1** shows estimates of the sibling recurrence risk for various conditions.

It is possible to identify subjects who have clinically severe disease, for example, severe enough symptoms to lead to total joint replacement (TJR), and to compare the prevalence of OA in their siblings (who have a genetic exposure) with that in controls who are matched as closely as possible to the siblings. A study in Nottingham[20] assessed the prevalence of hip OA in siblings of individuals undergoing total hip replacement (THR) to the prevalence of radiographic hip OA in controls. A similar study was performed using total knee replacement (TKR) as the selection criterion.[17] Similar data but using self-reported TJR data in a smaller sample set was found in a study in Oxford.[18] The data presented in **Table 1** indicate a strong familial aggregation, even by comparison to some autoimmune conditions known to have an important genetic component. In addition familial aggregation of specific knee OA phenotypes, such as anteromedial OA, which correspond to lesions in the tibial plateau and preservation of cartilage of other compartments of the knee, have also been reported in United Kingdom populations.[19] Unlike other patterns of OA, cartilage degeneration in

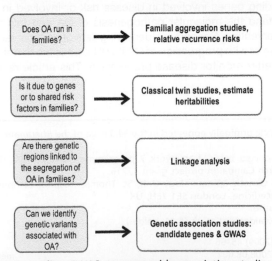

Fig. 1. Types of genetic studies. GWAS, genome-wide association studies.

Table 1
Familial aggregation of osteoarthritis and of other disorders

Type of Disorder	Condition	Ascertained by	Sibling Recurrence Risk λ_s	Reference
Autoimmune	Rheumatoid arthritis	Sibs with condition	5	[12]
	Juvenile rheumatoid arthritis	Sibs with condition	15	[13]
	Celiac disease	Sibs with condition	7.5–30	[14]
Metabolic	Obesity	Sibs with condition	1.60–1.91	[15]
	Hyperglycemia	Sibs with condition	1.39–1.81	[15]
	Type 2 diabetes	Sibs with condition	1.2–1.6	[16]
Cardiovascular	Hypertension	Sibs with condition	1.22–1.34	[15]
Osteoarthritis	Tibiofemoral OA	Sibs with TKR	2.13	[17]
	Patellofemoral OA	Sibs with TKR	1.66	[17]
	Knee OA (TF and/or PF)	Sibs with TKR	2.08	[17]
	TKR	Sibs with TKR	4.81	[18]
	Anteromedial OA	Sibs with UKR	3.21	[19]
	Hip osteophytes grade 3	Sibs with THR	4.27	[20]
	THR	Sibs with THR	1.87–8.53	[18,20]
	Hip KL grade ≥3	Sibs with THR	4.99	[20]
	Hip JSW ≤1.5 mm	Sibs with THR	5.07	[20]

Abbreviations: JSW, joint space width; KL, Kellgren–Lawrence grade; PF, patellofemoral; TF, tibio-femoral; THR, total hip replacement; TKR, total knee replacement; UKR, unicompartmental knee replacement.

anteromedial OA is consistent with increased loading and thus could be assumed to be attributable mostly to mechanical causes, rather than genetic factors. Yet the high familial aggregation reported suggests a genetic contribution even for this particular type of OA.

Familial Aggregation of Generalized Osteoarthritis and Progression of Osteoarthritis

Early studies by Kellgren and colleagues[21] in the 1950s reported in families of probands who had generalized OA involving six or more joint groups a twofold excess of OA among first-degree relatives compared with population controls, and the recurrence risk was highest among the relatives of female probands. These recurrence risks are comparable to those for knee or hip OA shown in **Table 1**.

Among participants of the Genetics, Arthrosis, and Progression study (GARP) in the Netherlands where probands were diagnosed with primary OA at multiple sites, familial aggregation has been investigated by assessing concordance rates with their siblings. The odds ratio (OR) adjusted for age, sex, and body mass index (BMI) for siblings to be affected in the same joint sites as the proband were increased in osteoarthritis of the hand (OR = 4.4, 95% CI 2.0–9.5), hip (OR = 3.9, 95% CI 1.8–8.4), spine (OR = 2.2, 95% CI 1.0–5.1), hip–spine (OR = 4.7, 95% CI 2.1–10.4), and hand–hip (OR = 3.4, 95% CI 1.1–10.4). Siblings of probands who had osteoarthritis in the knee (affected also at other joints) did not have an increased likelihood of knee OA.[22] Familial aggregation of OA radiographic progression has also been investigated. Radiographic progression is measured by comparing the joint space narrowing (JSN) and osteo-phyte grades at baseline and follow-up in the same joint. These radiographic grades, which can range from absent to severe, yield a semiquantitative measure of cartilage loss and of bony growths in a degenerating joint, respectively. Familial aggregation on progression was measured in the GARP study[23] by evaluating concordance in the change in JSN and in osteophyte grade at various anatomic sites The odds ratios (95% confidence intervals), adjusted for age, sex, and BMI, of a sibling having radio-graphic progression if the proband had progression were 3.0 (1.2–7.8) for JSN pro-gression and 1.5 (0.6–3.6) for osteophyte progression. A dose-response relationship was found between the amount of increase in JSN total scores among probands and the progression of JSN in siblings.

The reference control population drawn on to estimate the odds ratios in the GARP study were other probands and their siblings who had OA, although not OA at that specific site or without progression at that site. Such measures of familial aggregation are thus not recurrence risks and are not directly comparable to those shown in **Table 1**. The data from the GARP study indicate that in middle-aged patients who have familial osteoarthritis at multiple sites, familial aggregation of osteoarthritis is most striking for hand and hip, and that changes in joint space narrowing are signifi-cantly correlated between siblings.

Familial aggregation does not result exclusively from genetic factors and may reflect environmental exposures that are shared by family members. If only a weak familial aggregation is observed it may not in itself constitute convincing evidence of the con-tribution of genetic as opposed to environmental factors to a disease.[24] An alternative method to assess the actual genetic contribution to a condition, in this case OA, is the use of classic twin studies, which enable investigators to quantify the environmental and genetic factors that contribute to a trait or disease.

CLASSIC TWIN STUDIES

The classic twin study compares resemblances of identical, or monozygotic (MZ), and nonidentical, or dizygotic (DZ), twins. MZ twins derive from a single fertilized egg and therefore inherit identical genetic material, unlike DZ twins who on average share only 50% of their genetic material. Comparing the resemblance of MZ twins for a trait or disease with the resemblance of DZ twins offers the first estimate of the extent to which genetic variation determines variation of that trait. If MZ twins resemble each other more than DZ twins do, then the heritability of the trait can be estimated from twice the difference between MZ and DZ correlations.[25] In this context then heritability refers specifically to how much of the variance in the distribution of the trait under study might be attributable to genetic, rather than constitutional or environmental, factors that might be shared by individuals from the same family.

The heritability of OA has been calculated in twin sets after adjustment of the data for other known risk factors, such as age, sex, and BMI. The correlations of radio-graphic osteophytes and joint space narrowing at most sites and the presence of Heberden nodes and knee pain have been found to be higher in the MZ pairs than in the DZ pairs.[26] Such findings show that the influence of genetic factors in radio-graphic OA of the hand, hip, and knee in women is between 39% and 65%, indepen-dent of known environmental or demographic confounding factors. Classic twin studies and familial aggregation studies have also investigated the genetic contribu-tion to cartilage volume and progression of disease.

Genetic Contribution to Disease Progression

Cartilage loss is the hallmark of established osteoarthritis.[27] Recent twin and sibling studies have indicated that the heritability of cartilage volume is high (**Table 2**).[28] Comparing the offspring of people who have severe OA to controls, however, Jones and colleagues[29] were able to identify no difference in cartilage volume, suggesting that it is cartilage loss later in life that influences OA pathogenesis but not a lower cartilage volume in itself.

Using longitudinal radiographic data, heritability estimates of 62% for progression of osteophytes and 72% for progression of JSN of the knee, independent of age and BMI, have been reported.[33] Genetic influence on radiographic disease progression over 2 years in a separate study was also assessed in a sibling pair design with generalized symptomatic OA (the GARP study).[23] Moreover, a longitudinal sibpair study using MRI also demonstrated that longitudinal changes in knee structures of relevance to later OA, such as medial tibial cartilage volume, lateral tibial bone size, and progression of chondral defects, have a high heritability.[32] The MRI sib pair study and the twin radiograph study found that the heritability of change in medial compartments had a much stronger genetic component than those in lateral compartments. These results highlighted a strong genetic influence on progression of OA and provide a logical basis for the next step to identify specific genetic factors responsible for incidence and progression of OA.

Few studies to date have attempted to test candidate genes involved in longitudinal changes (eg, see Ref.;[34] Section 4). The past few years, however have seen the advent of prospective studies designed specifically to investigate factors affecting the incidence and progression of knee OA. The two most notable examples are the Multicenter Osteoarthritis Study (MOST[35]) and the Osteoarthritis Initiative (OAI; www.oai.ucsf.edu), both of which are funded by the US National Institutes of Health.

These cohorts have recruited individuals who have clinically significant knee OA or are at high risk for developing new clinical knee OA and are obtaining appropriate images and biospecimens at various time points on these subjects. Although no genetic studies have been performed on these collections yet, these cohorts present

Table 2
Heritability of various osteoarthritis-associated traits

Trait	Heritability (%)	Reference
Radiographic knee OA	39	30
Radiographic hip OA	60	26
Radiographic hand OA	59	31
Femoral cartilage volume	61	28
Tibial cartilage volume	76	28
Patellar cartilage volume	66	28
Change in medial cartilage volume[a]	73	32
Change in lateral cartilage volume[a]	40	32
Change in medial knee osteophyte grade	69	33
Change in lateral knee osteophyte grade	33	33
Change in knee JSN grade	74	33

Abbreviation: JSN, joint space narrowing.
[a] From a sib pair, not twin study.

an ideal opportunity to investigate the role of genetic variation on incidence and progression of disease.

Genes may affect the incidence, progression, or severity of OA through several pathways (**Fig. 2**). It is important then to investigate, of the pathways known to affect progression, which ones are also influenced by genes. Based on data from multiple high-quality studies, Belo and colleagues[36] concluded that sex, knee injury, quadriceps strength, and regular sport activities are not associated with radiographic progression of knee OA and knee pain at baseline and radiographic severity of OA at baseline seems to be at best only weakly associated with the progression. Evidence from multiple high-quality studies[36] shows that the level of hyaluronic acid (HA) in serum and the presence of generalized OA are associated with radiographic progression of knee OA. There is strong evidence for a genetic contribution to generalized OA. To date, however, no studies exploring the genetic contribution to serum levels of HA are available. Other factors that have been implicated in knee OA progression include synovial fluid volume, medial bone marrow edema lesions, adduction moment, alignment of the joint (varus/valgus), bone density, low serum levels, and dietary intake of vitamin D, among others. Some of these, such as bone density, are known to be strongly influenced by genes.

Bone is not structurally normal in OA. Periarticular bone in OA has increased turnover, decreased bone mineral content and stiffness, and decreased trabecular numbers. Individuals who have OA exhibit striking increases in bone mass for affected sites, such as the knee and hip, and nonsynovial sites, such as the lumbar spine.[37] This increase in bone mass is attributable to an abnormal metabolism of osteoblasts particularly in the subchondral bone tissue that seem to be a response to altered local signals.[38] It has been hypothesized[39] that enhanced bone remodeling is the initiating event triggering the cartilage damage. The attempt to repair the cartilage then leads to several biochemical adaptations in bone and cartilage that may overwhelm the attempts to repair cartilage and lead to further sclerosis and damage.

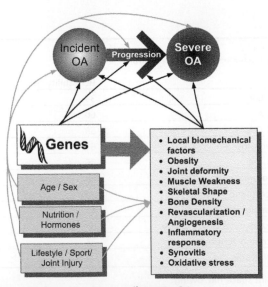

Fig. 2. Mechanisms by which genes can contribute to OA.

Bone mineral density (BMD) and bone remodeling are under strong genetic control[40] and genetic variation at genes strongly and consistently involved in determining BMD and fractures has also been involved in risk for OA. Most notably the genes encoding the low-density lipoprotein receptor–related protein (*LRP5*)[41] and osteoprotegerin (*OPG*)[42] have repeatedly been associated with BMD and are also associated with OA.

Certain alterations in the mechanical environment of the joint adversely affect load distribution. Knee alignment is knee position in reference to the hip and ankle. Alignment at the knee (the hip–knee–ankle angle as measured by full-limb radiography) can either be varus (bow-legged), valgus (knock-knee), or neutral.[4] Varus–valgus alignment has been shown to influence the risk for patellofemoral[43] and tibiofemoral osteoarthritis progression.[44]

Malalignment predicts worse surgical outcomes, but its role in the natural history of OA has been minimally considered. The magnitude of the torque that adducts the knee during the stance phase of gait correlates with disease severity in knee OA[4] and may predict the natural rate of disease progression. Further, in a longitudinal MRI-based study, Cicuttini and colleagues[45] found that baseline knee angle is associated with the rate of cartilage loss in the knee. Two recent studies from the United States and Australia have shown, however, that knee malalignment is not associated with disease incidence and that it is more likely to be a marker of disease progression or severity.[46] On the other hand, an increasing degree of varus alignment was associated not only with progression of radiographic knee OA but also with development of knee OA in the Rotterdam study.[44] This association seemed particularly applicable to overweight and obese people.

Other mechanical factors that may affect risk for incidence or progression of OA include knee laxity[47] and proprioception.[4] Studies assessing the role that genetics plays in these factors have not been published to date.

Another possible route of genetic control of risk for OA could be through skeletal shape. Studies in animal models have shown how skeletal development and skeletal shape are under tight genetic control[48] and some studies have indicated a role for skeletal shape in the risk for OA. For example, Lane and colleagues,[49] examining baseline and 8-year follow-up radiographs, found that an abnormal center-edge angle and acetabular dysplasia were each associated with an increased risk for incident hip osteoarthritis, adjusting for age, current weight, BMI, affected side, and investigational site (adjusted OR 3.3, 95% CI 1.1–10.1 for center-edge angle and adjusted OR 2.8, 95% CI 1.0–7.9 for acetabular dysplasia). In a cross-sectional study Shepstone and colleagues[50] found a statistically significant difference in the shape of the intercondylar notch between the OA and non-OA groups. The observed difference in shape might have been congenital and one that increases the risk for anterior cruciate ligament damage or perhaps alters knee mechanics through some other route and, therefore, a genuine risk factor for knee OA. Given the cross-sectional nature of the study, however, it could also be a result of OA.

In a recent study of radiographic progression of hip OA in the Rotterdam cohort significant changes in shape of the proximal femur occurred within the OA group from baseline to follow-up[51] apparently as a result of OA.

Several of the genes known to control skeletal development in animal model systems, such as bone morphogenetic proteins and Wnt signaling genes (discussed later), have indeed been associated with risk for OA, but whether this is because of an effect on skeletal shape has not been investigated.

Another aspect shown to contribute to disease risk and progression is inflammation, in particular synovitis. There is a growing body of evidence that synovial inflammation is implicated in many of the signs and symptoms of OA, including joint swelling and effusion.[52] Histologically, the OA synovium shows hyperplasia with an increased number of lining cells and a mixed inflammatory infiltrate consisting mainly of macrophages.[53]

The low-grade OA synovitis is cytokine driven, although the levels of proinflammatory cytokines are lower than in rheumatoid arthritis. In particular, tumor necrosis factor (TNF)–α and interleukin (IL-1) have been suggested as key players in OA pathogenesis[54] in synovial inflammation and in activation of chondrocytes. These cytokines can stimulate their own production and can induce synovial cells and chondrocytes to produce IL-6, IL-8, and leukocyte inhibitory factor. They can also stimulate protease and prostaglandin production. Progression of tibiofemoral cartilage damage is more severe in patients who have synovial inflammation. Ayral and coworkers[55] assessed changes in tibiofemoral cartilage damage over a 1-year period in 422 patients who had knee OA. Their results indicated that the extent of cartilage damage of the medial tibia after 1 year was statistically more severe in the group of patients who had an inflammatory perimeniscal synovial membrane at baseline than in patients who had normal synovium. An individual's inflammatory response is known to be under genetic control[56] and several variants in genes encoding for cytokines or proteins involved in inflammation have been reported to be associated with OA.

LINKAGE ANALYSES

In genetics, a locus refers to a particular location on a chromosome or the DNA at that position. It can be present in the population in one or more forms, called alleles. If more than one allele exists for a locus, it is termed polymorphic. When the specific alleles at two or more loci in the same chromosome are being studied, the particular combination of alleles is called a haplotype. A polymorphic locus genotyped solely because its inheritance can be monitored and not because it may be involved in a clinical or phenotypic trait is called a genetic marker. A single nucleotide polymorphism (SNP) is a polymorphic locus consisting of a change at a single nucleotide base. When comparing alleles at a locus between two individuals, the alleles may be identical by descent, if the allele came from the same parent (or ancestor), or only by state, if for example one patient obtained the allele from her mother and her sibling obtained an identical allele from their father.

Genetic linkage then occurs when a locus involved in the trait of interest (in this case OA) and alleles at nearby markers are inherited jointly, indicating that the genetic markers and the disease locus map relatively close to each other in the same chromosome. Genetic markers can therefore be used as tools to track the inheritance pattern of a gene involved in a specific trait or disease. Consequently, to identify chromosomal regions harboring OA genes, researchers have used pairs of siblings in which both siblings are affected with OA. When the proportion of alleles identical by descent that sibs concordant for OA share at a given marker is higher than expected, then it is concluded that marker is close in chromosomal location to an OA-related gene, or that significant linkage with OA has been found.

At least five genome-wide linkage scans have been published to date based on small families or twins of affected relatives collected in the United Kingdom,[57–59] Finland,[60] Iceland,[61,62] and the United States.[63,64] These genome-wide linkage scans have been performed on patients ascertained for hip, knee, or hand OA and have identified a large number of relatively broad genomic intervals that may harbor OA susceptibility in chromosomes 2, 4, 6, 7, 11, 16, 19, and the X. Recently, Lee and colleagues[65] conducted a meta-analysis of OA whole-genome scans from 893 families who had

3000 affected individuals taking part in three studies (Iceland, United Kingdom, and United States). Their analysis provided summarized linkage loci of OA across whole-genome scan studies and based on their data they concluded that genetic regions such as 7q34–7q36.3, 11p12–11q13.4, 6p21.1–6q15, 2q31.1–2q34, and 15q21.3–15q26.1 were the most likely to harbor OA susceptibility genes.

A summary of the chromosomal regions identified by linkage analyses is presented in **Table 3**. Some of the intervals identified from genome-wide linkage scans have subsequently been subjected to association analyses, principally candidate-gene based studies, specifically: the interleukin 1 (*IL1*) gene cluster chr 2q11-q13; matrilin 3 (*MATN3*), chromosome 2p24.1; interleukin 4 receptor (*IL4R*), chromosome 16p12.1; secreted frizzled-related protein 3 (*FRZB*), chromosome 2q32.1; and bone morphogenetic protein 5 (*BMP5*), chromosome 6p12.1. These have been reviewed in detail by Loughlin.[8] The genetic associations found at these and other genes are discussed in the next section (**Table 4**).

Table 3

Chromosomal region identified from genome-wide linkage scans that have been performed on families containing osteoarthritis-affected relatives

Chromosome	Cytogenetic Location	Genes in Region Associated with OA	Linkage Study	Linkage with Trait	Reference
1	1p32–p22		United States	Hand OA	63,64
2	2q12–2q21	IL1	Finland	Hand/knee/ hip OA	60
	2q31.1–2q34	FRZB	United Kingdom	Hip OA	57,58
	2p23.2–2p16.2	MATN3	Iceland, United States	Hand OA	61–64
3	3p22.2–3p14.1		Iceland	Hand OA	61,62
4	4q26–4q32.1		Finland, Iceland	Hand OA	60,61
6	6p21.1–6q15	BMP5, HLA	United Kingdom	Hip OA	57,58
7	7q34–7q36.3		United States	Hand OA	63,64
	7p15–7p21		Finland	Hand OA	60
11	11p12–11q13.4	LRP5	United Kingdom	Hip OA	57,58
13	13q33.1–13q34		United States	Hand OA	63,64
15	15q21.3–15q26.1		United States	Hand OA	63,64
16	16p13.1–16q12.1	IL4R	United Kingdom, Iceland	Hip OA	57,58,61,62
	16q22.1–q23.1		United Kingdom	Knee OA/ Hip OA	57,58
19	19q13		United States, United Kingdom	Hand OA	57,58,63,64
X	X cen		Finland	Hand OA	60

Also listed are those instances in which a gene within a linked interval has subsequently been shown to be associated with OA.

Table 4
Selected published genetic associations with osteoarthritis

Symbol	Gene Name	Reported Significant Associations	Negative Reports	Trait Associated with	In Linkage Region?	Known or Putative Function
AACT	Alpha1 antiproteinase antitrypsin	34,66		Knee OA	No	Natural inhibitor of serine proteinase involved in the degradation of cartilage proteoglycan
ADAM12	A disintegrin and metalloproteinase domain 12	34,66		Knee OA	No	Metalloproteinase involved in osteoclast formation and cell–cell fusion
ASPN	Asporin	67-71		Hip OA/ knee OA	No	Cartilage extracellular protein that regulates the activity of TGF-β
BMP2	Bone morphogenetic protein 2	34,66		Knee OA	No	Growth factor involved in chondrogenesis and osteogenesis
BMP5	Bone morphogenetic protein 5	72		Hip OA	Yes	Regulator of articular chondrocyte development
CALM1	Calmodulin 1	73	67,74	Hip OA	No	Intracellular protein, interacts with proteins involved in signal transduction
CILP	Cartilage intermediate layer protein	34,67,75		Knee OA, LDD	No	Inhibits TGFβ1–mediated induction of cartilage matrix genes
COL2A1	Type II collagen	67,76		Knee OA	No	Major cartilage collagen, structural cartilage component
COMP	Cartilage oligomeric matrix protein	67		Knee OA	No	Cartilage matrix macromolecule
COX2 (PTGS2)	Prostaglandin	34,66,77,78		Knee OA, spine OA	No	COX-2–produced PGE(2) modulates cartilage proteoglycan degradation in OA
DIO2	Iodothyronine-deiodinase enzyme type 2	79		Hip OA, GOA	No	Regulates intracellular levels of active thyroid hormones in target tissues

Gene	Gene name	References	OA type	Meta-analysis	Function
ESR1	Estrogen receptor alpha	34,61,80,81	Knee OA, GOA	No	In chondrocytes, modulator of proteoglycan degradation and matrix metalloproteinase mRNA expression
FRZB	Secreted frizzled-related protein 3	67,82–85 86	Hip /knee OA, GOA,	Yes	Wnt antagonist and modulator of chondrocyte maturation
GDF5	Growth differentiation factor 5	87,88	Hip OA	No	Member of the bone morphogenetic family, regulator of growth and differentiation
HLA	Human leukocyte antigen system	89–92	Hand/hip/ knee OA, GOA	Yes	Antigen presentation and binding of HLA/antigen complex to the T cell receptor determining specificity of immune response
IL1 gene cluster	Interleukin 1-α, -β and interleukin 1 receptor antagonist (Knee OA)	93–95 95	(Knee OA) Hip/knee OA	Yes	Regulation of metalloproteinase gene expression in synovium and chondrocytes
IL4R	Interleukin 4 receptor	96	Hip OA	Yes	Putative role in cartilage chondrocyte response to mechanical signals
IL6	Interleukin 6	97,98	Hip /knee OA	No	Proinflammatory cytokine, involved in the cartilage degradation but also induces ILRa
IL10	Interleukin 10	99,100	Knee/hand OA	No	Anti-inflammatory cytokine inhibits the synthesis of IL-1

(continued on next page)

Table 4
(continued)

Symbol	Gene Name	Reported Significant Associations	Negative Reports	Trait Associated with	In Linkage Region?	Known or Putative Function
LRCH1	Leucine-rich repeats and calponin homology (CH) domain containing 1	101	102	Hip/knee OA	No	Unknown
LRP5	Low-density lipoprotein receptor-related protein 5	103	86	Knee OA	Yes	Receptor involved in Wnt signaling by way of the canonical β-catenin pathway
MATN3	Matrilin 3	61,104		Hand OA		
Spine OA	Yes	Extracellular matrix macromolecule				
OPG	Osteoprotegerin	34,66		Knee OA	No	Regulation of osteoclastogenesis
RHOB	Ras homolog gene family, member B	105	106	Hip OA, knee OA	No	GTPase with tumor suppressor activity (antagonist of the PI3K/Akt pathway)
TXNDC3	Thioredoxin domain containing 3	105	106	Knee OA	No	Protein disulfide reductase participating in several cellular processes by way of redox-mediated reactions
TNA	Tetranectin	34,66		Knee OA	No	Plasminogen binding protein, mediates degradation of extracellular matrix
VDR1	Vitamin D receptor	34,67,107		Knee OA	No	Nuclear receptor, mediates effects of vitamin D whose serum levels affect incidence severity and progression of OA

Abbreviations: GOA, generalized osteoarthritis; ILRa, interleukin receptor antagonist; LDD, lumbar disc degenerative disease; PGE2, prostaglandin 2.

GENETIC ASSOCIATIONS

Genetic association studies provide a means of quantifying the effects of specific gene variants on disease occurrence. It is important to distinguish between a genetic association and the role of a gene or its encoded product in disease. For example, matrix metalloproteinases (MMPs) are of key importance in OA yet genetic variants in these genes have not been reported to be associated with susceptibility to disease. This finding can be explained if over- or underexpression of the gene encoding MMPs during disease is attributable to other factors (inflammation, aging, injury) but not to an individual carrying a particular genetic variant. On the other hand, if a variant at a gene is associated with disease risk, there is a high probability that the gene is involved in disease pathogenesis.

Early candidate gene studies concentrated on cartilage components, such as COL2A1, which encodes for the alpha1 polypeptide chain of type II collagen, the principal collagenous component of articular cartilage. Other extracellular matrix (ECM)–related genes that were considered included type IX and type XI collagen genes and the aggrecan gene. These studies did not yield convincing evidence to support a role for common, nonsynonymous mutations in cartilage ECM structural protein genes as risk factors for primary OA.[8] Other candidates were some of the genes associated with osteoporosis and bone density, such as the genes encoding estrogen receptor alpha (ESR1) and the vitamin D receptor (VDR). Various variants at these two genes have been reported to be associated with OA[66] (see **Table 4**).

A different approach was taken by our own group. We compared human cDNA libraries from OA-affected and normal cartilage and synovium and selected 22 genes that showed significantly different expression. One or two SNPs per gene were then tested for association with cross-sectional and longitudinal radiographic features of knee OA. SNPs at 9 of the 22 genes were found to be associated with OA in a population-based cohort. Variants at 7 of those 9 were also associated with clinical knee OA in either men, women, or both in an independent population.[66]

Genes falling under linkage peaks have also been tested with varying results. Replication studies for genes derived from linkage studies have yielded mixed results, with FRZB being the gene most replicated in association studies. The genes in **Table 4** represent, broadly speaking, at least five different molecular pathways or classes of molecules: inflammation (IL1, IL4R, COX2, IL6, IL10, HLA), ECM molecules (ASPN, MATN3, COL2A1, COMP, CILP), Wnt signaling (FRZB, LRP5), bone morphogenetic proteins (BMP2, BMP5, and GDF5), and proteases or their inhibitors (ADAM12, TNA, AACT), in addition to genes related to modulation of osteocyte or chondrocyte differentiation or proteolytic activity as would be ESR1, VDR, and OPG. The genes that have been replicated in the largest number of independent populations to date are GDF5 and FRZB; therefore, it is worth discussing in more detail the BMP and Wnt signaling pathways and their genetic association with OA.

Wnt Signaling, FRZB Variants, and Gender-Specific Associations

Wnt proteins form a family of highly conserved secreted signaling molecules. As currently understood, Wnt proteins bind to receptors of the Frizzled and LRP families on the cell surface. Through several cytoplasmic relay components, the signal is transduced to the cell nucleus to activate transcription of Wnt target genes, some of which include TIMP1 (stromelysin, inhibitor of MMPs), RANK ligand, COX-2, osteocalcin, BMP4, NOS2, and FGF.[108] Evidence in the literature shows that the Wnt signaling pathway is involved in cartilage degeneration and OA.[109]

The *FRZB* gene is one of the frizzled transmembrane receptors. The loss of Frzb in Frzb(−/−) knockout mice has been recently shown to contribute to cartilage damage by increasing the expression and activity of MMPs. *FRZB* deficiency in mice also resulted in thicker cortical bone, with increased stiffness and higher cortical appositional bone formation after loading, which may contribute to the development of OA by producing increased strain on the articular cartilage during normal locomotion.[110]

Several studies have explored the relationship between OA and two polymorphisms in the *FRZB* gene: the Arg200Trp and Arg324Gly variants. In three studies, the relationship between the rare *FRZB* Trp^{200}-Gly^{324} haplotype (frequency of 0.6%–5.0%) and OA has been examined.[67,82–84] It was found that female carriers of this haplotype have an increased risk for THR,[82,84] severe JSN of the hip,[83] and clinical knee OA,[67] further supporting a role for *FRZB* variants in OA. In a Dutch study the association of the Arg324Gly was also seen with generalized OA, but not with radiographic hip OA.[85] Although strongly associated in females, these variants did not seem to be associated with hip or knee OA in males,[67,82] suggesting a gender-specific effect. A meta-analysis for hip or knee OA in women yielded an OR of the effect of less than 1.4.[67]

In contrast with the above, a recent study, sufficiently powered to find evidence of association between *FRZB* variants and radiographic OA in two large independent cohorts, failed to do so. Kerkhof and colleagues[86] did not study individuals who had symptoms of OA or severe OA requiring TJA, as was done in previous studies, but focused on markers of cartilage degradation and on radiographic features of knee and hip OA. Their data, along with previous results,[85] suggest that *FRZB* genetic variants may play a role in OA limited to severe (joint replacement phenotype) or symptomatic OA, but not in radiographic OA. The clinical phenotype is not restricted to people who have radiographic OA, so its clinical relevance is still inherent.

Bone Morphogenetic Proteins

BMPs are members of the transforming growth factor (TGF)–β superfamily of signal molecules that mediate many diverse biologic processes. BMPs trigger cellular responses mainly through the Smad pathway, although the signal molecules can also activate the mitogen-activated protein kinase pathway.[111] In model organisms a remarkable array of long-distance, modular regulatory elements surrounding the genes that encode BMPS has been identified. These sequences correspond to individual "anatomy" elements that help control the size, shape, and number of individual bones and joints. For example, regulatory elements from the *GDF5* gene can be used to inactivate other genes specifically in joints, making It possible to identify genes and signals required for maintenance or repair of articular cartilage.[112]

Among the BMP genes reported to be associated with OA are *BMP5* (not replicated to date), *BMP2*, which has been associated in two United Kingdom populations, and *GDF5*. An association with hip and knee OA of a single SNP (rs143383, T/C) located in the 5′-UTR of the growth and differentiation factor 5 gene, *GDF5*, was reported in Japanese and in Chinese case-control cohorts.[87] The major T allele of the SNP was common in the Asian populations, with frequencies greater than 70% in controls, and was at an elevated frequency in OA cases, with ORs ranging from 1.30 to 1.79 for knee and hip cases. In vitro cell transfection studies revealed that the T allele mediated a moderate but significant reduction in the activity of the *GDF5* promoter. The same T allele was found to be increased in hip and knee OA cases from Spain and the United Kingdom relative to controls with a modest odds ratio of 1.10. Although the effect size in European samples was extremely modest in RNA extracted from the cartilage of patients who had OA who had undergone joint replacement surgery, the T allele showed up to a 27% reduction in expression relative to the C allele $(P<7 \times 10^{-5})$[88] suggesting that a small but persistent imbalance of GDF5 expression throughout life might render an individual more susceptible to OA.

From the above discussion regarding the FRZB and GDF5 genes it is clear that even genetic variants that are replicated in many populations have fairly modest effects and that the associations may be limited to certain phenotypes.

WHAT CAN WE EXPECT IN THE YEARS TO COME IN GENETIC RESEARCH IN OSTEOARTHRITIS?

Genome-wide association studies (GWAS) are a result of the human genome and HapMap projects (http://www.hapmap.org), and, if successful, can find variants in specific genes, or narrow genomic regions, that are associated with the presence or severity of a specific clinical condition. The information conveyed by these studies is unlikely to influence clinical practice in the immediate future, yet represents an important advance in medicine.[113] The GWAS approach enables a genome-wide comparison of gene variant prevalence between cases and controls, avoiding the need to guess which genes are likely to harbor variants affecting risk. Although the same was true of genome-wide linkage analyses the association approach uses three orders of magnitude more genetic markers and thorough coverage of the genome than the linkage scans did. If a marker is found to be associated it will be much closer or even in the gene actually involved in disease.

These studies have the potential to convey novel, unbiased information about the heritable basis of OA at a level of detail that has not been possible previously. The results of such genome-wide association scans will tell us that a particular genetic variant is located at a gene or—more likely—is in linkage disequilibrium with a gene that is important in the pathogenesis of OA. This kind of analysis cannot tell us the mechanisms responsible, however. Some of the other major weaknesses and pitfalls of this approach have been highlighted already.[114] For example, even the newest assays do not cover all genetic variation in the genome, thus false positives and false negatives can be expected. More importantly, to correct for 5×10^5 comparisons extremely large sample sizes are needed. Investigators can thus find themselves with low power to detect modest effects. Further, an independent replication of findings becomes absolutely necessary. In fact, the only assurance that scientists can have that a genetic association found in this manner is real is to find the same marker to be consistently associated in independent studies.

Few large case-control association scans have been reported to date. Mototani and colleagues[73] tested 72,000 markers for association with hip OA, and identified a variant in the CALM1 gene to be strongly associated in the Japanese population. Studies in United Kingdom samples failed to show an association of this variant with hip[74] or knee OA, however.[67] Spector and colleagues[101] examined 25,000 SNPs for association with radiographic knee osteoarthritis in whites and identified an SNP in a gene of unknown function. Association with this gene—LRCH1—failed to replicate in two sufficiently powered large studies from East Asia of knee and hip OA samples from China and Japan.[102]

A pooled large-scale (500,000 markers) GWAS has been recently published[77] on knee OA. The variants identified by this scan, which were subsequently replicated in independent cohorts, fell in the 5' region of the gene encoding the COX-2 and the cytosolic phospholipase enzymes (both involved in prostaglandin synthesis), in the 2q33 linkage region, and near a gene involved in transcriptional repression of thyroid hormone receptors. In addition a large consortium in the United Kingdom funded by the arthritis research campaign is underway to determine variants associated with TKR and THR in a total of 8000 cases. Other large cohorts (eg, Rotterdam, Framingham, TwinsUK, Iceland) with radiographic OA features are also currently being tested. Once we identify the individual genes involved, we will probably have a relatively long list of genes relating to various processes that may relate to the health of joint tissues. Because GWAS is a position-based approach many genes will hold no prior association with osteoarthritis. Those genes might be developmental and not be disease specific.[9]

A greater understanding of the pathogenesis of OA is not the only valuable contribution of GWAS results. To date no single large genetic effect has been found. Rather, the increased risks for carrying a predisposing genetic variant seem to be fairly modest, with most of them having odds ratios between 1.1 and 1.6 (eg, GDF5 and FRZB). One obvious question then is: if an individual carries risk variants at several genes does his or her risk for OA increase in proportion? Our group has investigated this by computing a genetic risk variable combining variants from 10 different genes that had been implicated in risk for knee or hip OA in other populations. When the top and bottom quartiles of this variable were used the odds ratios became 8.68 (95% CI 5.20–14.49, $P<2 \times 10^{-16}$) for women and 5.06 (95% CI 3.10–8.27, $P<1 \times 10^{-10}$) for men.[115] The odds ratios obtained using the genetic risk variable were comparable to those reported for obesity or knee injury by some studies. Such data indicate that it is possible to identify individuals at high risk for knee OA by combining genotype data from several loci and that the genetic risk for knee OA is likely to be due to the sum of many loci making a small contribution each. The same may hold true for hip or generalized OA. The next step, once GWAS results appear, will be gene–gene and gene–environment interaction studies that will be needed to enlarge our understanding of the manner in which the individual genes implicated in OA exert their effect. Fully understanding the genetic basis for OA will require the availability of large cohorts of extremely well-characterized individuals who have hip OA, knee OA, or multiple joint OA,[5] such as the OAI and MOST cohorts.

REFERENCES

1. Dieppe P, Kirwan J. The localization of osteoarthritis. Br J Rheumatol 1994;33: 201–3.
2. Lawrence RC, Felson DT, Helmick CG, et al. National Arthritis Data Workgroup. Estimates of the prevalence of arthritis and other rheumatic conditions in the United States. Part II. Arthritis Rheum 2008;58(1):26–35.
3. Stoddard S, Jans L, Ripple J, et al. Chartbook on work and disability in the United States, 1998: an InfoUse report. US National Institute on Disability and Rehabilitation Research. Available at: www.infouse.com/disabilitydata/workdisability/3_2.php. Accessed June 3, 2008.
4. Sharma L, Kapoor D, Issa S. Epidemiology of osteoarthritis: an update. Curr Opin Rheumatol 2006;18(2):147–56.
5. Doherty M. How important are genetic factors in osteoarthritis? J Rheumatol Suppl 2004;70:22–7.
6. Stecher RM. Heberden's nodes: heredity in hypertrophic arthritis of the finger joints. Am J Med Sci 1941;210:801–9.
7. Kellgren JH, Lawrence JS, Bier F. Genetic factors in generalized osteoarthritis. Ann Rheum Dis 1963;22:237–55.

8. Loughlin J. Polymorphism in signal transduction is a major route through which osteoarthritis susceptibility is acting. Curr Opin Rheumatol 2005;17(5):629–33.
9. Ikegawa S. New gene associations in osteoarthritis: what do they provide, and where are we going? Curr Opin Rheumatol 2007;19(5):429–34.
10. Risch N. Linkage strategies for genetically complex traits. Multilocus models. Am J Hum Genet 1990;46:222–8.
11. Guo S-W. Sibling recurrence risk ratio as a measure of genetic effect: caveat emptor!. Am J Hum Genet 2002;70(3):818–9.
12. Del Junco D, Luthra HS, Annegers JF, et al. The familial aggregation of rheumatoid arthritis and its relationship to the HLA-DR4 association. Am J Epidemiol 1984;119(5):813–29.
13. Moroldo MB, Chaudhari M, Shear E, et al. Juvenile rheumatoid arthritis affected sibpairs: extent of clinical phenotype concordance. Arthritis Rheum 2004;50(6): 1928–34.
14. Peña AS, Wijmenga C. Genetic factors underlying gluten-sensitive enteropathy. Curr Allergy Asthma Rep 2001;1(6):526–33.
15. Chen WJ, Liu PH, Ho YY, et al. Sibling recurrence risk ratio analysis of the metabolic syndrome and its components over time. BMC Genet 2003;4(Suppl 1): S33:1–6.
16. Weijnen CF, Rich SS, Meigs JB, et al. Risk of diabetes in siblings of index cases with Type 2 diabetes: implications for genetic studies. Diabet Med 2002;19(1): 41–50.
17. Neame RL, Muir K, Doherty S, et al. Genetic risk of knee osteoarthritis: a sibling study. Ann Rheum Dis 2004;63(9):1022–7.
18. Chitnavis J, Sinsheimer JS, Clipsham K, et al. Genetic influences in end-stage osteoarthritis. Sibling risks of hip and knee replacement for idiopathic osteoarthritis. J Bone Joint Surg Br 1997;79:660–4.
19. McDonnell SM, Sinsheimer J, Price AJ, et al. Genetic influences in the aetiology of anteromedial osteoarthritis of the knee. J Bone Joint Surg Br 2007;89(7): 901–3.
20. Lanyon P, Muir K, Doherty S, et al. Assessment of a genetic contribution to osteoarthritis of the hip: sibling study. BMJ 2000;321(7270):1179–83.
21. Kellgren J, Moore R. Generalised osteoarthritis and Heberden's nodes. BMJ 1952;1:181–7.
22. Riyazi N, Meulenbelt I, Kroon HM, et al. Evidence for familial aggregation of hand, hip, and spine but not knee osteoarthritis in siblings with multiple joint involvement: the GARP study. Ann Rheum Dis 2005;64(3):438–43.
23. Botha-Scheepers SA, Watt I, Slagboom E, et al. Influence of familial factors on radiologic disease progression over two years in siblings with osteoarthritis at multiple sites: a prospective longitudinal cohort study. Arthritis Rheum 2007; 57(4):626–32.
24. Khoury MJ, Beaty TH, Liang KY. Can familial aggregation of disease by explained by familial aggregation of environmental risk factors? Am J Epidemiol 1988;127:674–83.
25. Boomsma D, Busjahn A, Peltonen L. Classical twin studies and beyond. Nat Rev Genet 2002;3(11):872–82.
26. MacGregor AJ, Antoniades L, Matson M, et al. The genetic contribution to radiographic hip osteoarthritis in women: results of a classic twin study. Arthritis Rheum 2000;43:2410–6.
27. Maroudas A, Venn MF. Chemical composition and swelling of normal and osteoarthritic femoral head cartilage. Ann Rheum Dis 1973;32:1–9.

28. Hunter DJ, Snieder H, March L, et al. Genetic contribution to cartilage volume in women: a classical twin study. Rheumatology 2003;42:1495–500.
29. Jones G, Ding C, Scott F, et al. Genetic mechanisms of knee osteoarthritis: a population based case-control study. Ann Rheum Dis 2004;63(10):1255–9.
30. Spector TD, Cicuttini F, Baker J, et al. Genetic influences on osteoarthritis in women: a twin study. BMJ 1996;312:940–3.
31. Doherty M. Genetics of hand osteoarthritis. Osteoarthritis Cartilage 2000; 8(Suppl A):S8–10.
32. Zhai G, Ding C, Stankovich J, et al. The genetic contribution to longitudinal changes in knee structure and muscle strength: a sibpair study. Arthritis Rheum 2005;52:2830–4.
33. Zhai G, Hart DJ, Kato BS, et al. Genetic influence on the progression of radiographic knee osteoarthritis: a longitudinal twin study. Osteoarthritis Cartilage 2007;15(2):222–5.
34. Valdes AM, Hart DJ, Jones KA, et al. Association study of candidate genes for the prevalence and progression of knee osteoarthritis. Arthritis Rheum 2004; 50(8):2497–507.
35. Englund M, Niu J, Guermazi A, et al. Effect of meniscal damage on the development of frequent knee pain, aching, or stiffness. Arthritis Rheum 2007;56(12): 4048–54.
36. Belo JN, Berger MY, Reijman M, et al. Prognostic factors of progression of osteoarthritis of the knee: a systematic review of observational studies. Arthritis Rheum 2007;57(1):13–26.
37. Hunter DJ, Spector TD. The role of bone metabolism in osteoarthritis. Curr Rheumatol Rep 2003;5(1):15–9.
38. Burr DB. The importance of subchondral bone in osteoarthrosis. Curr Opin Rheumatol 1998;10:256–62.
39. Lajeunesse D. Altered subchondral osteoblast cellular metabolism in osteoarthritis: cytokines, eicosanoids, and growth factors. J Musculoskelet Neuronal Interact 2002;2(6):504–6.
40. Kiel DP, Demissie S, Dupuis J, et al. Genome-wide association with bone mass and geometry in the Framingham Heart Study. BMC Med Genet 2007;8 (Suppl 1): S14:1–13.
41. Giroux S, Elfassihi L, Cardinal G, et al. LRP5 coding polymorphisms influence the variation of peak bone mass in a normal population of French-Canadian women. Bone 2007;40(5):1299–307.
42. Arko B, Prezelj J, Kocijancic A, et al. Association of the osteoprotegerin gene polymorphisms with bone mineral density in postmenopausal women. Maturitas 2005;51(3):270–9.
43. Cahue S, Dunlop D, Hayes K, et al. Varus-valgus alignment in the progression of patellofemoral osteoarthritis. Arthritis Rheum 2004;50(7):2184–90.
44. Brouwer GM, van Tol AW, Bergink AP, et al. Association between valgus and varus alignment and the development and progression of radiographic osteoarthritis of the knee. Arthritis Rheum 2007;56:1204–11.
45. Cicuttini F, Wluka A, Hankin J, et al. Longitudinal study of the relationship between knee angle and tibiofemoral cartilage volume in subjects with knee osteoarthritis. Rheumatology 2004;43(3):321–4.
46. Hunter DJ, Niu J, Felson DT, et al. Knee alignment does not predict incident osteoarthritis: the Framingham osteoarthritis study. Arthritis Rheum 2007;56(4):1212–8.
47. Sharma L, Lou C, Felson DT, et al. Laxity in healthy and osteoarthritic knees. Arthritis Rheum 1999;42(5):861–70.

48. Wagner EF, Karsenty G. Genetic control of skeletal development. Curr Opin Genet Dev 2001;11(5):527–32.
49. Lane NE, Lin P, Christiansen L, et al. Association of mild acetabular dysplasia with an increased risk of incident hip osteoarthritis in elderly white women: the Study of Osteoporotic Fractures. Arthritis Rheum 2000;43:400–4.
50. Shepstone L, Rogers J, Kirwan JR, et al. Shape of the intercondylar notch of the human femur: a comparison of osteoarthritic and non-osteoarthritic bones from a skeletal sample. Ann Rheum Dis 2001;60(10):968–73.
51. Gregory JS, Waarsing JH, Day J, et al. Early identification of radiographic osteoarthritis of the hip using an active shape model to quantify changes in bone morphometric features: can hip shape tell us anything about the progression of osteoarthritis? Arthritis Rheum 2007;56(11):3634–43.
52. Benito MJ, Veale DJ, FitzGerald O, et al. Synovial tissue inflammation in early and late osteoarthritis. Ann Rheum Dis 2005;64(9):1263–7.
53. Farahat MN, Yanni G, Poston R, et al. Cytokine expression in synovial membranes of patients with rheumatoid arthritis and osteoarthritis. Ann Rheum Dis 1993;52(12):870–5.
54. Goldring MB, Berenbaum F. The regulation of chondrocyte function by proinflammatory mediators: prostaglandins and nitric oxide. Clin Orthop Relat Res 2004;427(Suppl):S37–46.
55. Ayral X, Pickering EH, Woodworth TG, et al. Synovitis: a potential predictive factor of structural progression of medial tibiofemoral knee osteoarthritis—results of a 1 year longitudinal arthroscopic study in 422 patients. Osteoarthritis Cartilage 2005;13(5):361–7.
56. Wörns MA, Victor A, Galle PR, et al. Genetic and environmental contributions to plasma C-reactive protein and interleukin-6 levels—a study in twins. Genes Immun 2006;7(7):600–5.
57. Chapman K, Mustafa Z, Irven C, et al. Osteoarthritis-susceptibility locus on chromosome 11q, detected by linkage. Am J Hum Genet 1999;65(1):167–74.
58. Loughlin J, Mustafa Z, Irven C, et al. Stratification analysis of an osteoarthritis genome screen—suggestive linkage to chromosomes 4, 6, and 16. Am J Hum Genet 1999;65(6):1795–8.
59. Livshits G, Kato B, Zhai G, et al. Genomewide linkage scan of hand osteoarthritis in female twin pairs showing replication of quantitative trait loci on chromosomes 2 and 19. Ann Rheum Dis 2007;66:623–7.
60. Leppävuori J, Kujala U, Kinnunen J, et al. Genome scan for predisposing loci for distal interphalangeal joint osteoarthritis: evidence for a locus on 2q. Am J Hum Genet 1999;65(4):1060–7.
61. Stefánsson SE, Jónsson H, Ingvarsson T, et al. Genomewide scan for hand osteoarthritis: a novel mutation in matrilin-3. Am J Hum Genet 2003;72(6):1448–59.
62. Ingvarsson T, Stefánsson SE, Gulcher JR, et al. A large Icelandic family with early osteoarthritis of the hip associated with a susceptibility locus on chromosome 16p. Arthritis Rheum 2001;44(11):2548–55.
63. Demissie S, Cupples LA, Myers R, et al. Genome scan for quantity of hand osteoarthritis: the Framingham Study. Arthritis Rheum 2002;46(4):946–52.
64. Hunter DJ, Demissie S, Cupples LA, et al. A genome scan for joint-specific hand osteoarthritis susceptibility: The Framingham Study. Arthritis Rheum 2004;50(8):2489–96.
65. Lee YH, Rho YH, Choi SJ, et al. Osteoarthritis susceptibility loci defined by genome scan meta-analysis. Rheumatol Int 2006;26(11):996–1000.

66. Valdes AM, Van Oene M, Hart DJ, et al. Reproducible genetic associations between candidate genes and clinical knee osteoarthritis in men and women. Arthritis Rheum 2006;54(2):533–9.

67. Valdes AM, Loughlin J, Oene MV, et al. Sex and ethnic differences in the association of ASPN, CALM1, COL2A1, COMP, and FRZB with genetic susceptibility to osteoarthritis of the knee. Arthritis Rheum 2007;56(1):137–46.

68. Kizawa H, Kou I, Iida A, et al. An aspartic acid repeat polymorphism in asporin inhibits chondrogenesis and increases susceptibility to osteoarthritis. Nat Genet 2005;37(2):138–44.

69. Kaliakatsos M, Tzetis M, Kanavakis E, et al. Asporin and knee osteoarthritis in patients of Greek origin. Osteoarthritis Cartilage 2006;14(6):609–11.

70. Mustafa Z, Dowling B, Chapman K, et al. Investigating the aspartic acid (D) repeat of asporin as a risk factor for osteoarthritis in a UK Caucasian population. Arthritis Rheum 2005;52(11):3502–6.

71. Rodriguez-Lopez J, Pombo-Suarez M, Liz M, et al. Lack of association of a variable number of aspartic acid residues in the asporin gene with osteoarthritis susceptibility: case-control studies in Spanish Caucasians. Arthritis Res Ther 2006;8(3):1–4.

72. Southam L, Dowling B, Ferreira A, et al. Microsatellite association mapping of a primary osteoarthritis susceptibility locus on chromosome 6p12.3-q13. Arthritis Rheum 2004;50(12):3910–4.

73. Mototani H, Mabuchi A, Saito S, et al. A functional single nucleotide polymorphism in the core promoter region of CALM1 is associated with hip osteoarthritis in Japanese. Hum Mol Genet 2005;14(8):1009–17.

74. Loughlin J, Sinsheimer JS, Carr A, et al. The CALM1 core promoter polymorphism is not associated with hip osteoarthritis in a United Kingdom Caucasian population. Osteoarthritis Cartilage 2006;14(3):295–8.

75. Seki S, Kawaguchi Y, Chiba K, et al. A functional SNP in CILP, encoding cartilage intermediate layer protein, is associated with susceptibility to lumbar disc disease. Nat Genet 2005;37(6):607–12.

76. Ikeda T, Mabuchi A, Fukuda A, et al. Association analysis of single nucleotide polymorphisms in cartilage-specific collagen genes with knee and hip osteoarthritis in the Japanese population. J Bone Miner Res 2002;17(7):1290–6.

77. Valdes AM, Loughlin J, Timms KM, et al. Genome-wide association scan identifies a PTGS2 (prostaglandin-endoperoxide synthase 2) variant involved in risk of knee osteoarthritis. Am J Hum Genet 2008;82(6):1231–40.

78. Valdes AM, Hassett G, Hart DJ, et al. Radiographic progression of lumbar spine disc degeneration is influenced by variation at inflammatory genes: a candidate SNP association study in the Chingford cohort. Spine 2005;30(21):2445–51.

79. Meulenbelt I, Min JL, Bos S, et al. Identification of DIO2 as new susceptibility locus for symptomatic osteoarthritis. Hum Mol Genet 2008 Mar 11; [Epub ahead of print].

80. Fytili P, Giannatou E, Papanikolaou V, et al. Association of repeat polymorphisms in the estrogen receptors alpha, beta, and androgen receptor genes with knee osteoarthritis. Clin Genet 2005;68(3):268–77.

81. Jin SY, Hong SJ, Yang HI, et al. Estrogen receptor-alpha gene haplotype is associated with primary knee osteoarthritis in Korean population. Arthritis Res Ther 2004;6(5):R415–21.

82. Loughlin J, Dowling B, Chapman K, et al. Functional variants within the secreted frizzled-related protein 3 gene are associated with hip osteoarthritis in females. Proc Natl Acad Sci U S A 2004;101(26):9757–62.

83. Lane NE, Lian K, Nevitt MC, et al. Frizzled-related protein variants are risk factors for hip osteoarthritis. Arthritis Rheum 2006;54(4):1246–54.
84. Rodriguez-Lopez J, Pombo-Suarez M, Liz M, et al. Further evidence of the role of frizzled-related protein gene polymorphisms in osteoarthritis. Ann Rheum Dis 2007;66(8):1052–5.
85. Min JL, Meulenbelt I, Riyazi N, et al. Association of the Frizzled-related protein gene with symptomatic osteoarthritis at multiple sites. Arthritis Rheum 2005; 52(4):1077–80.
86. Kerkhof JM, Uitterlinden AG, Valdes AM, et al. Radiographic osteoarthritis at three joint sites and FRZB, LRP5, and LRP6 polymorphisms in two population-based cohorts. Osteoarthritis Cartilage 2008;16(10):1141–9.
87. Miyamoto Y, Mabuchi A, Shi D, et al. A functional polymorphism in the 5′-UTR of GDF5 is associated with susceptibility to osteoarthritis. Nat Genet 2007;39: 529–33.
88. Southam L, Rodriguez-Lopez J, Wilkins JM, et al. An SNP in the 5′-UTR of GDF5 is associated with osteoarthritis susceptibility in Europeans and with in vivo differences in allelic expression in articular cartilage. Hum Mol Genet 2007;16(18): 2226–32.
89. Rovetta G, Buffrini L, Monteforte P, et al. HLA-DRB1alleles and osteoarthritis in a group of patients living in Liguria-Italy. Minerva Med 2006;97(3):271–5.
90. Riyazi N, Spee J, Huizinga TW, et al. HLA class II is associated with distal interphalangeal osteoarthritis. Ann Rheum Dis 2003;62(3):227–30.
91. Moos V, Menard J, Sieper J, et al. Association of HLA-DRB1*02 with osteoarthritis in a cohort of 106 patients. Rheumatology (Oxford) 2002;41(6):666–9.
92. Wakitani S, Imoto K, Mazuka T, et al. Japanese generalised osteoarthritis was associated with HLA class I—a study of HLA-A, B, Cw, DQ, DR in 72 patients. Clin Rheumatol 2001;20(6):417–9.
93. Smith AJ, Keen LJ, Billingham MJ, et al. Extended haplotypes and linkage disequilibrium in the IL1R1-IL1A-IL1B-IL1RN gene cluster: association with knee osteoarthritis. Genes Immun 2004;5(6):451–60.
94. Loughlin J, Dowling B, Mustafa Z, et al. Association of the interleukin-1 gene cluster on chromosome 2q13 with knee osteoarthritis. Arthritis Rheum 2002; 46(6):1519–27.
95. Meulenbelt I, Seymour AB, Nieuwland M, et al. Association of the interleukin-1 gene cluster with radiographic signs of osteoarthritis of the hip. Arthritis Rheum 2004;50(4):1179–86.
96. Forster T, Chapman K, Loughlin J. Common variants within the interleukin 4 receptor alpha gene (IL4R) are associated with susceptibility to osteoarthritis. Hum Genet 2004;114(4):391–5.
97. Pola E, Papaleo P, Pola R, et al. Interleukin-6 gene polymorphism and risk of osteoarthritis of the hip: a case-control study. Osteoarthritis Cartilage 2005;13(11): 1025–8.
98. Nicklas BJ, Mychaleckyj J, Kritchevsky S, et al. Physical function and its response to exercise: associations with cytokine gene variation in older adults with knee osteoarthritis. J Gerontol A Biol Sci Med Sci 2005;60(10):1292–8.
99. Fytili P, Giannatou E, Karachalios T, et al. Interleukin-10G and interleukin-10R microsatellite polymorphisms and osteoarthritis of the knee. Clin Exp Rheumatol 2005;23(5):621–7.
100. Riyazi N, Kurreeman FA, Huizinga TW, et al. The role of interleukin 10 promoter polymorphisms in the susceptibility of distal interphalangeal osteoarthritis. J Rheumatol 2005;32(8):1571–5.

101. Spector TD, Reneland RH, Mah S, et al. Association between a variation in LRCH1 and knee osteoarthritis: a genome-wide single-nucleotide polymorphism association study using DNA pooling. Arthritis Rheum 2006;54(2):524–32.
102. Jiang Q, Shi D, Nakajima M, et al. Lack of association of single nucleotide polymorphism in LRCH1 with knee osteoarthritis susceptibility. J Hum Genet 2008; 53(1):42–7.
103. Smith AJ, Gidley J, Sandy JR, et al. Haplotypes of the low-density lipoprotein receptor-related protein 5 (LRP5) gene: are they a risk factor in osteoarthritis? Osteoarthritis Cartilage 2005;13(7):608–13.
104. Min JL, Meulenbelt I, Riyazi N, et al. Association of matrilin-3 polymorphisms with spinal disc degeneration and osteoarthritis of the first carpometacarpal joint of the hand. Ann Rheum Dis 2006;65(8):1060–6.
105. Mahr S, Burmester GR, Hilke D, et al. Cis- and trans-acting gene regulation is associated with osteoarthritis. Am J Hum Genet 2006;78(5):793–803.
106. Loughlin J, Meulenbelt I, Min J, et al. Genetic association analysis of RHOB and TXNDC3 in osteoarthritis. Am J Hum Genet 2007;80(2):383–6.
107. Uitterlinden AG, Fang Y, Van Meurs JB, et al. Genetics and biology of vitamin D receptor polymorphisms. Gene 2004;338(2):143–56.
108. Huelsken J, Behrens J. The Wnt signalling pathway. J Cell Sci 2002;115(Pt 21): 3977–8.
109. Enomoto-Iwamoto M, Kitagaki J, Koyama E, et al. The Wnt antagonist Frzb-1 regulates chondrocyte maturation and long bone development during limb skeletogenesis. Dev Biol 2002;251(1):142–56.
110. Lories RJ, Peeters J, Bakker A, et al. Articular cartilage and biomechanical properties of the long bones in FRZB-knockout mice. Arthritis Rheum 2007;56(12): 4095–103.
111. Li X, Cao X. BMP Signaling and skeletogenesis. Ann N Y Acad Sci 2006;1068: 26–40.
112. Rountree RB, Schoor M, Chen H, et al. BMP receptor signaling is required for postnatal maintenance of articular cartilage. PLoS Biol 2004;2(11):e355: 1816–27.
113. Drazen JM, Phimister EG. Publishing genomewide association studies. N Engl J Med 2007;357(5):496.
114. Hunter DJ, Kraft P. Drinking from the fire hose—statistical issues in genomewide association studies. N Engl J Med 2007;357(5):436–9.
115. Valdes AM, Doherty M, Spector TD. The additive effect of individual genes in predicting risk of knee osteoarthritis. Ann Rheum Dis 2008;67(1):124–7.

The Measurement of Joint Mechanics and Their Role in Osteoarthritis Genesis and Progression

David R. Wilson, DPhil[a,b,*], Emily J. McWalter, MASc[b,c], James D. Johnston, MSc[b,c]

KEYWORDS

• Osteoarthritis • Biomechanics • Knee • Hip • Kinematics

Mechanics play a role in the initiation, progression, and successful treatment of osteoarthritis. However, we don't yet know enough about which specific mechanical parameters are most important and what their impact is on the disease process to make comprehensive statements about how mechanics should be modified to prevent, slow, or arrest the disease process. The idea of a mechanical role in osteoarthritis is often made clear to the patient: Osteoarthritis is "wear and tear" arthritis and joint surfaces need to be replaced because of wear in advanced stages of the disease, much like bearing surfaces in an engine that have worn down after too many revolutions. The parallels with machines are sometimes (at least superficially) obvious: obese people load their joints more and have a higher prevalence of osteoarthritis, which seems analogous to higher loads on a bearing increasing the rate of wear on its surfaces, a well-known mechanical phenomenon. High enough loads can destroy any tissue, so it seems clear that there is a level of joint loading that can injure cartilage irreversibly, leading to erosion from the joint surface. However, the utility of drawing

A version of this article originally appeared in the 34:3 issue of the *Rheumatic Disease Clinics of North America*.

This work was supported by grants from the Canadian Institutes of Health Research and the Natural Sciences and Engineering Research Council of Canada.

[a] Department of Orthopaedics, University of British Columbia, UBC Orthopaedics, Room 3114, 910 West 10th Avenue, Vancouver, BC, V5Z 4E3 Canada

[b] Vancouver Coastal Health Research Institute, Vancouver, Canada

[c] Departments of Orthopaedics and Mechanical Engineering, University of British Columbia, UBC Orthopaedics, Room 3114, 910 West 10th Avenue, Vancouver, BC, V5Z 4E3 Canada

* Corresponding author. UBC Orthopaedics, Room 3114, 910 West 10th Avenue, Vancouver, BC, V5Z 4E3 Canada.

E-mail address: dawilson@interchange.ubc.ca (D.R. Wilson).

parallels with machines is limited. Cartilage, though avascular and aneural, is a living tissue with capacity to adapt to its mechanical environment. It endures apparently un-scathed through the most active decades of life in most people. Currently, many sur-gical procedures and other treatment and prevention approaches are based implicitly or explicitly on the assumption that they improve or correct joint mechanics, and that this improvement or correction is required to protect the joint from osteoarthritis. Jus-tifying and improving mechanically based treatment and prevention approaches re-quires a critical understanding of the methods used to study joint mechanics and the current evidence for the role of mechanics in osteoarthritis. The objectives of this review are (1) to summarize methods for assessing joint mechanics and their rel-ative merits and limitations, (2) to describe current evidence for the role of mechanics in osteoarthritis initiation and progression, and (3) to describe some current treatment approaches that focus on modifying joint mechanics.

MECHANICAL HYPOTHESES ABOUT OSTEOARTHRITIS

Many of the hypotheses proposed to explain why osteoarthritis begins and progresses center on mechanics. The most prevalent and researched hypothesis regarding oste-oarthritis pathogenesis is that acute trauma, overuse, or altered mechanics destroy chondrocytes and disrupt the extracellular matrix, resulting in proteoglycan deple-tion[1,2] (proteoglycans are essential to maintaining the load-bearing role of cartilage). Prolonged loading results in further cartilage breakdown and subsequent osteoarthri-tis. Surface damage, proteoglycan loss,[3] and chondrocyte death[1] are commonly seen in osteoarthritis, and similar observations have been made with in vitro impact studies on human and animal specimens.[4–6] One hypothesis is that osteoarthritis progresses because of mechanical changes in subchondral bone.[7] According to this hypothesis, impulse loading and cumulative trauma create microfractures in the trabeculae, which are repaired by fracture callus. As the trabeculae become thicker and new trabeculae are added, the repair process stiffens the subchondral bone, in effect acting as a sup-port for the endplate. This causes the subchondral region to lose its shock-absorbing capabilities, resulting in increased cartilage stresses and eventual degradation.[8,9] A more recent hypothesis, which has been generally accepted, speculates that micro-fractures *within* the subchondral cortical endplate, as opposed to adjacent trabeculae, result in subchondral thickening. These microfractures, attributed to impulse loading and repetitive stress, increase biological activity at the site of injury and result in in-creased bone turnover and reactivation of the secondary center of ossification, ac-cording to this hypothesis.[10] While evidence is emerging from animal studies in support of some of these hypotheses, little work testing these hypotheses has been done in humans. Studies using traditional bone mineral density measures are emerg-ing to examine the role of bone in osteoarthritis. For example, cartilage thinning cor-relates with bone structure losses in the contralateral compartment in subjects with tibiofemoral osteoarthritis.[11] Ratios of medial to lateral compartment bone mineral density have also been associated with compartmental tibiofemoral osteoarthritis.[12] In particular, higher bone mineral density in the medial compartment was associated with medial joint space narrowing (a radiographic measure of osteoarthritis progres-sion) and medial sclerosis. Meanwhile, higher bone mineral density in the lateral com-partment was associated with lateral joint space narrowing and lateral sclerosis.[12] Improved tools for measuring bone, cartilage, and joint mechanics may ultimately al-low us to test these and other hypotheses in vivo in humans.

METHODS FOR ASSESSING JOINT MECHANICS
The Challenges of Study Design

It is difficult to test hypotheses about the role of mechanics in osteoarthritis initiation and progression and the effects of a change in mechanics on osteoarthritis because appropriate in vivo human studies present major challenges. First, studies require a well-characterized population that has osteoarthritis or is at risk for osteoarthritis, and such populations can be difficult to identify. Identifying more specific populations of interest, such as those with acute injuries associated with osteoarthritis, those with rapid progression of the disease, or those at risk of early disease onset, adds to the difficulty. Large populations are generally needed for studies to have appropriate statistical power, which adds to costs and makes managing the study more difficult. Second, studies require a means of assessing osteoarthritis incidence or progression. Radiographic measurements of osteoarthritis (eg, Kellgren-Lawrence grade)[13] are often insensitive to early osteoarthritis and to small increments of progression. More recently, advanced MRI techniques have shown some potential for more sensitive, quantitative measurement of osteoarthritis progression,[14] but these measures are more time-consuming and expensive than radiographic approaches and they have not often been used in conjunction with mechanical assessments. Finally and most critically, such studies require in vivo assessments of joint mechanics. Standard clinical measurements used as surrogates for mechanics have been used in a number of studies, but they have many limitations. More advanced mechanical measurement methods have been developed, but studies have generally only been done in small populations because the measurements are expensive and time consuming.

What Would We Like To Measure and Why Can't We Do It?

There are a number of hypotheses about the links between mechanics and osteoarthritis, and these hypotheses define the mechanical quantities of primary interest to researchers: force, force distribution, loading rate, stress, strain, and kinematics. Unfortunately, the most interesting quantities are among the most difficult to measure. Force on the joint surfaces is a key quantity in many hypotheses, but it can only be measured directly by implanting a measurement device into the joint, which is far too interventional (in the case of the natural joint) for most in vivo studies of humans. Force distribution on the cartilage surface is also widely believed to be important because the ability of the cartilage to support force without damage varies across the joint surface due to differences in such factors as cartilage thickness and subchondral bone properties. While there are sensors available to measure force distribution,[15] they must also be implanted, which carries the same limitations in vivo as direct measurements of force. Loading rate has been postulated to play a role in osteoarthritis.[16] Assessing loading rate requires very rapid measurements of force (typically every 100th of a second or faster), which is considerably more challenging than static force measurements. There is also substantial interest in how force is transmitted through joint structures, such as cartilage and bone (stress). Stress describes the amount of force transmitted per unit of area, and is considered important because, for example, moderate force transmitted through a small contact area may cause cartilage damage, while the same force transmitted through a large contact area would produce no cartilage injury. Measuring stress in simple machines and structures is a challenge, and stress has not been measured in human joints in vivo to our knowledge. Some approaches are emerging for measuring strain, or deformation of the joint tissues in response to stress,[17] but the relationship between stress and strain is much more complex in joint tissues than in, say, steel, which makes it difficult to use strain measurements to predict stress. Kinematics (joint movements) are easier to measure and several methods for accurately quantifying joint kinematics in vivo have been developed in recent years. Kinematics describe how the bones that make up the joint move relative to each other, which can reflect where load is transmitted through the surfaces and the lines of action of structures that transmit forces.

Ex Vivo Studies and Joint Models

Our current understanding of joint mechanics is founded on ex vivo studies, which are inappropriate for linking mechanics with clinical symptoms. In ex vivo studies, kinematics and contact mechanics have been measured in cadaver specimens loaded in mechanical rigs.[18–25] While studies of this type have helped us to understand biomechanics of healthy joints, their central limitation for studying osteoarthritis is that morphologic adaptations due to the disease process or the healing process and mechanical links to clinical symptoms, such as pain, and to ongoing processes, such as cartilage degeneration, cannot be studied in cadavers. An alternative that avoids some of the limitations of mechanical measurements that can be made in vivo is to predict joint mechanics using mathematical models. Models are limited primarily by the assumptions that must be made to formulate them, such as the orientation of muscle and ligament lines of action, shapes of bones, and the deformation of tissues in response to load. Models incorporating sophisticated descriptions of joint structures have been developed, validated,[26–31] and used to answer specific clinically motivated questions.[32–36] Two primary limitations of mathematical models are that (1) many simplifying assumptions must be made about the properties of the joint, which limits the models' validity and applicability, and (2), like ex vivo studies, mathematical models are inappropriate for studying links with ongoing in vivo symptoms and processes, unless these changes are measured and incorporated into the model.

Radiographic Measures of Alignment

Most of the measures used clinically to quantify joint mechanics assess joint alignment. For example, tibiofemoral alignment is often quantified with the femorotibial angle, or hip-knee-ankle angle.[37] A range of measures have emerged for quantifying patellofemoral alignment, with particular emphasis on medial-lateral position and patellar tilt. A central limitation of this approach is that the measures describe the joint (for which movement is the primary function) at only one static position. In addition, while it is intuitive that these alignment measures are related to how load is transmitted in the joint, it is unclear how for most measures any given change in alignment measure would change force distribution in the joint. A further limitation is that the accuracy and repeatability of these measures are affected by their two-dimensional nature. Two-dimensional radiographic measurements are prone to errors due to magnification and subject positioning. MRI and CT collect three-dimensional information about joint anatomy, which has been used, for example, to quantify femoral neck deformities thought to be associated with hip osteoarthritis.[38] In many cases, however, the three-dimensional data are still reduced to a two-dimensional measurement, which does not describe three-dimensional deformities adequately.

Gait Analysis

Gait analysis (often more generally referred to as motion analysis) is an important modality for estimating joint mechanics in activity. In motion analysis, movement of the joint segments is tracked with an optical, magnetic, or optoelectronic system and loads applied to the body (eg, ground-reaction forces) are measured. Mechanical analysis can then be used to assess the resultant forces and moments at the joints.

The resultant forces and moments at the joints, which are output by the majority of commercial motion analysis systems, are entirely different from the contact forces in the joint. To determine contact forces, joint models must be used. Generally these models require resultant forces and moments obtained from motion analysis as inputs.[39] The advantage of gait analysis is that movement is relatively unconstrained by the measurement system. Therefore, a large range of activities can be analyzed. One key limitation of gait analysis is that joint movement is typically measured with markers fixed to the skin. These markers move substantially relative to the bones and can therefore introduce significant error. The use of large groups of skin-mounted markers has reduced the error due to skin movement.[40] A second key limitation is that the models and analysis required to determine joint contact loads require many simplifications and assumptions, which limits accuracy. Typically, only general, rather than subject-specific models, are used. This limits the utility of these methods when pathologic joints are involved.

In Vivo Radiography

Some of the limitations of motion analysis have been addressed with x-ray–based methods of measuring motion, including biplanar radiography and fluoroscopy. Three-dimensional knee kinematics have been measured during activity in vivo using fluoroscopy and subsequent image processing. This has been done in joints after arthroplasty[41] and in natural joints.[42] A limitation of this approach is that measurement errors are quite large out of the imaging plane. The most accurate measurements of kinematics are made with biplanar radiography, which has been used to study kinematics in a number of joints.[43,44] While many biplanar radiography studies are done with a series of static positions, recent work using high-speed biplanar radiography has made accurate measurements of kinematics during dynamic activity possible.[45] Because these measurements are so accurate, combining kinematics with known joint geometry yields predictions of joint contact interactions.[46] One key limitation of these approaches is that markers (typically small tantalum spheres) need to be implanted into the bones, an invasive procedure. The second key limitation is that these approaches expose patients to ionizing radiation, which always carries some risk and limits the number of repeat assessments that can be made.

MRI Measurements of Kinematics

A number of different approaches have been described that use MRI to assess joint kinematics. They are distinguished from each other by whether they measure two-dimensional or three-dimensional movement, whether kinematics are measured when the joint is actively loaded or unloaded, and whether the movement is measured continuously or at selected static positions. Some two-dimensional measurements of patellar tracking have been made in loaded flexion, but these do not describe the movement of the patella completely because the measurements are planar.[47,48] Two-dimensional studies of the patellofemoral joint have shown that patterns of patellar tracking are different in loaded flexion from those in unloaded flexion. However, the studies found that patterns measured in very slow flexion are not different from those measured in rapid flexion.[48] The primary limitation of two-dimensional studies is that they neglect at least half of the movement. Planar studies can measure at most three of the six quantities of movement (typically three rotations and three translations) required to completely describe any joint's movement. One three-dimensional kinematic approach includes cine-phase contrast MRI[49–54] and fast-phase contrast MRI,[55] in which velocity information is extracted from magnetic resonance scans and used to measure three-dimensional tracking of the joint. Applications have focused on the knee. Although promising, these techniques have some limitations. The most notable limitation is the requirement that subjects must flex their knees through many cycles, limiting the magnitude of load that can be applied and the applicability of the technique in symptomatic subjects. Subject interexamination variability ranges from 0.8° to 2.4° for fast-phase contrast MRI and 1.3° to 6.1° for cine-phase contrast MRI.[55] Another approach involves imaging the joint statically at a number of positions of loaded flexion. For some variations of this method,[56,57] accuracy has not been quantified in real knees. For other variations, however, the accuracy and repeatability have been measured.[58–60] A limitation of this approach is that movement is not measured during continuous flexion. One of the limitations of all of these MRI-based approaches is that kinematics are measured when participants are supine in the confined cylindric bore of a magnetic resonance scanner. Some very recent work has explored using open configuration magnetic resonance scanners with a vertical gap, in which participants can stand and load their weight-bearing joints while being scanned.[61] While this configuration provides a superior simulation of active weight-bearing to that simulated in closed-bore scanners, open scanners have lower field strengths than standard closed-bore scanners, which limits the image quality that can be obtained.

MRI Measurements of Contact Area

A number of methods for assessing cartilage contact area from MRI in vivo have been described, although most methods have not yet been validated extensively. Contact area can be used to infer force distribution and some measurement approaches describe where contact occurs in the joint, which may also be relevant in osteoarthritis. While MRI has been used to measure contact area in animals, the applicability of measurements in cats[62] and dogs[63] to humans is difficult because of differences in geometry. In one study in humans, knees of healthy volunteers were imaged in a 1.5-T scanner at several angles of flexion while they pressed against a weighted foot pedal to simulate standing load.[56] Area was assessed by constructing B-spline curves along the contact boundary of the patellofemoral joint in each slice and integrating across all of the slices to calculate area. A simplified version of this technique[64] defined cartilage contact with straight-line segments along the patellofemoral joint and then multiplied this contact length by the slice thickness, which was summed across all slices to determine total contact area. An in vitro validation study of this method using pressure-sensitive film in cadavers[65] found an average measurement difference of 10.9% between the methods and no consistent directional difference between the MRI and pressure-sensitive film techniques. The same group has used the technique in other studies,[66,67] and a second group applied the method to standing volunteers in a 0.5-T open scanner.[68] This group validated their measurements using a phantom model with known contact areas and reported a coefficient of variation of 3%. In a study using a 0.2-T open magnetic resonance scanner to examine the knees of healthy volunteers at 30° and 90° of flexion while an external torque was applied distal to the knee joint, the coefficient of variation was less than 9% for contact areas in repeated scans.[69] Most approaches have focused on the patellofemoral joint. While contact areas in the elbow have been studied,[70] there is little work on the hip, shoulder, wrist, or the tibiofemoral joint (due in part to the presence of the meniscus). Most contact area measurement techniques have not been adequately validated with assessments of accuracy, which limits their utility.

The Future

Technological advances hold promise for more and better in vivo mechanical measurements. Many of the methods described in this review are only now reaching maturity, and more widespread use and further development present the real possibility of accelerating results. One area with promise is MRI mapping of cartilage strain, which has been done ex vivo.[17] Very high field strength scanners are required to achieve the resolution needed to detect small changes in cartilage thickness in a short imaging time. Such scanners at these field strengths for clinical use are becoming available, raising the possibility of widespread assessment of strain in vivo. CT scans are becoming very fast and require relatively small doses of ionizing radiation, which raises the possibility of their use in assessing joint kinematics. Developments in nanotechnology suggest the feasibility of developing implantable transducers that transmit measurements through telemetry.

CURRENT EVIDENCE FOR THE ROLE OF MECHANICS IN OSTEOARTHRITIS INITIATION AND PROGRESSION
Alignment

There is strong evidence that altered mechanics play a role in osteoarthritis incidence and progression, and recent studies are beginning to isolate specific mechanical factors that may be of particular importance. A review to 1999 presented the evidence for the role of obesity; laxity, proprioception and alignment; joint injury and deformity; occupation and sports participation; and muscle weakness in osteoarthritis.[71] Since that time, the importance of joint alignment has become even more clear. Tibiofemoral alignment has been extensively studied in individuals with tibiofemoral or patellofemoral osteoarthritis. Although one study found that tibiofemoral alignment did not predict incident tibiofemoral osteoarthritis,[72] it was important in tibiofemoral osteoarthritis progression. The effect of increased body mass index on osteoarthritis progression was seen only in knees with moderate malalignment.[73] A study of bone marrow lesions also highlighted the role of joint alignment: medial bone marrow lesions were seen mostly in patients with varus limbs, and lateral lesions were seen mostly in those with valgus limbs.[74] In this study, approximately 69% of knees that progressed medially had medial lesions, and lateral lesions conferred a marked risk for lateral progression. Imaging of cartilage glycosaminoglycan concentration using delayed gadolinium-enhanced MRI of cartilage showed that participants in varus malalignment had evidence of medial tibiofemoral osteoarthritis incidence and participants in valgus malalignment had evidence of lateral tibiofemoral osteoarthritis incidence.[75] The importance of tibiofemoral alignment has also been highlighted in a study that found that differences in tibiofemoral alignment between Chinese and Caucasians may explain differences in the incidence of lateral tibiofemoral osteoarthritis in these populations.[76] Tibiofemoral alignment has also been shown to be associated with patellofemoral osteoarthritis. Valgus tibiofemoral malalignment was associated with incidence and progression of lateral patellofemoral osteoarthritis and varus tibiofemoral malalignment was associated with incidence and progression of medial patellofemoral osteoarthritis.[77–80] However, a substantial number of subjects did not follow the prevailing pattern of patellofemoral osteoarthritis progression with tibiofemoral malalignment.[79] This finding was supported by a biomechanical study that found that tibiofemoral alignment alone did not predict patellar kinematics.[81] These inconsistencies have led researchers to study patellar alignment independently of tibiofemoral alignment. One study found that patellar alignment measures were associated with markers of patellofemoral osteoarthritis.[82] Medial displacement and tilt of the patella was associated with medial compartment osteoarthritis progression and lateral displacement was associated with lateral compartment osteoarthritis progression.[83] Overall, it appears that a malaligned joint is likely to get osteoarthritis or to have osteoarthritis progress if already affected, but a complete understanding of the interaction of malalignment with other mechanical factors requires further research.

Other Surrogates for High Joint Forces

A number of studies have found associations between surrogate measures of high joint forces and osteoarthritis. As discussed previously, joint forces cannot be measured directly, but estimates based on anthropometry, gait analysis, and activities of daily living can be used to study the effect of higher joint forces. A static measure of greater knee height, which contributes to increased moments about the knee and associated higher theoretical contact forces in the joints, was associated with an increasing prevalence of incident symptomatic and radiographic knee osteoarthritis.[84] Prolonged squatting (which theoretically produces high forces in the knee) in elderly Chinese men was associated with higher risk for incident knee osteoarthritis.[85] Gait analysis, a very widely used tool to study links between mechanics and osteoarthritis, has the potential to determine which compensatory mechanisms are helpful and which are harmful to the joints. One gait analysis study found links between a higher knee adduction moment and incident tibiofemoral osteoarthritis, and that adduction moment varies according to osteoarthritis severity.[86] This finding provides some support for the hypothesis that higher joint moments lead to osteoarthritis.[87] Medial tibiofemoral compartment knee osteoarthritis is also associated with increased external knee and hip adduction moments and higher axial loading rates at the hip, knee, and ankle.[88] Interestingly, another study found that a greater hipabduction moment was protective against medial tibiofemoral osteoarthritis progression.[89] It has also been shown that gait parameters at the hip, knee, and ankle vary according to osteoarthritis severity.[90] It has been suggested that the changes in gait mechanics may be a compensatory mechanism to reduce pain by reducing joint loads at the affected joint.[91,92] Asymmetric knee loading has been seen in subjects with advanced hip osteoarthritis: The healthier leg experienced higher peak external knee adduction moment and peak medial compartment loads both before and after total hip replacement.[93] Ankle mechanics have been studied to a lesser extent than mechanics of the knee and hip. However, it has been shown that a greater toe-out angle is associated with medial tibiofemoral osteoarthritis progression.[94] All of these surrogate measures of joint loading provide information about the relative magnitudes of force being transmitted through the joint, but they do not tell us where in the joints these loads are being transmitted. Advances in weight-bearing imaging may elucidate this in the future.

Injury

Acute injury is clearly associated with the development of osteoarthritis. Forty-three percent of subjects who had undergone meniscectomy because of meniscal tears had radiographic evidence of osteoarthritis after 16 years,[95] 51% of female soccer players with anterior cruciate ligament (ACL) injury had radiographic evidence of osteoarthritis after 12 years,[96] and 41% of male soccer players with ACL injury had radiographic evidence of osteoarthritis after 14 years.[97] A study of ACL injury in a population of individuals with symptomatic knee osteoarthritis found that a complete ACL tear increased the risk for medial tibiofemoral cartilage thinning as compared with those with intact ACL or partial ACL tears (odds ratio 1.8, adjusted for age, body mass index, and gender).[98] However, once an adjustment for medial meniscal tears was included in the regression model, a complete ACL tear was not an independent risk factor of cartilage thinning (odds ratio 1.1).[98] Bone marrow lesions were associated with ACL tears in the same cohort.[99] From these studies, it is clear that acute injury is associated with osteoarthritis. However, the mechanism by which this occurs is unclear. Researchers have proposed hypotheses detailing the cascade of events involving the effect of ACL injury on knee mechanics, the resulting change in loading patterns, and the cartilage response.[100]

Deformity

In contrast with knee osteoarthritis, hip osteoarthritis is generally associated with either instability or deformity, with primary hip osteoarthritis considered rare. While the association between severe hip deformity and osteoarthritis has been understood for decades, interest has recently focused on the role of more subtle deformities. It has been suggested that most cases of "idiopathic" hip osteoarthritis can be attributed to bony deformity.[101] The hypothesis that femoroacetabular impingement (FAI) is a major etiologic factor leading to osteoarthritis is gaining support in the orthopedic literature. Two mechanisms by which the cartilage and labrum are affected by FAI have been described: cam impingement and pincer impingement[102] Cam impingement is a result of a nonspherical femoral head abutting against the acetabular rim in flexion and internal rotation. The abutment creates shear forces resulting in damage to the anterosuperior acetabular cartilage. Pincer impingement occurs as a result of linear contact between the femoral head-neck junction and the acetabular rim. Repeated abutment leads to degeneration of the labrum and circumferential cartilage damage. In a study of 149 hips with mild or no radiographic osteoarthritis, patients with radiological features of cam impingement (26 hips) had damage to the anterosuperior acetabular cartilage, while patients with radiological features of pincer impingement (16 hips) had a narrow strip of circumferential cartilage damage.[103] In 25 patients diagnosed with FAI (including both cam and pincer mechanisms), histologic examination showed degeneration of the acetabular labrum and radiographic examination showed that most had mild to moderate osteoarthritis.[104] A histologic study of cartilage taken from the femoral heads of 22 young patients diagnosed with FAI showed degenerative changes similar to those seen in osteoarthritis.[105] Although hip deformity appears to be related to osteoarthritis, it is not clear how many patients with the symptoms of FAI have cartilage changes, at what stage osteoarthritic changes begin in FAI, how they progress, and whether they can be prevented or reversed. Therefore, more work in this area is warranted.

THE ROLE OF MECHANICS IN OSTEOARTHRITIS TREATMENT

Given the clear role of mechanical factors in osteoarthritis incidence and progression, it makes sense that some treatment approaches focus on modifying joint mechanics. Approaches include surgery, bracing, shoe wedging, and muscle stretching and strengthening exercises. ACL repair is the treatment of choice for ligament rupture, with the primary justification for the procedure being protection of the joint from osteoarthritis. Similarly, joint reconstruction, including repair of the posterior cruciate ligament, medial collateral ligament, menisci, acetabular labrum, and many smaller structures, is now widespread, and cartilage repair using grafts or engineered tissue is used to treat small lesions in young patients with traumatic damage to the cartilage. High tibial osteotomy is a surgical procedure used to treat tibiofemoral osteoarthritis associated with abnormal tibiofemoral malalignment. In high tibial osteotomy, a wedge of bone from the proximal tibia is resected (closing-wedge) or added (opening-wedge) to realign the lower limb, placing more force on the lateral compartment of the knee (generally) in an effort to reduce pain and delay cartilage degeneration in the medial compartment.[106] Several groups have reported that high tibial osteotomy either arrests cartilage degeneration[107] or leads to cartilage regeneration[37,108] in the diseased compartment. A number of investigators have sought to link cartilage degeneration to correction of the mechanical axis, a crude measurement of knee alignment. However, cartilage regeneration is not explained by the degree of mechanical axis correction. While one group has suggested that this arrested degeneration or regeneration is only related to "overcorrection" of the axis,[108] another group has shown that cartilage is regenerated in knees with "undercorrected" axes.[109] These results suggest that restoring the mechanical axis to normal is not sufficient for restoring joint mechanics to normal. Surgical correction of hip deformity associated with femoroacetabular impingement syndrome reduced pain and appeared to limit osteoarthritis progression in patients whose cartilage was not severely degenerated at the time of surgery.[103] Bracing increased patellar contact areas and reduced pain in subjects with patellofemoral pain.[66] Shoe insoles have been assessed. Two different sizes of lateral-wedged insole reduced varus torque,[110] and a lateral-wedge insole with a subtalar strap improved femorotibial angle and pain more effectively than a conventional wedge insole in female patients with knee osteoarthritis.[111] Shoes with variations in both angle and stiffness reduced knee adduction moments, and subjects with higher knee adduction moments before intervention had larger reductions in the peak knee adduction moment.[112] However, a controlled study focusing on knee pain and function found that the effect of treatment with a lateral-wedged insole for knee osteoarthritis was neither statistically significant nor clinically important.[113]

There is no simple explanation for why more mechanically based interventions are not being pursued. Weight loss is difficult, and exercise regimens require dedication. Insoles and braces can be uncomfortable and cumbersome. Joint reconstruction surgery aims to protect the joint from osteoarthritis in many instances, but its success is generally judged more on return to joint function in the short term rather than long-term incidence of osteoarthritis. High tibial osteotomy is technically demanding, requires a relatively long recovery, has yielded only mixed clinical success,[114] and has unicompartmental arthroplasty as an appealing alternative. Hip deformity correction is rapidly gaining interest, but is technically demanding. More generally, many surgeons are reluctant to operate on asymptomatic or mildly symptomatic joints, but intervening to restore joint integrity or correct a joint deformity may prove effective at heading off the osteoarthritis disease process.

SUMMARY

We have learned a lot about the links between mechanics and osteoarthritis in recent years. We should not be surprised that the findings are not all necessarily straightforward (osteoarthritis and joint biomechanics are both complex), nor should we be deterred from pursuing more knowledge in this area. New and better methods for measuring joint mechanics offer substantial promise to accelerate the pace of discovery. There is substantial scope for improving our understanding of mechanically based treatments for osteoarthritis and for developing new ones that better address this prevalent and disabling condition.

REFERENCES

1. Blanco FJ, Guitian R, Vazquez-Martul E, et al. Osteoarthritis chondrocytes die by apoptosis. A possible pathway for osteoarthritis pathology. Arthritis Rheum 1998; 41(2):284–9.
2. Aigner T, McKenna L. Molecular pathology and pathobiology of osteoarthritic cartilage. Cell Mol Life Sci 2002;59(1):5–18.

3. Mankin HJ, Dorfman H, Lippiello L, et al. Biochemical and metabolic abnormalities in articular cartilage from osteo-arthritic human hips. II. Correlation of morphology with biochemical and metabolic data. J Bone Joint Surg Am 1971; 53(3):523–37.
4. Green DM, Noble PC, Ahuero JS, et al. Cellular events leading to chondrocyte death after cartilage impact injury. Arthritis Rheum 2006;54(5):1509–17.
5. Huser CA, Davies ME. Validation of an in vitro single-impact load model of the initiation of osteoarthritis-like changes in articular cartilage. J Orthop Res 2006;24(4):725–32.
6. Whiteside RA, Jakob RP, Wyss UP, et al. Impact loading of articular cartilage during transplantation of osteochondral autograft. J Bone Joint Surg Br 2005; 87(9):1285–91.
7. Radin EL, Rose RM. Role of subchondral bone in the initiation and progression of cartilage damage. Clin Orthop Relat Res 1986;213:34–40.
8. Radin EL, Paul IL, Rose RM. Role of mechanical factors in pathogenesis of primary osteoarthritis. Lancet 1972;1(7749):519–22.
9. Radin EL, Parker HG, Pugh JW, et al. Response of joints to impact loading. 3. Relationship between trabecular microfractures and cartilage degeneration. J Biomech 1973;6(1):51–7.
10. Burr DB, Radin EL. Microfractures and microcracks in subchondral bone: are they relevant to osteoarthrosis? Rheum Dis Clin North Am 2003;29(4):675–85.
11. Lindsey CT, Narasimhan A, Adolfo JM, et al. Magnetic resonance evaluation of the interrelationship between articular cartilage and trabecular bone of the osteoarthritic knee. Osteoarthritis Cartilage 2004;12(2):86–96.
12. Lo GH, Zhang Y, McLennan C, et al. The ratio of medial to lateral tibial plateau bone mineral density and compartment-specific tibiofemoral osteoarthritis. Osteoarthritis Cartilage 2006;14(10):984–90.
13. Kellgren JH, Lawrence JS. Radiological assessment of osteo-arthrosis. Ann Rheum Dis 1957;16(4):494–502.
14. Burstein D, Gray ML. Is MRI fulfilling its promise for molecular imaging of cartilage in arthritis? Osteoarthritis Cartilage 2006;14(11):1087–90.
15. Wilson DR, Apreleva MV, Eichler MJ, et al. Accuracy and repeatability of a pressure measurement system in the patellofemoral joint. J Biomech 2003;36(12): 1909–15.
16. Radin EL, Ehrlich MG, Chernack R, et al. Effect of repetitive impulsive loading on the knee joints of rabbits. Clin Orthop Relat Res 1978;131:288–93.
17. Song Y, Greve JM, Carter DR, et al. Articular cartilage MR imaging and thickness mapping of a loaded knee joint before and after meniscectomy. Osteoarthritis Cartilage 2006;14(8):728–37.
18. Ahmed AM, Burke DL, Yu A. In-vitro measurement of static pressure distribution in synovial joints–part II: retropatellar surface. J Biomech Eng 1983;105(3): 226–36.
19. Ahmed AM, Duncan NA. Correlation of patellar tracking pattern with trochlear and retropatellar surface topographies. J Biomech Eng 2000;122(6):652–60.
20. Ahmed AM, Duncan NA, Tanzer M. In vitro measurement of the tracking pattern of the human patella. J Biomech Eng 1999;121(2):222–8.
21. Huberti HH, Hayes WC. Contact pressures in chondromalacia patellae and the effects of capsular reconstructive procedures. J Orthop Res 1988;6(4): 499–508.
22. Huberti HH, Hayes WC. Patellofemoral contact pressures. The influence of q-angle and tendofemoral contact. J Bone Joint Surg Am 1984;66(5):715–24.

23. Ateshian GA, Kwak SD, Soslowsky LJ, et al. A stereophotogrammetric method for determining in situ contact areas in diarthrodial joints, and a comparison with other methods. J Biomech 1994;27(1):111–24.
24. Brown TD, Shaw DT. In vitro contact stress distributions in the natural human hip. J Biomech 1983;16(6):373–84.
25. Apreleva M, Hasselman CT, Debski RE, et al. A dynamic analysis of glenohumeral motion after simulated capsulolabral injury. A cadaver model. J Bone Joint Surg Am 1998;80(4):474–80.
26. Blankevoort L, Huiskes R. Validation of a three-dimensional model of the knee. J Biomech 1996;29(7):955–61.
27. Elias JJ, Wilson DR, Adamson R, et al. Evaluation of a computational model used to predict the patellofemoral contact pressure distribution. J Biomech 2004; 37(3):295–302.
28. Wismans J, Veldpaus F, Janssen J, et al. A three-dimensional mathematical model of the knee-joint. J Biomech 1980;13(8):677–85.
29. Blankevoort L, Kuiper JH, Huiskes R, et al. Articular contact in a three-dimensional model of the knee. J Biomech 1991;24(11):1019–31.
30. van der Helm FC. A finite element musculoskeletal model of the shoulder mechanism. J Biomech 1994;27(5):551–69.
31. Brown TD, DiGioia AM III. A contact-coupled finite element analysis of the natural adult hip. J Biomech 1984;17(6):437–48.
32. Ahmad CS, Kwak SD, Ateshian GA, et al. Effects of patellar tendon adhesion to the anterior tibia on knee mechanics. Am J Sports Med 1998;26(5):715–24.
33. Kwak SD, Ahmad CS, Gardner TR, et al. Hamstrings and iliotibial band forces affect knee kinematics and contact pattern. J Orthop Res 2000;18(1):101–8.
34. Cohen ZA, Henry JH, McCarthy DM, et al. Computer simulations of patellofemoral joint surgery. Patient-specific models for tuberosity transfer. Am J Sports Med 2003;31(1):87–98.
35. Cohen ZA, Roglic H, Grelsamer RP, et al. Patellofemoral stresses during open and closed kinetic chain exercises. An analysis using computer simulation. Am J Sports Med 2001;29(4):480–7.
36. Hadley NA, Brown TD, Weinstein SL. The effects of contact pressure elevations and aseptic necrosis on the long-term outcome of congenital hip dislocation. J Orthop Res 1990;8(4):504–13.
37. Kanamiya T, Naito M, Hara M, et al. The influences of biomechanical factors on cartilage regeneration after high tibial osteotomy for knees with medial compartment osteoarthritis: clinical and arthroscopic observations. Arthroscopy 2002; 18(7):725–9.
38. Ito K, Minka MA II, Leunig M, et al. Femoroacetabular impingement and the cam-effect. A MRI-based quantitative anatomical study of the femoral head-neck offset. J Bone Joint Surg Br 2001;83(2):171–6.
39. Morrison JB. The mechanics of the knee joint in relation to normal walking. J Biomech 1970;3(1):51–61.
40. Andriacchi TP, Alexander EJ, Toney MK, et al. A point cluster method for in vivo motion analysis: applied to a study of knee kinematics. J Biomech Eng 1998; 120(6):743–9.
41. Delport HP, Banks SA, De Schepper J, et al. A kinematic comparison of fixed- and mobile-bearing knee replacements. J Bone Joint Surg Br 2006;88(8): 1016–21.
42. Komistek RD, Dennis DA, Mahfouz M. In vivo fluoroscopic analysis of the normal human knee. Clin Orthop Relat Res 2003;410:69–81.

43. Karrholm J, Brandsson S, Freeman MA. Tibiofemoral movement 4: changes of axial tibial rotation caused by forced rotation at the weight-bearing knee studied by RSA. J Bone Joint Surg Br 2000;82(8):1201–3.
44. Fleming BC, Peura GD, Abate JA, et al. Accuracy and repeatability of Roentgen stereophotogrammetric analysis (RSA) for measuring knee laxity in longitudinal studies. J Biomech 2001;34(10):1355–9.
45. You BM, Siy P, Anderst W, et al. In vivo measurement of 3-D skeletal kinematics from sequences of biplane radiographs: application to knee kinematics. IEEE Trans Med Imaging 2001;20(6):514–25.
46. Anderst WJ, Tashman S. A method to estimate in vivo dynamic articular surface interaction. J Biomech 2003;36(9):1291–9.
47. Powers CM, Ward SR, Fredericson M, et al. Patellofemoral kinematics during weight-bearing and non-weight-bearing knee extension in persons with lateral subluxation of the patella: a preliminary study. J Orthop Sports Phys Ther 2003;33(11):677–85.
48. Muhle C, Brossmann J, Heller M. Kinematic CT and MR imaging of the patellofemoral joint. Eur Radiol 1999;9(3):508–18.
49. Sheehan FT, Drace JE. Quantitative MR measures of three-dimensional patellar kinematics as a research and diagnostic tool. Med Sci Sports Exerc 1999; 31(10):1399–405.
50. Sheehan FT, Zajac FE, Drace JE. In vivo tracking of the human patella using cine phase contrast magnetic resonance imaging. J Biomech Eng 1999;121(6): 650–6.
51. Sheehan FT, Zajac FE, Drace JE. Using cine phase contrast magnetic resonance imaging to non-invasively study in vivo knee dynamics. J Biomech 1998;31(1):21–6.
52. Barrance PJ, Williams GN, Novotny JE, et al. A method for measurement of joint kinematics in vivo by registration of 3-D geometric models with cine phase contrast magnetic resonance imaging data. J Biomech Eng 2005;127(5):829–37.
53. Barrance PJ, Williams GN, Snyder-Mackler L, et al. Altered knee kinematics in ACL-deficient non-copers: a comparison using dynamic MRI. J Orthop Res 2006;24(2):132–40.
54. Barrance PJ, Williams GN, Snyder-Mackler L, et al. Do ACL-injured copers exhibit differences in knee kinematics?: An MRI study. Clin Orthop Relat Res 2007;454:74–80.
55. Rebmann AJ, Sheehan FT. Precise 3D skeletal kinematics using fast phase contrast magnetic resonance imaging. J Magn Reson Imaging 2003;17(2): 206–13.
56. Patel VV, Hall K, Ries M, et al. Magnetic resonance imaging of patellofemoral kinematics with weight-bearing. J Bone Joint Surg Am 2003;85-A(12):2419–24.
57. Patel VV, Hall K, Ries M, et al. A three-dimensional MRI analysis of knee kinematics. J Orthop Res 2004;22(2):283–92.
58. Fellows RA, Hill NA, Gill HS, et al. Magnetic resonance imaging for in vivo assessment of three-dimensional patellar tracking. J Biomech 2005;38(8): 1643–52.
59. Fellows RA, Hill NA, Macintyre NJ, et al. Repeatability of a novel technique for in vivo measurement of three-dimensional patellar tracking using magnetic resonance imaging. J Magn Reson Imaging 2005;22(1):145–53.
60. Lerner AL, Tamez-Pena JG, Houck JR, et al. The use of sequential MR image sets for determining tibiofemoral motion: reliability of coordinate systems and accuracy of motion tracking algorithm. J Biomech Eng 2003;125(2):246–53.

61. McWalter EJW, Wilson DC, Kacher DF, et al. Three-dimensional patellar kinematics in weightbearing flexion using open MRI. Munich (Germany): World Congress of Biomechanics; 2006.
62. Ronsky JL, Herzog W, Brown TD, et al. In vivo quantification of the cat patellofemoral joint contact stresses and areas. J Biomech 1995;28(8):977–83.
63. Tashman S, Anderst W. In-vivo measurement of dynamic joint motion using high speed biplane radiography and CT: application to canine ACL deficiency. J Biomech Eng 2003;125(2):238–45.
64. Brechter JH, Powers CM. Patellofemoral joint stress during stair ascent and descent in persons with and without patellofemoral pain. Gait Posture 2002; 16(2):115–23.
65. Heino Brechter J, Powers CM, Terk MR, et al. Quantification of patellofemoral joint contact area using magnetic resonance imaging. Magn Reson Imaging 2003;21(9):955–9.
66. Powers CM, Ward SR, Chan LD, et al. The effect of bracing on patella alignment and patellofemoral joint contact area. Med Sci Sports Exerc 2004;36(7): 1226–32.
67. Salsich GB, Ward SR, Terk MR, et al. In vivo assessment of patellofemoral joint contact area in individuals who are pain free. Clin Orthop 2003;417:277–84.
68. Gold GE, Besier TF, Draper CE, et al. Weight-bearing MRI of patellofemoral joint cartilage contact area. J Magn Reson Imaging 2004;20(3):526–30.
69. von Eisenhart-Rothe R, Siebert M, Bringmann C, et al. A new in vivo technique for determination of 3D kinematics and contact areas of the patello-femoral and tibio-femoral joint. J Biomech 2004;37(6):927–34.
70. Goto A, Moritomo H, Murase T, et al. In vivo elbow biomechanical analysis during flexion: three-dimensional motion analysis using magnetic resonance imaging. J Shoulder Elbow Surg 2004;13(4):441–7.
71. Felson DT, Lawrence RC, Dieppe PA, et al. Osteoarthritis: new insights. Part 1: the disease and its risk factors. Ann Intern Med 2000;133(8):635–46.
72. Hunter DJ, Niu J, Felson DT, et al. Knee alignment does not predict incident osteoarthritis: the Framingham osteoarthritis study. Arthritis Rheum 2007;56(4): 1212–8.
73. Felson DT, Goggins J, Niu J, et al. The effect of body weight on progression of knee osteoarthritis is dependent on alignment. Arthritis Rheum 2004;50(12): 3904–9.
74. Felson DT, McLaughlin S, Goggins J, et al. Bone marrow edema and its relation to progression of knee osteoarthritis. Ann Intern Med 2003;139(5 Pt 1):330–6.
75. Williams A, Sharma L, McKenzie CA, et al. Delayed gadolinium-enhanced magnetic resonance imaging of cartilage in knee osteoarthritis: findings at different radiographic stages of disease and relationship to malalignment. Arthritis Rheum 2005;52(11):3528–35.
76. Harvey WF, Niu J, Zhang Y, et al. Knee alignment differences between Chinese and Caucasians subjects without osteoarthritis. Ann Rheum Dis 2008 [Epub ahead of print].
77. Elahi S, Cahue S, Felson DT, et al. The association between varus-valgus alignment and patellofemoral osteoarthritis. Arthritis Rheum 2000;43(8):1874–80.
78. Sharma L, Song J, Felson DT, et al. The role of knee alignment in disease progression and functional decline in knee osteoarthritis. JAMA 2001;286(2): 188–95.
79. Cahue S, Dunlop D, Hayes K, et al. Varus-valgus alignment in the progression of patellofemoral osteoarthritis. Arthritis Rheum 2004;50(7):2184–90.

80. Cerejo R, Dunlop DD, Cahue S, et al. The influence of alignment on risk of knee osteoarthritis progression according to baseline stage of disease. Arthritis Rheum 2002;46(10):2632–6.
81. McWalter EJ, Cibere J, MacIntyre NJ, et al. Relationship between varus-valgus alignment and patellar kinematics in individuals with knee osteoarthritis. J Bone Joint Surg Am 2007;89(12):2723–31.
82. Kalichman L, Zhang Y, Niu J, et al. The association between patellar alignment on magnetic resonance imaging and radiographic manifestations of knee osteoarthritis. Arthritis Res Ther 2007;9(2):R26.
83. Hunter DJ, Zhang YQ, Niu JB, et al. Patella malalignment, pain and patellofemoral progression: the Health ABC Study. Osteoarthritis Cartilage 2007;15(10): 1120–7.
84. Hunter DJ, Niu J, Zhang Y, et al. Knee height, knee pain, and knee osteoarthritis: the Beijing Osteoarthritis Study. Arthritis Rheum 2005;52(5):1418–23.
85. Zhang Y, Hunter DJ, Nevitt MC, et al. Association of squatting with increased prevalence of radiographic tibiofemoral knee osteoarthritis: the Beijing Osteoarthritis Study. Arthritis Rheum 2004;50(4):1187–92.
86. Mundermann A, Dyrby CO, Hurwitz DE, et al. Potential strategies to reduce medial compartment loading in patients with knee osteoarthritis of varying severity: reduced walking speed. Arthritis Rheum 2004;50(4):1172–8.
87. Baliunas AJ, Hurwitz DE, Ryals AB, et al. Increased knee joint loads during walking are present in subjects with knee osteoarthritis. Osteoarthritis Cartilage 2002;10(7):573–9.
88. Mundermann A, Dyrby CO, Andriacchi TP. Secondary gait changes in patients with medial compartment knee osteoarthritis: increased load at the ankle, knee, and hip during walking. Arthritis Rheum 2005;52(9):2835–44.
89. Chang A, Hayes K, Dunlop D, et al. Hip abduction moment and protection against medial tibiofemoral osteoarthritis progression. Arthritis Rheum 2005; 52(11):3515–9.
90. Astephen JL, Deluzio KJ, Caldwell GE, et al. Gait and neuromuscular pattern changes are associated with differences in knee osteoarthritis severity levels. J Biomech 2008;41(4):868–76.
91. Hurwitz DE, Hulet CH, Andriacchi TP, et al. Gait compensations in patients with osteoarthritis of the hip and their relationship to pain and passive hip motion. J Orthop Res 1997;15(4):629–35.
92. McGibbon CA, Krebs DE. Compensatory gait mechanics in patients with unilateral knee arthritis. J Rheumatol 2002;29(11):2410–9.
93. Shakoor N, Hurwitz DE, Block JA, et al. Asymmetric knee loading in advanced unilateral hip osteoarthritis. Arthritis Rheum 2003;48(6):1556–61.
94. Chang A, Hurwitz D, Dunlop D, et al. The relationship between toe-out angle during gait and progression of medial tibiofemoral osteoarthritis. Ann Rheum Dis 2007;66(10):1271–5.
95. Englund M, Roos EM, Lohmander LS. Impact of type of meniscal tear on radiographic and symptomatic knee osteoarthritis: a sixteen-year followup of meniscectomy with matched controls. Arthritis Rheum 2003;48(8):2178–87.
96. Lohmander LS, Ostenberg A, Englund M, et al. High prevalence of knee osteoarthritis, pain, and functional limitations in female soccer players twelve years after anterior cruciate ligament injury. Arthritis Rheum 2004;50(10):3145–52.
97. von Porat A, Roos EM, Roos H. High prevalence of osteoarthritis 14 years after an anterior cruciate ligament tear in male soccer players: a study of radiographic and patient relevant outcomes. Ann Rheum Dis 2004;63(3):269–73.

98. Amin S, Guermazi A, Lavalley MP, et al. Complete anterior cruciate ligament tear and the risk for cartilage loss and progression of symptoms in men and women with knee osteoarthritis. Osteoarthritis Cartilage 2008;16(8):897–902.
99. Hernandez-Molina G, Guermazi A, Niu J, et al. Central bone marrow lesions in symptomatic knee osteoarthritis and their relationship to anterior cruciate ligament tears and cartilage loss. Arthritis Rheum 2008;58(1):130–6.
100. Chaudhari AM, Briant PL, Bevill SL, et al. Knee kinematics, cartilage morphology, and osteoarthritis after ACL injury. Med Sci Sports Exerc 2008;40(2): 215–22.
101. Harris WH. Etiology of osteoarthritis of the hip. Clin Orthop 1986;213:20–33.
102. Beck M, Kalhor M, Leunig M, et al. Hip morphology influences the pattern of damage to the acetabular cartilage: femoroacetabular impingement as a cause of early osteoarthritis of the hip. J Bone Joint Surg Br 2005;87(7):1012–8.
103. Beck M, Leunig M, Parvizi J, et al. Anterior femoroacetabular impingement: part II. Midterm results of surgical treatment. Clin Orthop 2004;418:67–73.
104. Ito K, Leunig M, Ganz R. Histopathologic features of the acetabular labrum in femoroacetabular impingement. Clin Orthop Relat Res 2004;429:262–71.
105. Wagner S, Hofstetter W, Chiquet M, et al. Early osteoarthritic changes of human femoral head cartilage subsequent to femoro-acetabular impingement. Osteoarthritis Cartilage 2003;11(7):508–18.
106. Coventry MB. Osteotomy of the upper portion of the tibia for degenerative arthritis of the knee. A preliminary report. J Bone Joint Surg Am 1965;47:984–90.
107. Wakabayashi S, Akizuki S, Takizawa T, et al. A comparison of the healing potential of fibrillated cartilage versus eburnated bone in osteoarthritic knees after high tibial osteotomy: an arthroscopic study with 1-year follow-up. Arthroscopy 2002;18(3):272–8.
108. Odenbring S, Egund N, Lindstrand A, et al. Cartilage regeneration after proximal tibial osteotomy for medial gonarthrosis. An arthroscopic, roentgenographic, and histologic study. Clin Orthop 1992;277:210–6.
109. Bergenudd H, Johnell O, Redlund-Johnell I, et al. The articular cartilage after osteotomy for medial gonarthrosis. Biopsies after 2 years in 19 cases. Acta Orthop Scand 1992;63(4):413–6.
110. Kerrigan DC, Lelas JL, Goggins J, et al. Effectiveness of a lateral-wedge insole on knee varus torque in patients with knee osteoarthritis. Arch Phys Med Rehabil 2002;83(7):889–93.
111. Toda Y, Tsukimura N. A six-month followup of a randomized trial comparing the efficacy of a lateral-wedge insole with subtalar strapping and an in-shoe lateral-wedge insole in patients with varus deformity osteoarthritis of the knee. Arthritis Rheum 2004;50(10):3129–36.
112. Fisher DS, Dyrby CO, Mundermann A, et al. In healthy subjects without knee osteoarthritis, the peak knee adduction moment influences the acute effect of shoe interventions designed to reduce medial compartment knee load. J Orthop Res 2007;25(4):540–6.
113. Baker K, Goggins J, Xie H, et al. A randomized crossover trial of a wedged insole for treatment of knee osteoarthritis. Arthritis Rheum 2007;56(4):1198–203.
114. Rinonapoli E, Mancini GB, Corvaglia A, et al. Tibial osteotomy for varus gonarthrosis. A 10- to 21-year followup study. Clin Orthop 1998;353:185–93.

The Symptoms of Osteoarthritis and the Genesis of Pain

David J. Hunter, MBBS, MSc, PhD[a],*, Jason J. McDougall, BSc, PhD[b],
Francis J. Keefe, PhD[c]

KEYWORDS

• Osteoarthritis • Symptoms • Pain

Symptomatic osteoarthritis (OA) causes substantial physical and psychosocial disability.[1] In the early 1990s, more than 7 million Americans were limited in their ability to participate in their main daily activities, such as going to school or work or maintaining their independence, simply because of their arthritis.[2] The risk for disability (defined as needing help walking or climbing stairs) attributable to knee OA is as great as that attributable to cardiovascular disease and greater than that due to any other medical condition in elderly people.[1] Like arthritis prevalence, the prevalence of arthritis-related disability is also expected to increase by the year 2020, when an estimated 11.6 million people will be affected.[2]

Compounding this picture are the enormous financial costs that our nation bears for treating arthritis and its complications, and the disability that results from uncontrolled disease. The total annual cost in the United States is almost $65 billion—a figure equivalent to a moderate national recession.[3] This amount includes an estimated medical bill of $15 billion each year for such expenses as 39 million physician visits and more than half a million hospitalizations (Centers for Disease Control, unpublished data, 1999). OA accounts for 90% of hip and knee replacements.[4] The balance is largely due to indirect costs, such as those from wage losses.[3] Arthritis has thus

A version of this article originally appeared in the 34:3 issue of the *Rheumatic Disease Clinics of North America*.

Preparation of this article for Francis Keefe was supported in part by NIH grants AG026010, AR47218, AR049059, AR050245, and AR05462.

[a] Division of Research, New England Baptist Hospital, 125 Parker Hill Avenue, Boston MA 02120, USA

[b] Department of Physiology and Biophysics, Faculty of Medicine, University of Calgary, 3330 Hospital Drive NW, Calgary, Alberta T2N 4N1, Canada

[c] Pain Prevention and Treatment Research Program, Department of Psychiatry and Behavioral Sciences, Duke University Medical Center, Suite 340, 2200 West Main Street, Durham, NC 27705, USA

* Corresponding author. Division of Research, New England Baptist Hospital, 125 Parker Hill Avenue, Boston MA 02120.

E-mail address: djhunter@caregroup.harvard.edu (D.J. Hunter).

Med Clin N Am 93 (2009) 83–100
doi:10.1016/j.mcna.2008.08.008
0025-7125/08/$ – see front matter © 2008 Elsevier Inc. All rights reserved.

medical.theclinics.com

become one of our most pressing public health problems—a problem that is expected to worsen in the next millennium with the increasing prevalence of this disease.

This article delineates the characteristic symptoms and signs associated with OA and how they can be used to make the clinical diagnosis. The predominant symptom in most patients is pain. The remainder of the article focuses on what we know causes pain in OA and contributes to its severity. Much has been learned over recent years; however, for the budding researcher much of this puzzle remains unexplored or inadequately understood.

WHAT IS OSTEOARTHRITIS?

OA can be viewed as the clinical and pathologic outcome of a range of disorders that result in structural and functional failure of synovial joints.[5] OA occurs when the dynamic equilibrium between the breakdown and repair of joint tissues is overwhelmed.[6] This progressive joint failure may cause pain, physical disability, and psychologic distress,[1] although many people who have structural changes consistent with OA are asymptomatic.[7] The reason for this disconnect between disease severity and the level of reported pain and disability is unknown.

Typically OA presents as joint pain. During a 1-year period, 25% of people older than 55 years have a persistent episode of knee pain, of whom about one in six consult their general practitioner about it.[8] Approximately 50% of these people have radiographic knee OA. The usefulness of radiographs relates more importantly to the exclusion of other diagnostic possibilities rather than confirmation of osteoarthritic disease.[9] Factors differentiating symptomatic OA from asymptomatic radiographic disease are largely unknown. Symptomatic knee OA (pain on most days and radiographic features consistent with OA) occurs in approximately 12% of those older than age 55.[8]

Although OA is common in the knee, it is even more prevalent in the hands, especially the distal (DIP) and proximal (PIP) interphalangeal joints and the base of the thumb. When symptomatic, especially so for the base of thumb joint, hand OA is associated with functional impairment.[10,11] OA of the thumb carpometacarpal (CMC) joint is a common condition that can lead to substantial pain, instability, deformity, and loss of motion.[12] After the age of 70 years, approximately 5% of women and 3% of men have symptomatic OA affecting this joint with impairment of hand function.[10]

The prevalence of hip OA is about 9% in Caucasian populations.[13] In contrast, studies in Asian, black, and East Indian populations indicate a low prevalence of hip OA.[14] The prevalence of symptomatic hip OA is approximately 4%.[15]

WHAT ARE THE CHARACTERISTIC SYMPTOMS OF OSTEOARTHRITIS?

The joint pain of OA is typically described as exacerbated by activity and relieved by rest. More advanced OA can cause rest and night pain leading to loss of sleep, which further exacerbates pain. The cardinal symptoms that suggest a diagnosis of OA include:

Pain (typically described as activity related or mechanical, may occur with rest in advanced disease; often deep, aching and not well localized; usually of insidious onset)
Reduced function
Stiffness (of short duration, also termed "gelling" [ie, short-lived stiffness after inactivity])
Joint instability, buckling, or giving way

Reduced movement, deformity, swelling, crepitus, and increased age (OA is unusual before age 40) in the absence of systemic features (such as fever)
Pain-related psychologic distress if pain persists.

TAILORING THE PHYSICAL EXAMINATION: WHAT SIGNS ARE ASSOCIATED WITH OSTEOARTHRITIS?

Physical examination should include an assessment of body weight and body mass index, joint range of motion, the location of tenderness, muscle strength, and ligament stability. For lower limb joint involvement, this should include assessment of body mass and postural alignment in standing and walking.[16] A goniometer can be used to permit the examiner to visually bisect the thigh and lower leg along their lengths. The centers of the patella and ankle should be located and marked with a pen. The center of the goniometer is placed on the center of the patella, and the arms of this goniometer are extended along the center of the thigh and along the axis of the lower leg to the center of the ankle.

The features on physical examination that suggest a diagnosis of OA include:

Tenderness, usually located over the joint line
Crepitus with movement of the joint
Bony enlargement of the joint, (eg, Heberden and Bouchard nodes, squaring of the first CMC, typically along the affected joint line in the knee)
Restricted joint range of motion
Pain on passive range of motion
Deformity, (eg, angulation of the DIP and PIP joints, varus [bowed legs] deformity of the knees)
Instability of the joint
Altered gait
Muscle atrophy or weakness
Joint effusion

THE DIAGNOSIS OF OSTEOARTHRITIS

Bearing in mind that radiographs are notoriously insensitive to the earliest pathologic features of OA, the absence of positive radiographic findings should not be interpreted as confirming the complete absence of symptomatic disease. Conversely, the presence of positive radiographic findings does not guarantee that an osteoarthritic joint is also the active source of the patient's current knee or hip symptoms; other sources of pain, including periarticular sources, such as pes anserine bursitis at the knee and trochanteric bursitis at the hip, often contribute.[7] According to the American College of Rheumatology criteria for classification of hand OA (unlike the hip and knee, in which radiographs enhance the sensitivity and specificity), radiographs are less sensitive and specific than physical examination in the diagnosis of symptomatic hand OA.[17]

In clinical practice the diagnosis of OA should be made on the basis of the history and physical examination; the role of radiography is to confirm this clinical suspicion and rule out other conditions.

When disease is advanced, it is visible on plain radiographs, which show narrowing of joint space, osteophytes, and sometimes changes in the subchondral bone. MRI can be used in infrequent circumstances to facilitate the diagnosis of other causes of joint pain that can be confused with OA (osteochondritis dissecans, avascular necrosis). An unfortunate consequence of the frequent use of MRI in clinical practice is the frequent detection of meniscal tears. In the interest of preserving menisci, be cautioned that meniscal tears are nearly universal in people who have knee OA and are not necessarily a cause of increased symptoms.[18] The penchant to remove menisci is to be avoided, unless there are symptoms of locking or extension blockade.[19]

Do not rely on laboratory testing to establish the diagnosis of OA. Because OA is a noninflammatory arthritis, laboratory findings are expected to be normal.

WHAT ARE THE DIAGNOSTIC CRITERIA FOR OSTEOARTHRITIS?

When making the diagnosis of OA, consider using the criteria of the American College of Rheumatology for diagnostic purposes and classification of OA of the hip, knee, and hands in patients who have pain in these joints.[17,20] These are the criteria that are used in research studies and should be used to inform your diagnosis in individuals; not limiting your information gathering to these criteria and considering the wealth of other information that patients who have OA may provide can help to either confirm or refute an OA diagnosis.

In the process of taking a history it is important to ask how the pain has affected the person's ability to function at home, at work, and in recreational activities. Also, ask about how the person is coping with pain and how well that is going. It is important to look for signs of psychologic distress (eg, signs of anxiety, such as excessive pain-avoidant posturing, sleep-onset insomnia, or signs of depression, such as early morning wakening, weight loss, irritability, or a marked in increase in memory/concentration problems).

FACTORS THAT CONTRIBUTE TO PAIN

The source of pain is not particularly well understood and is best framed in a biopsychosocial framework, which posits that biologic, psychologic, and social factors all play a significant role in pain in OA.[21] **Fig. 1** is a schematic representing some of this complexity.

From a biologic perspective, neuronal activity in the pain pathway is responsible for the generation and ultimate exacerbation of the feeling of joint pain. During inflammation chemical mediators are released into the joint, which sensitize primary afferent nerves such that normally innocuous joint movements (such as increased physical activity, high-heeled shoes, weather changes) now elicit a painful response. This response is the neurophysiologic basis of allodynia (ie, the sensation of pain in response to a normally nonpainful stimulus, such as walking). Over time this increased neuronal activity from the periphery can cause plasticity changes in the central nervous system (CNS) by a process termed "wind-up." In this instance, second-order neurones in the spinal cord increase their firing rate such that the transmission of pain information to the somatosensory cortex is enhanced. This central sensitization phenomenon intensifies pain sensation and can even lead to pain responses from regions of the body remote from the inflamed joint (ie, referred pain).

Constitutional factors that can predispose to symptoms include self-efficacy, pain catastrophizing, and the social context of arthritis (social support, pain communication); all are important considerations in understanding the pain experience.

LOCAL TISSUE PATHOLOGY

The structural determinants of pain and mechanical dysfunction in OA are also not well understood, but are believed to involve multiple interactive pathways. Articular cartilage is aneural and avascular. As such, cartilage is incapable of directly generating pain, inflammation, stiffness, or any of the symptoms that patients who have OA

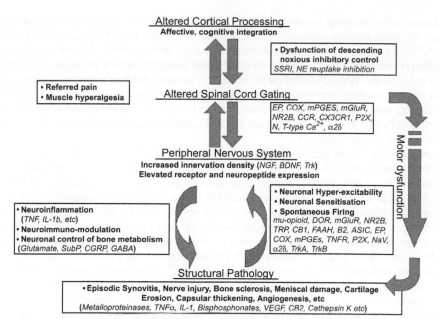

Altered Cortical Processing
Affective, cognitive integration

• Dysfunction of descending
  noxious inhibitory control
  SSRI, NE reuptake inhibition

• Referred pain
• Muscle hyperalgesia

Altered Spinal Cord Gating

*EP, COX, mPGES, mGluR,
NR2B, CCR, CX3CR1, P2X,
N, T-type Ca²⁺, α2δ*

Peripheral Nervous System
Increased innervation density (*NGF, BDNF, Trk*)
Elevated receptor and neuropeptide expression

• Neuronal Hyper-excitability
• Neuronal Sensitisation
• Spontaneous Firing
  *mu-opioid, DOR, mGluR, NR2B,
  TRP, CB1, FAAH, B2, ASIC, EP,
  COX, mPGEs, TNFR, P2X, NaV,
  α2δ, TrkA, TrkB*

• Neuroinflammation
  (*TNF, IL-1b, etc*)
• Neuroimmuno-modulation
• Neuronal control of bone metabolism
  (*Glutamate, SubP, CGRP, GABA*)

Motor dysfunction

Structural Pathology

• Episodic Synovitis, Nerve injury, Bone sclerosis, Meniscal damage, Cartilage
  Erosion, Capsular thickening, Angiogenesis, etc
  (*Metalloproteinases, TNFα, IL-1, Bisphosphonates, VEGF, CB2, Cathepsin K etc*)

Fig. 1. Key elements of OA pain pathophysiology and examples of pharmacologic intervention points. Observations of pain resolution following intra-articular local anesthetic and following joint replacement would implicate a peripheral drive in most patients who have OA. In the periphery, the interaction between structural pathology and the immune and nervous systems perpetuate the pain experience. Over time, as structural pathology develops, the principle algogenic mechanisms and mediators change. Furthermore, the dysfunction in central processing of information at the spinal and cortical levels has also been observed in patients who have OA, affecting sensory and motor systems. This phenomenon, in combination with altered affective and cognitive functions, may underpin the pain experience in other patient subsets. ASIC, acid-sensing ion channel; BDNF, brain-derived neurotrophic factor; CB, cannabinoid receptor; CCR, chemokine receptor; CGRP, calcitonin gene-related peptide; COX, cyclooxygenase; DOR, delta opioid receptor; EP, E prostanoid receptor; FAAH, fatty acid amide hydrolysis; GABA, γ-aminobutyric acid; IL, interleukin; mGluR, metabotropic glutamate receptor; mPGES, membrane or microsomal PGE synthase; N-type Ca²⁺, neuronal-type calcium channels; NE, noradrenaline; NGF, nerve growth factor; NR2B, N-methyl D-aspartate receptor 2B subunit; P2X, purinergic 2X ionotrophic receptor; SSRI, selective serotonin reuptake inhibitor; SubP, substance P; T-type Ca²⁺, transient type Ca²⁺ channels; TNF, tumor necrosis factor; TNFR, tumor necrosis factor receptor; Trk, tyrosine kinase; TRP, transient receptor potential; VEGF, vascular epidermal growth factor. (*From* Dray A, Read SJ, Dray A, et al. Arthritis and pain. Future targets to control osteoarthritis pain. Arthritis Res Ther 2007;9(3):212; with permission.)

typically describe.[22] Given its relative unimportance to OA's symptomatic presentation, it is ironic that articular cartilage has received so much attention, whereas other common symptom sources in the joint are ignored.

In contrast the subchondral bone, periosteum, periarticular ligaments, periarticular muscle spasm, synovium, and joint capsule are all richly innervated and are the source of nociception in OA.

In population studies there is a significant discordance between radiographically diagnosed OA and knee pain.[7] Although radiographic evidence of joint damage predisposes to joint pain, it is clear that the severity of the joint damage on the radiograph bears little relation to the severity of the pain experienced.

Using other imaging modalities, such as MRI, significant structural associations, such as bone marrow lesions,[23,24] subarticular bone attrition,[25] synovitis, and effusion,[26,27] have been related to knee pain. It remains unclear which of these local tissue factors predominate because until recently these analyses did not account for the fact that much of the structural change is collinear (a person who has more severe disease has worse structural change in multiple tissues, including the bone synovium, and so forth) and were not adjusting for other tissue changes. A recent analysis confirmed most beliefs that it is likely that changes in the subchondral bone and synovial activation/effusion predominate.[28]

Lesions in the bone marrow play an integral if not pivotal role in the symptoms that emanate from knee OA and its structural progression.[23] Bone marrow lesions were found in 272 of 351 (77.5%) people who had painful knees compared with 15 of 50 (30%) people who had no knee pain ($P<.001$). Large lesions were present almost exclusively in people who had knee pain (35.9% versus 2%; $P<.001$). After adjustment for severity of radiographic disease, effusion, age, and sex, lesions and large lesions remained associated with the occurrence of knee pain. More recently their relation to pain severity was also demonstrated.[24] Other bone-related causes of pain include periostitis associated with osteophyte formation,[29] subchondral microfractures,[30] and bone angina due to decreased blood flow and elevated intraosseous pressure.[31] The particular bone pathology most responsible for pain remains elusive; however, identifying this would be a major advance in delineating appropriate therapeutic targets. One likely source that remains underexplored is that of intraosseous hypertension. The pathophysiology remains unclear, although phlebographic studies in OA indicate impaired vascular clearance from bone and increased intraosseous pressure in the bone marrow near the painful joint.[31–34] What may subsequently cause pain is as yet unknown. Increased trabecular bone pressure, ischemia, and inflammation are all possible stimuli.

The synovial reaction in OA includes synovial hyperplasia, fibrosis, thickening of synovial capsule, activated synoviocytes, and in some cases lymphocytic infiltrate (B and T cells and plasma cells).[35] The site of infiltration of the synovium is of obvious relevance because one of the most densely innervated structures of the joint is the white adipose tissue of the fat pad, which also shows evidence of inflammation and can act as a rich source of inflammatory adipokines.[36] Synovial causes of pain include irritation of sensory nerve endings within the synovium from osteophytes and synovial inflammation that is due, at least in part, to the release of prostaglandins, leukotrienes, proteinases, neuropeptides, and cytokines.[37,38] Synovitis is frequently present in OA and may predict other structural changes in osteoarthritis and correlate with pain and other clinical outcomes.[26] Synovial thickening around the infrapatellar fat pad using noncontrast MRI has been shown on biopsy to represent mild chronic synovitis.[39] A semiquantitative measure of synovitis from the infrapatellar fat pad is associated with pain severity, and similarly, change in synovitis is associated with change in pain severity.[27]

Another source of joint pain in OA may be from the nerves themselves. Following joint injury in which there is ligamentous rupture, the nerves that reinnervate the healing soft tissues contain an overabundance of algesic chemicals, such as substance P and calcitonin gene-related peptide (CGRP). An interesting observation of these new nerves was that their overall morphology was abnormal with fibers appearing punctate and disorganized.[40,41] Because these phenomena are consistent with the innervation profiles described in nerve injury models, we speculate that injured joints may develop neuropathic pain posttrauma. Treatment of inflamed joints with the neuropathic pain analgesic gabapentin can also relieve arthritis pain.[42]

INNERVATION IN THE JOINT

The musculature, articular capsule, synovium, tendons, ligaments, and subchondral bone of the joint have a rich nerve supply, whereas the articular hyaline cartilage is aneural. In addition to postganglionic sympathetic efferents, joints are supplied by numerous sensory fibers whose subcategorization is based on distinct anatomic features.[43] Joint afferents that have a thick diameter and are myelinated are called Aβ (Group II) fibers, thin nerves with a myelin sheath that disappears in the terminal region to become a free nerve ending are termed Aδ (Group III) fibers, and the thin unmyelinated nerves are C (Group IV) fibers. Proprioceptive Aβ fibers of the joint terminate in the capsule, fat pad, ligaments, menisci, and periosteum, and nociceptive Aδ and C fibers innervate the capsule, ligaments, menisci, periosteum, and mineralized bone (in particular in regions of high mechanical load).[37,43–45]

Joint nociceptors are typically localized within specific articular structures and their receptive field is normally restricted to the joint. During inflammation, however, this receptive field can expand into adjacent areas such that mechanical stimuli in nonarticular tissues, such as the surrounding muscle, can suddenly become activated. A typical neuron in the spinal cord with a receptive field in the joint may now respond to physical stimulation of extra-articular muscle, for example.[46,47]

Under disease conditions, the innervation territories of the various nerve fibers are highly plastic. An example of such plasticity is the innervation of normally aneural tissues, such as cartilage, with substance P– and CGRP-positive nerves in patients who have OA.[48] The normally mechanically insensitive cartilage becomes potentially a candidate for tibiofemoral pain in OA, although this has never been shown electrophysiologically. Furthermore, these peptide-containing nerves may also accelerate disease progression by way of localized neurogenic inflammatory mechanisms.

Tissue injury activates the nociceptive system, which generates the subjective pain experience. Spontaneous pain and mechanical hypersensitivity can develop as a consequence of sensitization of primary afferents directly by locally released inflammatory mediators and following sensitization of neuronal processes in the spinal cord (central sensitization) or higher centers.[46]

In arthritis, inflammatory mediators, such as bradykinin, histamine, prostaglandins, lactic acid, substance P, vasoactive intestinal peptide (VIP), and CGRP, are released into the joint.[38] These mediators reduce the firing threshold of joint nociceptors, making them more likely to respond to both non-noxious and noxious painful stimuli. As the disease progresses, more and more of these mediators accumulate in the joint, thereby triggering a self-perpetuating cycle of pain generation. The first study to explore which chemical mediators are responsible for OA pain in an animal model focused on the neuropeptide VIP. VIP is a 28–amino acid peptide that was originally identified in the porcine intestine where it controls vascular tone and enzyme secretion.[49] More than 20 years ago, VIP was localized in the synovial fluid and serum of patients who had arthritis[50] and then the peptide was forgotten by the rheumatology field. Recently it was shown that local administration of VIP to rat knees causes synovial hyperemia[51] and sensitization of joint afferents leading to pain.[52,53] Treatment of OA knees with a VIP antagonist significantly attenuated peripheral sensitization and alleviated pain behavior in this animal model of degenerative joint disease. VIP inhibition may thus be a useful means of controlling OA pain.

In addition to sensitizing mediators being released into OA joints to elicit pain, evidence is beginning to emerge suggesting that naturally produced desensitizing agents may also contribute to pain modulation in the joint. For example, the endogenous opioid endomorphin is present in high concentration in arthritic knees[54,55] where it can reduce afferent firing rate in response to joint movement.[56] Similarly, endocannabinoid activity has been reported in OA knees and activation of the articular cannabinoid system can dramatically offset the hyperactivity of joint nociceptors.[57] Even though these endogenous analgesic agents are present in significant amounts in articular tissues, the question still remains as to why the body's natural pain killers are unable to provide any appreciable relief from the debilitating effects of joint pain.

Silent Nociceptors

Polymodal Aδ and C fibers that innervate the joint increase their firing rate in response to noxious mechanical stimuli and in the presence of various chemical agents, such as those released during inflammation. In addition to these classic nociceptors, there are also several fibers in the joint that are not normally activated by noxious stimulation but become responsive when damage or inflammation occurs in the joint. These fibers, called silent nociceptors, can make a major contribution to the pain sensation.[46]

The neuroanatomy of mineralized bone, bone marrow, and periosteum is well defined.[45] Aβ fibers, Aδ fibers, C fibers, and sympathetic fibers distribute densely throughout the periosteum, entering bone in close association with blood vessels.[58] Of these tissues, the periosteum has the greatest density of sensory and sympathetic innervation, which may be further enhanced during joint inflammation. Electrophysiologic studies of the mechanosensitivity of joint innervation indicate that generally Aβ fibres are activated by non-noxious normal working range joint movement, whereas approximately 50% of Aδ and 70% of C fibers are classified as high threshold units.[59] During inflammation, Aδ and C fibers show increased mechanosensitivity. Low threshold populations exhibit exaggerated responses, whereas high threshold populations and units that were initially mechanoinsensitive are sensitized and now respond to movements in the normal working ranges of the joint.[60] It is this increased activity of low threshold units and the awakening of the silent nociceptors that conspire to intensify joint pain sensation in arthritis.

CENTRAL MECHANISMS

The Aδ fibers transmit impulses centrally through the peripheral nerve up through the dorsal root and into the dorsal horn of the spinal cord. The C fibers conduct impulses relatively slowly through the same route to the CNS (see **Fig. 2**).[61] The Aδ fibers terminate in laminae I and V of the dorsal horn, and the C fibers terminate predominantly in lamina II. From the dorsal horn, the signals are carried along the ascending pain pathways to the brain stem, hypothalamus, thalamus, and cerebral cortex.

Descending pathways originating in supraspinal centers (somatosensory and limbic cortices) project through the periaqueductal gray area to the dorsal horn and modulate activity in the dorsal horn by controlling spinal pain transmission.[62]

Processing the Perception of Pain

Nociception is processed throughout the nervous system, but it reaches conscious levels and is interpreted through connections between the thalamus and cortex. There are two main systems in the brain that are responsible for the perception of pain: the lateral system and the medial system of the lateral spinothalamic tract.[63] The lateral system involves the activation of thalamic nuclei in the ventral lateral thalamus and the relay of information to the somatosensory cortex, where the noxious stimulus is analyzed for location, duration, intensity, and quality.

The medial system involves the relay of information by other (midline and intralaminar) thalamic nuclei to different parts of the brain, such as the amygdala. The medial

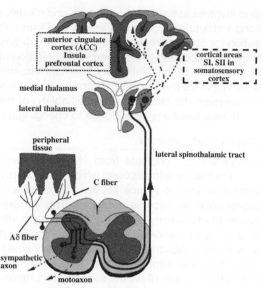

Fig. 2. Pain transmission. (*Reproduced from* Schaible H, Richter F. Pathophysiology of pain. Langenbecks Arch Surg 2004;389(4):238; with permission).

system comprises large areas of the brain that are responsible for pain perception and for functions in other contexts, such as affective responses, attention, and learning; this may explain the discrepancy between the degree of joint damage and the severity of pain. Because of the importance of the medial system in OA pain, a nonpharmacologic approach to management may be just as important as a pharmacologic strategy.

Finally, the perception of pain is modified by the patient's affective status (eg, level of depression, anxiety, or anger) and cognitive state (eg, pain beliefs, expectations, memories of pain). Age, gender, socioeconomic status, racial and cultural background, pain communication skills, and previous pain experiences can contribute to the way a patient perceives pain.

CENTRAL SENSITIZATION

The characteristic feature of most chronic pain is that hitherto non-noxious stimuli, such as walking or standing, are perceived as painful. It is now clear that pain pathways, far from being static or hardwired, exhibit marked plasticity and that sensitization at peripheral, spinal, and cortical levels accounts for many of the clinical features associated with chronic pain. Consistent with this, the three chronic pain categories currently recognized, including neuropathic pain, neuroplastic or inflammatory pain, and idiopathic pain, all exhibit features of an underlying central sensitization state.[38]

Like peripheral sensitization previously described, central nociceptive transmission in the dorsal horn also can be sensitized. Increased input from peripheral nociceptors modulates spinal cord pain-transmitting neurons and leads to increased synaptic excitability and decreased firing thresholds that outlast the initiating input, amplifying responses to both noxious and innocuous inputs.

Neuronal response to noxious input is thus exaggerated (hyperalgesia), or normally innocuous input is now perceived as painful (allodynia), and sensitivity is expanded, with pain experienced beyond the original site of tissue damage (secondary hyperalgesia).[64]

Central sensitization involves activation, modulation, and modification. Modification of dorsal horn neurons leads to changes in receptors and transmitters in addition to structural reorganization (or physical rearrangement of the neurons) and disinhibition of dorsal horn nociceptors. According to one theory, disinhibition of dorsal horn nociceptors results from the death of local inhibitory interneurons, which potentially are replaced by excitatory Aδ fibers that "sprout" from the dorsal horn. Peripheral and central sensitization represent the plasticity, or modifiability, of the nervous system, which can mold itself to new functions in response to changing inputs.[38,64]

Hyperexcitability of Spinal Cord Neurons

Spinal cord hyperexcitability can originate from either nociceptive or neuropathic types of pain, although the mechanisms through which this occurs may be different.[65] When a noxious stimulus is used to induce active inflammation, the sensitized area expands and additional neurons become activated. This process lowers the pain threshold and increases the sensitivity of adjacent neurons to stimulation.[65] Central sensitization occurs as a consequence of tissue damage and peripheral sensitization and also as a consequence of abnormal discharges from damaged nerve fibers. A spinal cord neuron that has been sensitized often has an expanded receptive field. In addition, as a result of the process of central sensitization, more neurons in a spinal segment respond to noxious stimuli. Central sensitization has been seen mainly in the wake of tissue damage. In some forms of neuropathy (eg, after sectioning of peripheral nerves) many spinal cord neurons are silent and have no receptive field. Only a few neurons are active and show abnormal discharges. Other parts of the CNS also have the capacity for plasticity. After denervation, cortical maps may be changed, and this cortical process may be responsible for the chronicity of pain. It is this plastic quality of the CNS that should enable us to reverse chronic pain in long-term diseases such as OA. By inhibiting the nociceptive input from the joint to the CNS it should be possible to rewire the brain gradually, such that the sensation of chronic joint pain can be unlearned. Peripherally restricted pharmacologic agents, perhaps in combination with a physical therapy approach, may help us ultimately to dismantle the neurophysiologic processes that were constructed during OA pain development.

Modulatory Mediators

Glutamate is the primary excitatory neurotransmitter in the CNS. It is the neurotransmitter in Aβ, Aδ, and C fibers. During repetitive noxious stimulation, glutamate activates N-methyl D-aspartate (NMDA) in the spinal cord, and neuropeptide receptors are activated by neuropeptides that are co-released with glutamate from synaptic endings.[65] Additionally, many modulatory mediators are present, including substance P, CGRP, opioids, neurotrophins, and prostaglandins, all of which also act in the CNS. Substance P, which is released in the superficial part of the dorsal horn into the gray matter, increases the pain response to noxious inputs from spinal cord neurons.[66]

Prostaglandins are also important, both in the periphery and in the spinal cord. They have a major impact on the sensitivity of neighboring spinal cord neurons.[67]

The Concept of Wind-Up

When action potentials reach the nerve terminal, the presynaptic membrane is depolarized. This process opens calcium channels, and calcium flows into the presynaptic ending, where it triggers the release of transmitters. The definition of wind-up is specific: In a classic situation, a peripheral nerve is stimulated repeatedly at C-fiber strength. This stimulation produces a response in a spinal neuron that grows from stimulus to stimulus; this is termed wind-up. Wind-up is short lived, surviving stimulation for only seconds to minutes. Wind-up intensifies pain during repetitive noxious stimulation. It is probably not produced by increased transmitter release but rather by postsynaptic changes, such as NMDA receptor activation and, possibly, by calcium influx into the postsynaptic neuron. Wind-up also occurs when the skin is stimulated repeatedly with short heat pulses.[65]

The Sympathetic Response

When a noxious stimulus is received, the sympathetic nervous system releases norepinephrine into the peripheral tissues, which decreases the firing threshold of peripheral nerve cells and makes them more sensitive to stimulation. During noxious painful movement, sympathetic postganglionic nerve activity increases leading to an increase in mean arterial pressure and heart rate.[68] Because sympathetic nerve stimulation leads to synovial vasoconstriction[69] it is possible that the resulting hypoxemia could contribute to joint pain. These findings indicate that activation of joint mechano-nociceptors causes reflex sympathetic discharges that could further augment joint pain sensitivity.

So far this article has focused on peripheral sensory input and central mechanisms, although clearly modulation through cognitive, genetic, affective, and environmental influences forms the net pain experience. The remainder of the article focuses on constitutional and environmental factors that may modulate the pain experience.

CONSTITUTIONAL FACTORS

Pain has long been recognized as a complex sensory and emotional experience.[70] Each individual has a unique experience of pain influenced by his or her life experience and genotypic profile. An individual's stable psychologic characteristics (trait) and the immediate psychologic context in which pain is experienced (state) both influence perception of pain.

A full understanding of pain requires consideration of psychologic and social environmental processes mediating a patient's response to his or her disease.[71] The biopsychosocial model is a useful approach to understanding and assessing the experience of pain in people who have OA.[72] Numerous studies have supported the importance of psychologic factors in understanding OA pain.[72] Two of the most important factors are self-efficacy and pain catastrophizing. Self-efficacy has been defined as an individual's confidence in their ability to accomplish a desired task (eg, control arthritis pain). Keefe and colleagues[73] found that patients who had OA who reported higher self-efficacy for pain control had higher thresholds and tolerance for thermal pain stimuli. Furthermore, increases in self-efficacy occurring over the course of a pain coping skills training protocol for patients who had OA was found to be one of the most important predictors of short- and long-term treatment outcome.[74,75] In fact, Lorig and colleagues[76] found that increases in self-efficacy that occurred following participation in an arthritis self-help intervention were related to improvements in pain and psychologic functioning at 4 years' follow-up. Pain catastrophizing refers to the tendency to focus on, ruminate on, and feel helpless in the face of pain. Patients who have OA who catastrophize report higher levels of pain, psychologic distress, and physical disability and also exhibit more pain behavior.[77] Pain catastrophizing has also been shown to relate to abnormal processing of pain signals in imaging studies, suggesting it may influence pain perception in a fundamental fashion.[78]

OA pain occurs in a social context and factors such as social support can play an important role in determining how patients adjust to arthritis pain.[79] Patients and their partners, however, may vary with respect to their abilities to communicate about and manage OA pain as a couple. In a recent study,[80] we examined key aspects of pain communication (self-efficacy for pain communication and holding back from discussing pain and arthritis-related concerns) in patients who had OA and their partners. Results indicated that patients who reported higher levels of self-efficacy for pain communication experienced much lower levels of pain and physical and psychologic disability, and their partners reported much lower levels of negative affect. Patients who reported holding back on discussions about pain and related arthritis concerns experienced much higher levels of psychologic disability. When partners reported they held back on discussions of pain and related arthritis concerns, they reported higher levels of caregiver strain and their patient-partners were more likely to report high levels of psychologic disability. Taken together, these findings suggest that patients' and partners' self-efficacy for pain communication and tendency to hold back on pain communication may be important in understanding patient and partner adjustment to OA pain. These findings also underscore the importance of involving spouses of patients who have OA in pain management efforts, something that has been shown to improve the outcomes of pain coping skills training.[74,75]

Further, CNS processing associated with pain perception is closely integrated with hypothalamic-pituitary axis and autonomic nervous system activity. Variations in pain perception within populations may reflect genetic polymorphisms in all three systems, with current attention being focused on serotonin transporter reuptake protein, alpha-2 receptor, and catechol-O-methyltransferase, although several other candidate genes are under review.[45]

ENVIRONMENTAL STIMULI

In the presence of OA local stimuli that typically would not be noxious can precipitate alteration in the severity of pain either through microstructural damage of the joint or by decreasing the pain threshold level. There is evidence that patients who have OA do experience fluctuations in pain severity or exacerbations of pain.[26,81] Some of the factors that could predispose to fluctuations in pain severity are discussed here.

Physical Activity

Numerous studies have assessed the relation of physical activity to the risk for radiographic knee OA with little or no attention paid to the relation of physical activity and OA symptoms. These include studies of runners,[82–84] heavy physical activity in daily life,[85] and occupational activities, including prolonged standing and knee-bending activities;[86–89] however, few if any of these studies have investigated the relation of these activities to symptom severity. There is a paucity of epidemiologic data to explain which particular activities are painful or more injurious than others; however, we know from clinical practice that different activities predispose to exacerbation of pain, whereas in a normal joint they typically would not. Identification of these factors that exacerbate pain is important because these are potentially modifiable.

Footwear

Appropriate supportive footwear is recommended in guidelines for treating symptomatic OA, although there are few data to support this recommendation.[90] There are several ways in which footwear can potentially modify impact loading through the lower limb and thus reduce impact that potentially may lead to pain in subjects who have OA. Impact force during locomotion increases with increasing age as a function of diminishing foot position awareness;[91] this impact force could be reduced through the addition of supportive shoes.[92]

Another link between footwear and knee loads comes from gait analysis studies demonstrating that high-heeled shoes increase compressive forces across the patellofemoral and medial tibiofemoral joints.[93] Women's shoes with even only moderately high heels (1.5 in) were found to increase the forces that strain the tibiofemoral and patellofemoral joints during walking.[94] Given the increased predilection for women experiencing symptomatic knee OA (female to male ratio is typically reported as 2:1) clarifying the impact high heeled shoes have on symptoms could have public health import.

Injury and Trauma

For both genders, a past history of injury to the stabilizing or load-bearing structures of the knee renders the joint highly vulnerable to radiographic OA in subsequent years.[95] People who have OA have quadriceps weakness[96] and impaired proprioception[97] that makes them more susceptible to falls[98] and injury risk. In contrast to the knowledge about the development of radiographic OA following injury, the relationship of pain exacerbation in subjects with pre-existing OA to joint injury/falls/trauma remains unknown and warrants further exploration.

Weather

Many people believe that weather conditions can influence joint pain, but science offers little proof.[99,100] If the phenomenon were real, cause-and-effect mechanisms might provide clues that would aid treatment of joint pain. Some theorize that alterations in barometric pressure and humidity can alter the synovial fluid (volume and content) in the joint and predispose to alteration in symptoms. The factors that have been considered include ambient temperature, barometric pressure, relative humidity, sunshine, wind speed, and precipitation; however, the literature on the subject is sparse, conflicting, and vulnerable to bias.[101,102] For patients who believe that weather can influence their pain, the biologic mechanisms may not be fully understood, but the effect seems to be real.

SUMMARY

The pathophysiology of pain in OA is complex and similarly the symptomatic presentation in OA is diverse and heterogeneous. Attention to the many modulating factors that alter the experience of pain may improve the way we treat this disease.

REFERENCES

1. Guccione AA, Felson DT, Anderson JJ, et al. The effects of specific medical conditions on the functional limitations of elders in the Framingham study. Am J Public Health 1994;84(3):351–8.
2. Arthritis prevalence and activity limitations—United States, 1990. MMWR–Morbidity & Mortality Weekly Report 1994;43(24):433–8.
3. Yelin E, Callahan LF. The economic cost and social and psychological impact of musculoskeletal conditions. National Arthritis Data Work Groups [see comments] [Review] [68 refs]. Arthritis Rheum 1995;38(10):1351–62.
4. Segal L, Day SE, Chapman AB, et al. Can we reduce disease burden from osteoarthritis? [see comment]. Med J Aust 2004;180(5 Suppl):S11–7.
5. Nuki G. Osteoarthritis: a problem of joint failure [Review] [55 refs]. Z Rheumatol 1999;58(3):142–7.

6. Eyre DR. Collagens and cartilage matrix homeostasis [Review] [37 refs]. Clin Orthop Relat Res 2004;427(Suppl):S118–22.

7. Hannan MT, Felson DT, Pincus T. Analysis of the discordance between radiographic changes and knee pain in osteoarthritis of the knee. J Rheumatol 2000;27(6):1513–7.

8. Peat G, McCarney R, Croft P. Knee pain and osteoarthritis in older adults: a review of community burden and current use of primary health care. Ann Rheum Dis 2001;60(2):91–7 [see comments] [Review] [45 refs].

9. Cibere J. Do we need radiographs to diagnose osteoarthritis? Best Pract Res Clin Rheumatol 2006;20(1):27–38 [Review] [60 refs].

10. Zhang Y, Niu J, Kelly-Hayes M, et al. Prevalence of symptomatic hand osteoarthritis and its impact on functional status among the elderly: the Framingham study. Am J Epidemiol 2002;156(11):1021–7.

11. Cunningham LS, Kelsey JL. Epidemiology of musculoskeletal impairments and associated disability. Am J Public Health 1984;74(6):574–9.

12. Armstrong AL, Hunter JB, Davis TR. The prevalence of degenerative arthritis of the base of the thumb in post-menopausal women. J Hand Surg [Br] 1994;19(3):340–1.

13. Felson DT, Zhang Y. An update on the epidemiology of knee and hip osteoarthritis with a view to prevention. Arthritis Rheum 1998;41(8):1343–55 [Review] [116 refs].

14. Nevitt MC, Xu L, Zhang Y, et al. Very low prevalence of hip osteoarthritis among Chinese elderly in Beijing, China, compared with whites in the United States: the Beijing osteoarthritis study. Arthritis Rheum 2002;46(7):1773–9.

15. Lawrence RC, Helmick CG, Arnett FC, et al. Estimates of the prevalence of arthritis and selected musculoskeletal disorders in the United States. Arthritis Rheum 1998;41(5):778–99 [see comments].

16. Kraus VB, Vail TP, Worrell T, et al. A comparative assessment of alignment angle of the knee by radiographic and physical examination methods. Arthritis Rheum 2005;52(6):1730–5.

17. Altman RD. Classification of disease: osteoarthritis. Seminars in. Arthritis Rheum 1991;20(6 Suppl 2):40–7 [Review] [38 refs].

18. Bhattacharyya T, Gale D, Dewire P, et al. The clinical importance of meniscal tears demonstrated by magnetic resonance imaging in osteoarthritis of the knee. J Bone Joint Surg Am 2003;85(1):4–9 [comment].

19. Englund M, Lohmander LS. Risk factors for symptomatic knee osteoarthritis fifteen to twenty-two years after meniscectomy. Arthritis Rheum 2004;50(9):2811–9.

20. Altman R, Asch E, Bloch D, et al. Development of criteria for the classification and reporting of osteoarthritis. Classification of osteoarthritis of the knee. Diagnostic and therapeutic criteria Committee of the American Rheumatism Association. Arthritis Rheum 1986;29(8):1039–49.

21. Dieppe PA, Lohmander LS. Pathogenesis and management of pain in osteoarthritis. Lancet 2005;365(9463):965–73 [Review] [100 refs].

22. Felson D. The sources of pain in knee osteoarthritis. Curr Opin Rheumatol 2005;17(5):624–8 [Review] [34 refs].

23. Felson DT, Chaisson CE, Hill CL, et al. The association of bone marrow lesions with pain in knee osteoarthritis. Ann Intern Med 2001;134(7):541–9 [see comments].

24. Hunter D, Gale D, Grainger G, et al. The reliability of a new scoring system for knee osteoarthritis MRI and the validity of bone marrow lesion assessment:

BLOKS (Boston Leeds Osteoarthritis Knee Score). Ann Rheum Dis 2008;67(2): 206–11.

25. Torres L, Dunlop DD, Peterfy C, et al. The relationship between specific tissue lesions and pain severity in persons with knee osteoarthritis. Osteoarthr Cartil 2006;14(10):1033–40.

26. Hill CL, Gale DG, Chaisson CE, et al. Knee effusions, popliteal cysts, and synovial thickening: association with knee pain in osteoarthritis. J Rheumatol 2001; 28(6):1330–7.

27. Hill CL, Hunter DJ, Niu J, et al. Changes in synovitis are associated with changes in pain in knee osteoarthritis. Annals of the Rheumatic Diseases 2007;66(12): 1599–603.

28. Lo G, McAlindon T, Niu J, et al. Strong association of bone marrow lesions and effusion with pain in osteoarthritis. Arthritis Rheum 2008;56(9):S790.

29. Cicuttini FM, Baker J, Hart DJ, et al. Association of pain with radiological changes in different compartments and views of the knee joint. Osteoarthr Cartil 1996;4(2):143–7.

30. Burr DB. The importance of subchondral bone in the progression of osteoarthritis. J Rheumatol Suppl 2004;70:77–80 [Review] [13 refs].

31. Simkin P. Bone pain and pressure in osteoarthritic joints. Novartis Found Symp 2004;260:179–86 [Review] [34 refs].

32. Arnoldi CC, Lemperg K, Linderholm H. Intraosseous hypertension and pain in the knee. J Bone Joint Surg Br 1975;57(3):360–3.

33. Arnoldi CC, Djurhuus JC, Heerfordt J, et al. Intraosseous phlebography, intraosseous pressure measurements and 99mTC-polyphosphate scintigraphy in patients with various painful conditions in the hip and knee. Acta Orthop Scand 1980;51(1):19–28.

34. Arnoldi CC. Vascular aspects of degenerative joint disorders. A synthesis. Acta Orthop Scand 1994;261(Suppl):1–82 [Review] [270 refs].

35. Roach HI, Aigner T, Soder S, et al. Pathobiology of osteoarthritis: pathomechanisms and potential therapeutic targets. Curr Drug Targets 2007;8(2):271–82 [Review] [138 refs].

36. Ushiyama T, Chano T, Inoue K, et al. Cytokine production in the infrapatellar fat pad: another source of cytokines in knee synovial fluids. Ann Rheum Dis 2003; 62(2):108–12.

37. McDougall J. Arthritis and pain. Neurogenic origin of joint pain. Arthritis Res Ther 2006;8(6):220 [Review] [138 refs].

38. Altman R. Management of osteoarthritis knee pain: the state of the science. Littleton (CO): Medical Education Resources; 2006.

39. Fernandez-Madrid F, Karvonen RL, Teitge RA, et al. Synovial thickening detected by MR imaging in osteoarthritis of the knee confirmed by biopsy as synovitis. Magn Reson Imaging 1995;13(2):177–83.

40. McDougall JJ, Bray RC, Sharkey KA. Morphological and immunohistochemical examination of nerves in normal and injured collateral ligaments of rat, rabbit, and human knee joints. Anat Rec 1997;248(1):29–39.

41. McDougall JJ, Yeung G, Leonard CA, et al. A role for calcitonin gene-related peptide in rabbit knee joint ligament healing. Can J Physiol Pharmacol 2000; 78(7):535–40.

42. Hanesch U, Pawlak M, McDougall JJ, et al. Gabapentin reduces the mechanosensitivity of fine afferent nerve fibres in normal and inflamed rat knee joints. Pain 2003;104(1–2):363–6.

43. Freeman MA, Wyke B. The innervation of the knee joint. An anatomical and histological study in the cat. J Anat 1967;101(Pt 3):505–32.
44. Schaible H, Richter F. Pathophysiology of pain. Langenbecks Arch Surg 2004; 389(4):237–43 [Review] [55 refs].
45. Dray A, Read SJ, Dray A, et al. Arthritis and pain. Future targets to control osteoarthritis pain. Arthritis Res Ther 2007;9(3):212 [Review] [176 refs].
46. Schaible H, Schmelz M, Tegeder I. Pathophysiology and treatment of pain in joint disease. Adv Drug Deliv Rev 2006;58(2):323–42 [Review] [226 refs].
47. Konttinen YT, Kemppinen P, Segerberg M, et al. Peripheral and spinal neural mechanisms in arthritis, with particular reference to treatment of inflammation and pain. Arthritis Rheum 1994;37(7):965–82 [Review] [55 refs].
48. Suri S, Gill SE, Massena dC, et al. Neurovascular invasion at the osteochondral junction and in osteophytes in osteoarthritis. Ann Rheum Dis 2007;66(11): 1423–8.
49. Said S, Mutt V. Polypeptide with broad biological activity: isolation from small intestine. Science 1970;169(951):1217–8.
50. Lygren I, Ostensen M, Burhol PG, et al. Gastrointestinal peptides in serum and synovial fluid from patients with inflammatory joint disease. Ann Rheum Dis 1986;45(8):637–40.
51. McDougall JJ, Barin AK. The role of joint nerves and mast cells in the alteration of vasoactive intestinal peptide (VIP) sensitivity during inflammation progression in rats. Br J Pharmacol 2005;145(1):104–13.
52. Schuelert N, McDougall JJ, Schuelert N, et al. Electrophysiological evidence that the vasoactive intestinal peptide receptor antagonist VIP6-28 reduces nociception in an animal model of osteoarthritis. Osteoarthr Cartil 2006;14(11):1155–62.
53. McDougall JJ, Watkins L, Li Z. Vasoactive intestinal peptide (VIP) is a modulator of joint pain in a rat model of osteoarthritis. Pain 2006;123(1–2):98–105.
54. McDougall JJ, Baker CL, Hermann PM. Attenuation of knee joint inflammation by peripherally administered endomorphin-1. J Mol Neurosci 2004;22(1–2):125–37.
55. McDougall JJ, Barin AK, McDougall CM. Loss of vasomotor responsiveness to the mu-opioid receptor ligand endomorphin-1 in adjuvant monoarthritic rat knee joints. Am J Physiol Regul Integr Comp Physiol 2004;286(4):R634–41.
56. Li Z, Proud D, Zhang C, et al. Chronic arthritis down-regulates peripheral mu-opioid receptor expression with concomitant loss of endomorphin 1 antinociception. Arthritis Rheum 2005;52(10):3210–9 [see comment].
57. Schuelert N, McDougall JJ, Schuelert N, et al. Cannabinoid-mediated antinociception is enhanced in rat osteoarthritic knees. Arthritis Rheum 2008;58(1): 145–53.
58. Mach DB, Rogers SD, Sabino MC, et al. Origins of skeletal pain: sensory and sympathetic innervation of the mouse femur. Neuroscience 2002;113(1):155–66.
59. Schaible HG, Grubb BD. Afferent and spinal mechanisms of joint pain. Pain 1993;55(1):5–54 [Review] [438 refs].
60. Schaible HG, Schmidt RF, Schaible HG, et al. Effects of an experimental arthritis on the sensory properties of fine articular afferent units. J Neurophysiol 1985; 54(5):1109–22.
61. Schwartzman RJ, Grothusen J, Kiefer TR, et al. Neuropathic central pain: epidemiology, etiology, and treatment options. Arch Neurol 2001;58(10):1547–50 [Review] [38 refs].
62. Basbaum AI. Spinal mechanisms of acute and persistent pain. Reg Anesth Pain Med 1999;24(1):59–67 [Review] [46 refs].

63. Treede RD, Kenshalo DR, Gracely RH, et al. The cortical representation of pain. Pain 1999;79(2-3):105–11 [see comment] [Review] [58 refs].
64. Woolf CJ, Salter MW. Neuronal plasticity: increasing the gain in pain. Science 2000;288(5472):1765–9 [Review] [73 refs].
65. Ollat H, Cesaro P. Pharmacology of neuropathic pain. Clin Neuropharmacol 1995;18(5):391–404 [Review] [62 refs].
66. Joshi GP, Ogunnaike BO. Consequences of inadequate postoperative pain relief and chronic persistent postoperative pain. Anesthesiol Clin North America 2005; 23(1):21–36 [Review] [94 refs].
67. Samad TA, Moore KA, Sapirstein A, et al. Interleukin-1beta-mediated induction of Cox-2 in the CNS contributes to inflammatory pain hypersensitivity. Nature 2001;410(6827):471–5 [see comment].
68. Sato Y, Schaible HG. Discharge characteristics of sympathetic efferents to the knee joint of the cat. J Auton Nerv Syst 1987;19(2):95–103.
69. McDougall J, Karimian SM, Ferrell WR. Prolonged alteration of vasoconstrictor and vasodilator responses in rat knee joints by adjuvant monoarthritis. Exp Physiol 1995;80(3):349–57.
70. Kane RL, Bershadsky B, Lin WC, et al. Efforts to standardize the reporting of pain. J Clin Epidemiol 2002;55(2):105–10.
71. Orbell S, Johnston M, Rowley D, et al. Cognitive representations of illness and functional and affective adjustment following surgery for osteoarthritis. Soc Sci Med 1998;47(1):93–102.
72. Keefe FJ, Smith SJ, Buffington AL, et al. Recent advances and future directions in the biopsychosocial assessment and treatment of arthritis. J Consult Clin Psychol 2002;70(3):640–55 [Review] [126 refs].
73. Keefe FJ, Lefebvre JC, Maixner W, et al. Self-efficacy for arthritis pain: relationship to perception of thermal laboratory pain stimuli. Arthritis Care Res 1997; 10(3):177–84.
74. Keefe FJ, Caldwell DS, Baucom D, et al. Spouse-assisted coping skills training in the management of osteoarthritic knee pain. Arthritis Care Res 1996;9(4): 279–91.
75. Keefe FJ, Caldwell DS, Baucom D, et al. Spouse-assisted coping skills training in the management of knee pain in osteoarthritis: long-term followup results. Arthritis Care Res 1999;12(2):101–11.
76. Lorig KR, Mazonson PD, Holman HR, et al. Evidence suggesting that health education for self-management in patients with chronic arthritis has sustained health benefits while reducing health care costs. Arthritis Rheum 1993;36(4): 439–46.
77. Keefe FJ, Lefebvre JC, Egert JR, et al. The relationship of gender to pain, pain behavior, and disability in osteoarthritis patients: the role of catastrophizing. Pain 2000;87(3):325–34.
78. Seminowicz DA, Davis KD. Cortical responses to pain in healthy individuals depends on pain catastrophizing. Pain 2006;120(3):297–306.
79. Penninx BW, van Tilburg T, Deeg DJ, et al. Direct and buffer effects of social support and personal coping resources in individuals with arthritis. Soc Sci Med 1997;44(3):393–402.
80. Porter L, Keefe F, Wellington C, et al. Pain communication in the context of osteoarthritis: patient and partner self-efficacy for pain communication and holding back from discussion of pain and arthritis-related concerns. Clinical Journal of Pain 2008;24(8):662–8.

81. McAlindon T, Formica M, LaValley M, et al. Effectiveness of glucosamine for symptoms of knee osteoarthritis: results from an internet-based randomized double-blind controlled trial. Am J Med 2004;117(9):643–9.

82. Panush RS, Schmidt C, Caldwell JR, et al. Is running associated with degenerative joint disease? JAMA 1986;255(9):1152–4.

83. Panush R, Hanson C, Caldwell J, et al. Is running associated with osteoarthritis? An eight year follow-up study. J Clin Rheumatol 1995;1:35–9.

84. Lane NE, Michel B, Bjorkengren A, et al. The risk of osteoarthritis with running and aging: a 5-year longitudinal study. J Rheumatol 1993;20(3):461–8.

85. McAlindon TE, Wilson PW, Aliabadi P, et al. Level of physical activity and the risk of radiographic and symptomatic knee osteoarthritis in the elderly: the Framingham study. Am J Med 1999;106(2):151–7.

86. Croft P, Cooper C, Wickham C, et al. Osteoarthritis of the hip and occupational activity. Scand J Work Environ Health 1992;18(1):59–63.

87. Maetzel A, Makela M, Hawker G, et al. Osteoarthritis of the hip and knee and mechanical occupational exposure—a systematic overview of the evidence. J Rheumatol 1997;24(8):1599–607.

88. Felson DT. Do occupation-related physical factors contribute to arthritis? Baillieres Clin Rheumatol 1994;8(1):63–77 [Review] [58 refs].

89. Vingard E, Alfredsson L, Goldie I, et al. Occupation and osteoarthrosis of the hip and knee: a register-based cohort study. Int J Epidemiol 1991;20(4):1025–31.

90. Anonymous. Recommendations for the medical management of osteoarthritis of the hip and knee: 2000 update. American College of Rheumatology Subcommittee on Osteoarthritis Guidelines. Arthritis Rheum 2000;43(9):1905–15.

91. Robbins S, Waked E, Allard P, et al. Foot position awareness in younger and older men: the influence of footwear sole properties. J Am Geriatr Soc 1997;45(1):61–6.

92. Robbins S, Waked E, Krouglicof N. Vertical impact increase in middle age may explain idiopathic weight-bearing joint osteoarthritis. Arch Phys Med Rehabil 2001;82(12):1673–7.

93. Kerrigan DC, Lelas JL, Karvosky ME. Women's shoes and knee osteoarthritis. Lancet 2001;357(9262):1097–8.

94. Kerrigan DC, Johansson JL, Bryant MG, et al. Moderate-heeled shoes and knee joint torques relevant to the development and progression of knee osteoarthritis. Arch Phys Med Rehabil 2005;86(5):871–5.

95. Davis MA, Ettinger WH, Neuhaus JM, et al. The association of knee injury and obesity with unilateral and bilateral osteoarthritis of the knee. Am J Epidemiol 1989;130(2):278–88.

96. Slemenda C, Brandt KD, Heilman DK, et al. Quadriceps weakness and osteoarthritis of the knee. Ann Intern Med 1997;127(2):97–104.

97. Hurley MV, Scott DL, Rees J, et al. Sensorimotor changes and functional performance in patients with knee osteoarthritis. Ann Rheum Dis 1997;56(11):641–8.

98. Pandya NK, Draganich LF, Mauer A, et al. Osteoarthritis of the knees increases the propensity to trip on an obstacle. Clin Orthop Relat Res 2005;431:150–6.

99. Quick DC. Joint pain and weather. A critical review of the literature. Minn Med 1997;80(3):25–9 [Review] [24 refs].

100. Wilder FV, Hall BJ, Barrett JP. Osteoarthritis pain and weather. Rheumatology 2003;42(8):955–8.

101. Laborde JM, Dando WA, Powers MJ. Influence of weather on osteoarthritics. Soc Sci Med 1986;23(6):549–54.

102. Strusberg I, Mendelberg RC, Serra HA, et al. Influence of weather conditions on rheumatic pain. J Rheumatol 2002;29(2):335–8.

Osteoarthritis: Current Role of Imaging

Ali Guermazi, MD[a],*, Felix Eckstein, MD[b],
Marie Pierre Hellio Le Graverand-Gastineau, MD, DSc, PhD[c],
Philip G. Conaghan, MBBS, PhD, FRACP, FRCP[d], Deborah Burstein, PhD[e],
Helen Keen, MBBS, FRACP[f], Frank W. Roemer, MD[a]

KEYWORDS

- Osteoarthritis • Magnetic resonance imaging • Radiography
- Knee • Computed tomography • Nuclear medicine
- Arthrography

Osteoarthritis (OA) is the most prevalent joint disease and is increasingly common in the aging population of Western society and has a major health economic impact. Despite surgery and symptom-oriented approaches there still is no efficient treatment for this complex and heterogeneous disease. Conventional radiography has played an important role in the past in confirming the diagnosis of OA and demonstrating late bony changes and joint space narrowing (JSN); it has been applied as an endpoint for disease progression in clinical trials. OA is a disease, however, of the whole joint, including cartilage, bone, and intra- and periarticular soft tissues. Magnetic resonance imaging (MRI), with its capability of visualizing bone, cartilage, and soft tissues, has become the method of choice in large research endeavors and may become important for individualized treatment planning in the future. This article focuses on radiography and MRI and gives insight into other modalities, such as ultrasound (US), scintigraphy, CT, and CT arthrography. Their role in the diagnosis, follow-up, and research in OA is discussed.

A version of this article originally appeared in the 34:3 issue of the *Rheumatic Disease Clinics of North America*.

[a] Department of Radiology, Boston University School of Medicine, 820 Harrison Avenue, FGH Building, Third Floor, Boston, MA 02118, USA
[b] Institute of Anatomy and Musculoskeletal Research, Paracelsus Medical University, Strubergasse 21, 5020 Salzburg, Austria
[c] Pfizer Global Research and Development, 50 Pequot Avenue, New London, CT 06320, USA
[d] Section of Musculoskeletal Disease, 2nd Floor, University of Leeds, Chapel Allerton Hospital, Chapel Town Road, Leeds LS7 4SA, UK
[e] Department of Radiology, Beth Israel Deaconess Medical Center, Harvard Medical School, 4 Blackfan Circle, Boston, MA 02115, USA
[f] Department of Medicine, School of Medicine and Pharmacology, University of Western Australia, Rear 50 Murray Street, Perth, WA 6000, Australia
* Corresponding author.
E-mail address: guermazi@bu.edu (A. Guermazi).

CONVENTIONAL RADIOGRAPHY

Conventional radiography is the simplest and least expensive imaging method for assessing knee OA. Radiography is able to directly visualize osseous features of OA, including marginal osteophytes (OPs), subchondral sclerosis, and subchondral cysts, but assessment of joint space width (JSW) provides only an indirect estimate of cartilage thickness and meniscal integrity. Radiography is used in clinical practice in patients to confirm the diagnosis of OA and to monitor progression of the disease. Current clinical research tends to focus on knee OA because of the prevalence of the disease in this joint; therefore, this article focuses on radiographic assessment of OA in the tibiofemoral compartment of the knee.

The radiographic definition of OA relies mainly on the evaluation of OPs and JSN. Because OPs are considered specific to OA, develop at an earlier stage than JSN, are more correlated with knee pain, and are easier to ascertain than other radiographic features, they represent the widely applied criterion to define the presence of OA.[1-3] Assessment of OA severity, however, relies mainly on JSN and subchondral bone lesions. Moreover, progression of JSN is the most commonly used criterion for the assessment of OA progression and the complete loss of JSW characterized by bone-on-bone contact is one of the factors considered in the decision for joint replacement.

Radiographs are a 2-D projection of a 3-D joint subject to problems with variability, in particular joint repositioning. Radiographs perform poorly in the detection of early OA and seem insensitive in the determination of disease progression. These limitations have been confirmed by concurrent investigations of joints using more sophisticated imaging method, including arthrography, CT, MRI, and arthroscopy.[4-9] Despite these limitations, conventional radiography commonly is used in clinical practice because radiographs are easily interpreted.

The severity of OA can be estimated using semiquantitative (SQ) scoring systems. Published atlases provide images that represent specific grades.[10,11] Several grading scales incorporating combinations of features also have been developed, including the most widely used, the Kellgren and Lawrence grade classification, which suffers from limitations based on the invalid assumptions that changes in radiographic features (eg, OPs and JSN) are linear over the course of the disease and that the relationship between these features is constant. In contrast, the Osteoarthritis Research Society International atlas classification grades separately the tibiofemoral JSN and OP in each compartment of the knee.

In routine clinical assessment of patients who have suspected OA, standing weight-bearing anteroposterior and lateral radiographs are sufficient imaging in most cases. Additional views may increase diagnostic sensitivity in cases of doubt.[12] Several standardized radiographic protocols have been introduced that are applied in clinical trials and epidemiologic studies. Radiographic protocols of the knee in flexion provide a more reliable image of JSW and bone changes in the tibiofemoral joint. This translates into greater sensitivity for detecting OA progression and more accurate identification of the location of JSN.[13] In particular, radiographs obtained using protocols with the knee in flexion are more sensitive for detecting JSN in the lateral femorotibial compartment. The appropriate identification of the location of JSN in the medial or lateral femorotibial compartment is important to consider for patient selection for longitudinal studies, especially in disease-modifying OA drug clinical trials, to ensure an accurate evaluation of JSN in the follow-up images.

An excellent specificity has been shown for radiography in the detection of longitudinal cartilage loss when compared with MRI as the reference standard. The reported sensitivity, however, is low.[14] Methods of measuring JSW can be manual, using callipers or a simple graduated ruler and a micrometric eyepiece, or semiautomated, using computer software (**Fig. 1**).[15–19] The smallest standard deviation of the difference between test-retest measurements of minimum JSW in pairs of radiographs reaches approximately 0.1 mm in the most reproducible methods, indicating that a smallest detectable difference of at least 0.2 mm, which remains relatively large considering the 0.10- to 0.15-mm expected average annual JSN of OA knee joints.[20–22] Conventional radiography does not visualize additional key features of OA (eg, subchondral bone marrow lesions [BMLs], the menisci, ligaments, and synovial tissue).

Lastly, reproducibility of positioning in longitudinal studies and large multicenter trials is still problematic, and variability of JSW resulting from the positioning protocol adds to the weaknesses of conventional radiography (**Fig. 2**). Several nonfluoroscopic radiographic protocols have been developed to assess joint space loss reliably and accurately in multicenter longitudinal studies of progression and treatment of knee OA. Examples of these protocols are the metatarsophalangeal protocol, the fixed flexion protocol, and the modified Lyon schuss protocol.[20,22–24]

ULTRASOUND

US increasingly is used in musculoskeletal medicine, as it has some advantages over other imaging techniques. These include the multiplanar nature of the modality, the ability to image dynamic structures in real time, and the lack of radiation allowing repeated imaging.[25] Additionally, it is inexpensive and does not routinely require contrast agents to image synovium. The major limitation is perhaps the operator-dependent nature of the modality.[25]

US has been demonstrated as a valid imaging modality in inflammatory arthritis, proved sensitive and specific to erosions and synovial pathology.[26–28] There is a small body of literature on the application of US in OA. The ability of US to detect OPs has been compared to scintigraphy and radiography (**Fig. 3**).[29,30] The subchondral

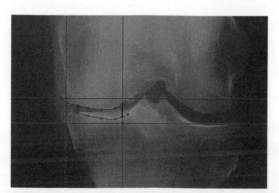

Fig. 1. Automated computer measurement of JSW of the medial tibial plateau (MTP) of the knee. Minimum JSW measured using a software (Holy's software, Lyon, France) in which the joint space contour detection is automatically performed by the computer with the help of an edge-based algorithm. The area of measurement of minimum JSW is defined by two vertical lines and two horizontal lines obtained by a single click on the nonosteophytic outer edge of the medial femoral condyle and a single click on the inner edge of the medial tibial plateau close to the articular surface. Within these landmarks, the delineation of the bone edges of both medial femoral condyle and medial tibial plateau floor and the minimum JSW are automatically obtained.

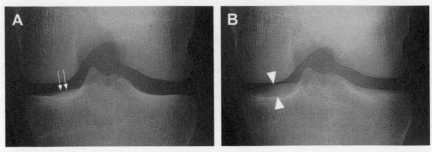

Fig. 2. Examples of good and poor alignment of the MTP with the x-ray beam. (*A*) Radiograph illustrates good alignment, as defined by virtual superimposition of the anterior and posterior margins at the center of the MTP (*arrows*). (*B*) Another radiograph of the knee shown in (*A*), showing poor alignment, as depicted by the wide separation (>1.5 mm) of the margins of the MTP (*arrow heads*).

features of OA detectable with radiographs, MRI, and CT are not detectable with US because of the physical properties of sound intrinsic to this imaging technique.

US easily can identify qualitative and quantitative cartilage pathology (**Fig. 4**). As visualization of central, load-bearing cartilage requires invasive techniques, however, and is not feasible in routine clinical practice,[31–35] the clinical relevance of US for imaging hyaline cartilage is uncertain. Meniscal pathologies also can be identified and US-detected meniscal extrusion and associated collateral ligament displacement are associated with pain in knee OA.[36]

Synovial pathologies may be identified readily with US and include macroscopic morphologic changes, vascularity, and synovial fluid (**Fig. 5**). US detects pathology more readily than clinical examination[37,38] and has been validated against MRI, arthroscopy, and histopathology.[37,39–42] The application of Doppler techniques allows assessment of synovial vascularity and generally is considered a surrogate of

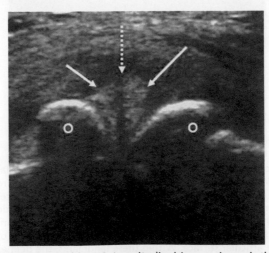

Fig. 3. OPs and meniscus imaged by US. Longitudinal image through the medial joint line demonstrates OPs (O) and meniscal extrusion (*solid arrows*). The mensicus has a horizontal cleavage tear (*dashed arrow*).

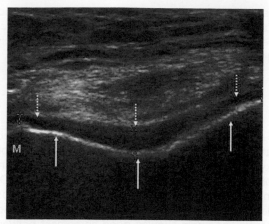

Fig. 4. Hyaline cartilage detected by US. Coronal image through the femoral condyles demonstrates cortical bone of the distal femur (*solid arrows*) and the overlying cartilage (*dashed arrows*). The cartilage is hypoechogenic and thinned laterally consistent with early osteoarthritis.

inflammatory activity.[39,40] Modern imaging techniques have demonstrated that synovial pathology is common in OA[36,38,43] and is associated with symptom parameters.[32,34,36,38,43–45] The importance of synovial pathology in symptom generation in OA or management strategies, however, is as yet not well understood and requires further investigation.

The use of US in rheumatology is likely to increase; however, the role it plays in assessment of OA is unclear. MRI has clear advantages over US in terms of structural imaging and proof of concept trials; however, US currently seems a more feasible tool

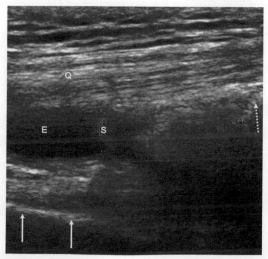

Fig. 5. Synovial inflammation as detected by US. Sagittal image through the suprapatellar pouch in the midline demonstrate the distal femoral cortex (*solid arrows*) patella (*dashed arrows*), anechoic effusion (E), hypoechoic synovial villi (S), and the quadriceps tendon (Q).

to be used in widespread clinical practice. Clinically it has been demonstrated as useful in guiding injections;[46] however, US potentially has wider clinical use. Potential roles for US may be in early diagnosis, predicting response to therapies, and objective monitoring of response.

NUCLEAR MEDICINE

Scintigraphy uses radiopharmaceuticals to visualize skeletal metabolism, to contribute to the localization of disease, and to assess severity of pathologic changes in OA. ^{99m}Tc-hydroxymethane diphosphonate scintigraphy shows increased activity during the bone phase in the subchondral region in nodal hand OA.[47] This finding was observed before the typical radiographic changes and reflects osteoblastic activity of early cartilage loss. A study that compared MRI findings with scintigraphy in patients who had chronic knee pain showed good agreement between MRI-detected subchondral BMLs and radionuclide uptake, but agreement between increased bone uptake and OP or cartilage defects was in general poor.[48] A prospective study proved the value of scintigraphy as a good predictor for disease progression in knee OA. A normal bone scan at baseline was highly predictive of a lack of progression over a 5-year period.[49] Two recent studies showed that scintigraphy may predict JSN but not superiorly to baseline radiographic or pain status (**Fig. 6**).[50,51]

Positron emission tomography (PET) demonstrates metabolic changes in target tissues and can detect foci of inflammation, infection, and tumors. PET uses 2-^{18}F-fluoro-2-deoxy-D-glucose (FDG) and reflects glucose metabolism in different tissues. A recent pilot study in knees with medial OA showed increased uptake in periarticular regions, the intercondylar notch, and areas of subchondral bone marrow corresponding to MRI detected BMLs (**Fig. 7**).[52]

In summary, scintigraphy may be a valuable additional tool in the assessment of OA as it has excellent sensitivity, is inexpensive, and is readily available. Drawbacks of the technique for the assessment of OA primarily are poor specificity and radiation concerns.[53] The value of FDG-PET for the assessment of OA in clinical and research

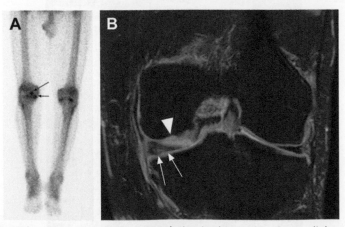

Fig. 6. Scintigraphy. (*A*) Radionuclide accumulation is observed in the medial compartment of the left knee (*black arrows*). (*B*) Coronal, T2-weighted, fat-suppressed MRI. Meniscal degeneration (*white arrows*) and cartilage damage (*arrowhead*) are seen on MRI of the same knee. (*Courtesy of* Dr. Gustavo Mercier, Boston, MA.)

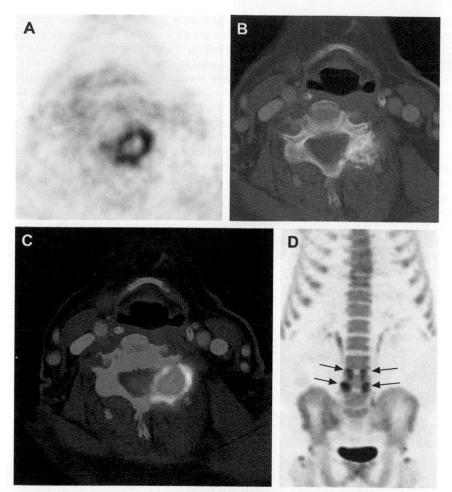

Fig. 7. FDG-PET and Fluoride PET of the spine. (*A*) Axial view FDG-PET. Inflammatory facet joint OA of the cervical spine. Strong glucose accumulation around the left facet joint is shown. (*B*) Axial CT. Hypertrophic left sided facet OA is depicted. (*C*) Fused PET-CT image. Correlation between metabolic changes depicted by PET and spatial localization by CT. (*D*) Coronal view Fluoride PET in the same patient. Bilateral facet joint OA L4/5 and L5/S1 (*arrows*). (*Courtesy of* Dr. Gustavo Mercier, Boston, MA.)

environment remains to be shown. Drawbacks of the method are its limited availability, radiation, and costs.

CT

CT is a cross-sectional digital imaging method based on advanced radiographic technology. Since the introduction of helical multidetector CT systems, multiplanar reconstructions in any given plane with equal quality to the original plane are possible. CT depicts cortical bone and soft tissue calcifications superiorly to MRI. CT has an established clinical role in assessing facet joint OA of the spine.[54]

Since the advent of multidetector CT systems, CT arthrography of the larger joints may play a larger role for the initial assessment and for longitudinal evaluation of OA.

This is true especially where access to MRI facilities is limited or a MRI examination is contraindicated. As cartilage is a nonradioopaque structure, its direct visualization by CT or radiographic technology is not possible. It has been shown, however, that spiral CT arthrography of the knee and shoulder is able to image the articular surface in an excellent manner.[55–58] Penetration of contrast medium (CM) within deeper layers of the cartilage surface indicates an articular-sided defect of the chondral surface (**Fig. 8**). Conspicuity of focal morphologic changes can be achieved as a result of the high spatial resolution and the high attenuation difference between the cartilage substance and the CM within the joint. In the assessment of dysplastic hips at risk for OA, the role of arthrography has been established for the assessment of the acetabular labrum.[59] Limitations of the technique are the insensitivity to changes of the deep layers of cartilage without surface alterations and its invasive nature. Qualitative assessment of the knee cartilage using CT arthrography is comparable to MRI.[56,58,60,61]

In summary, CT is a valuable additional imaging tool especially when detailed imaging of osseous changes or presurgical planning is required. In a routine clinical setting, however, CT plays a minor role in the assessment of patients who have established or suspected OA. Drawbacks of CT are low soft tissue contrast and exposure of patients to

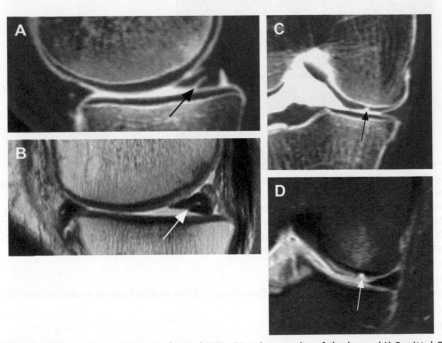

Fig. 8. Correlation of CT arthrography and MRI. CT arthrography of the knee. (*A*) Sagittal CT arthrography reformation of the medial knee compartment. Meniscal tear is depicted (*arrow*). Note superficial cartilage thinning at femoral condyle adjacent to meniscus. (*B*) Sagittal proton density–weighted image of the same knee. Meniscal tear is visualized on MRI (*arrow*). (*C*) CT arthrography. Coronal reformation of the medial compartment. Focal cartilage defect in the central medial condyle is shown (*arrow*). (*D*) Coronal, fat-suppressed, T2-weighted MRI shows the same defect (*arrow*). (*Courtesy of* B. Van de Berg, MD, PhD, Brussels, Belgium.)

ionizing radiation. CT arthrography is an alternative imaging method for indirect visualization of cartilage and other intrinsic joint structures, especially in the knee joint.

MRI

Although capable of detecting early changes of OA, MRI seldom is used in the routine assessment or initial diagnosis. In comparison to radiography, MRI offers several advantages for imaging of OA: MRI is 3-D and has a 3-D or tomographic viewing perspective, thus can provide cross-sectional images of the anatomy in any given plane free of the projectional limitations of radiography. Moreover, MRI is uniquely able to directly depict all anatomic structures of the joint, including the articular cartilage, menisci, intra-articular ligaments, synovium, capsular structures, bone contours, and bone marrow. This allows the joint to be evaluated as a whole organ and provides a more detailed picture of the changes associated with OA than is possible with other techniques.

Although MRI detects pathology of preradiographic OA at a very early stage of the disease,[62] at present the clinical importance of MRI for OA assessment lies in its ability to aid in the differential diagnosis and rule out other relevant pathology not detectable by radiography or other imaging methods. This article focuses on recent advances in MRI technology and on SQ whole-organ assessment of OA in clinical trials and epidemiologic studies. Techniques that may show with more detail the composition of the cartilage are discussed, such as T2 relaxation, T1 in the rotating frame (T1rho), sodium MRI, and proton-based delayed gadolinium-enhanced MRI of cartilage (dGEMRIC) technique. 3-D MRI morphometry used to quantify cartilage tissue is discussed, including its strengths and weaknesses over SQ 2-D MRI assessments.

Several magnetic resonance systems are available commercially that can be used for assessment of OA in a clinical setting and for research purposes. Most widely applied are 1.5-Tesla (T) large-bore MRI systems. The knee usually is imaged using a dedicated knee coil. Patients are imaged in the supine position and static images are acquired. Examination times vary depending on the purpose of the examination but usually last between 20 and 40 minutes, including patient positioning. Novel coil technology, such as commercially available 8-channel multiarray coils, offers improved image quality for 1.5-T systems. Examples of several osteoarthritic joints applying 1.5-T MRI are given in **Fig. 9**. Low-field MRI systems usually apply field strengths of 0.2 to 0.5 T and are offered by several manufacturers. Peripheral (extremity) magnets have advantages of installation, maintenance, and management costs that are lower than for whole-body systems and that they avoid the issue of claustrophobia.[63,64] Moreover, they potentially can be used in private offices and made widely available. As signal strength is a direct result of magnetic field strength, one drawback of low-field systems is longer acquisition times to achieve identical signal-to-noise ratios when compared with 1.5-T systems. One advantage of these systems is their usually open design that allows for examinations in claustrophobic subjects. Dedicated extremity systems have been introduced with field strengths of up to 1T and have been applied in large epidemiologic studies (eg, Multicenter Osteoarthritis Study [MOST]).[65,66] Open MRI systems that allow for dynamic studies under weight-bearing conditions also are available commercially, but their value remains to be established. These systems might be helpful in research environments, especially regarding questions of malalignment or whenever weight-bearing imaging is desirable. High-field MRI of 3 T was introduced for clinical application several years ago and experience has shown that these systems can be applied for imaging of knee OA in clinical and research environments. A clear advantage is the higher signal-to-noise ratio;

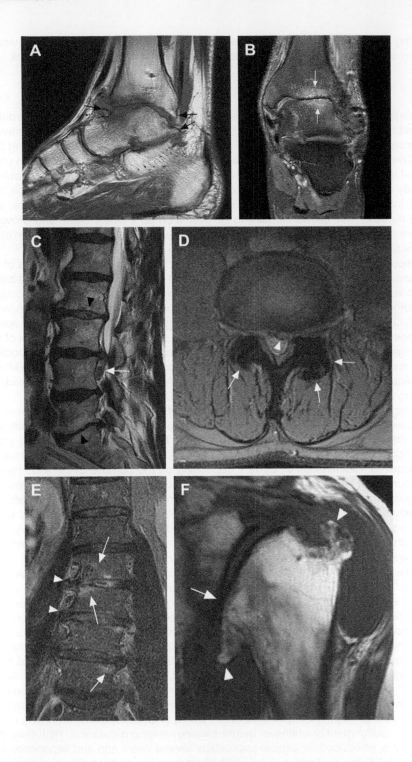

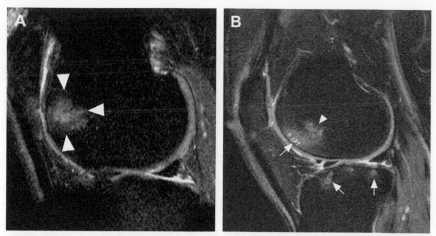

Fig. 10. Examples of 1.0-T and 3.0-T MRI of knee OA. (*A*) 1.0-T MRI. Sagittal, proton density–weighted, fat-suppressed image. Subchondral BML in anterior medial femur (*arrowheads*) associated with superficial cartilage damage. (*Courtesy* of the MOST study.) (*B*) 3.0-T MRI. Sagittal, proton density–weighted, fat-suppressed image. Subchondral BML in anterior lateral femur (*arrowhead*). Additional subchondral cysts are shown (*arrows*). (*Courtesy* of the MOST study.)

drawbacks are the associated costs, increased artifacts, and currently limited commercially available coils. Image examples of 1-T MRI and 3-T MRI are presented in **Fig. 10**. All described systems can be used for quantitative and SQ assessment of knee OA. Because of their wide availability and reliable image quality, most OA studies that include MRI are using 1.5-T MRI systems. To date only the Osteoarthritis Initiative (OAI), as one of the largest ongoing epidemiologic studies investigating OA, is applying 3-T systems. The role of contrast-enhanced MRI in clinical and research environments remains to be fully established. Visualization of synovitis in OA seems superior on contrast-enhanced scans using the intravenous paramagnetic agent, gadolinium (**Fig. 11**).[67,68]

SQ whole-organ scoring was introduced by Peterfy and colleagues[69] in 1999 and has been applied to many OA studies. The analyses based on SQ scoring have deeply added to the understanding of the pathophysiology and natural history of OA and the clinical implications of structural changes assessed. Examples are the associations of subchondral BMLs with cartilage loss in the same subregion with pain that were found in cross-sectional and longitudinal studies.[66,70–72] To date, three SQ scoring systems for the assessment of knee OA have been published and applied in epidemiologic studies: the whole-organ MRI score,[73] the knee osteoarthritis scoring system,[74] and

Fig. 9. 1.5-T MRI of advanced OA. (*A*) Post-traumatic ankle OA. Sagittal T1-weighted image. Note large periarticular OPs (*arrows*). (*B*) Periarticular subchondral BMLs (*white arrows*). Severe JSN. (*C*) OA of the spine. Sagittal T2-weighted image of the lumbar spine. Note disc space narrowing L2/3 and L5/S1. Additional inferiorly displaced disc herniation L3/4 (*white arrow*). (*D*) Axial, T2-weighted, gradient-echo image of segment L3/4. Hypertrophic facet joint OA (*white arrows*). Additional small medial disc herniation (*arrowhead*). (*E*) Coronal short tau inversion recovery (STIR) MRI of lumbar spine. Peridiscal edema-like lesions L2/3 and L4/5 (*arrows*). Note peridiscal lateral OPs (*arrowheads*). (*F*) Sagittal T1-weighted MRI of advanced shoulder OA. Large humeral OPs are depicted (*arrowheads*). Additional severe JSN and cartilage loss (*arrow*).

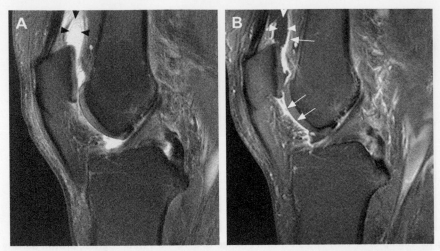

Fig. 11. Synovial activation in knee OA. (*A*) Sagittal, proton density–weighted, fat-suppressed image. Joint effusion is depicted as fluid-equivalent signal in the articular cavity. (*B*) Sagittal T1-weighted fat-suppressed image after intravenous contrast application of the same knee. Joint effusion is depicted as hypointense signal with in the articular cavity (*white arrowheads*). Supra- and infrapatellar synovial thickening is visualized (*white arrows*). Note that true extent of synovial thickening may be appreciated only on T1-weighted contrast-enhanced image.

the Boston-Leeds osteoarthritis knee score.[75] No study has been published that compares directly the different systems concerning longitudinal sensitivity to change and correlating the different systems to clinical outcomes. As no reference standard is available, true superiority of one system over another probably will not be proved. None of the scoring systems incorporates contrast-enhanced MRI. Inter- and intra-reader reliability results were published for all three systems. It has to be kept in mind, however, that these numbers are highly dependent on the MRI protocol used and experience of individual readers. Suggestions for useful MRI protocols for whole-organ assessment of knee OA have been published.[75,76] Examples of longitudinal SQ scoring of knee OA are presented in **Fig. 12**.

One of the promises of MRI in its usefulness for OA research and diagnosis is that it is sensitive to the molecular structure and content of tissue. One of the earliest recognitions of this was in the report of the laminar appearance that cartilage has on T2-weighted images (**Fig. 13**).[77] This laminar appearance is the result of the dipolar interaction of water with the depth-dependent orientation of the collagen matrix in cartilage. Over the past 20 years, much work has been done in further developing MRI for molecular imaging in OA. The majority of the studies have focused on cartilage, although there is more recent recognition for the future need for development of molecular imaging of other tissues, such as bone, ligament, and meniscus.

Perhaps the most studied parameter for molecular imaging of cartilage is T2. T2 is an MRI relaxation time reflecting interactions between water molecules and between water and surrounding macromolecules, with increasing interaction resulting in a decreased T2. Not surprisingly, T2 is affected by many physiologic and pathophysiologic processes that relate to the state of cartilage. In addition to the sensitivity of T2 to collagen orientation, T2 is sensitive to molecular concentration of proteoglycan and collagen.[78] Several reports demonstrate increased T2 with cartilage degeneration[79–81] and in individuals who have OA relative to healthy volunteers.[82,83] Other data,

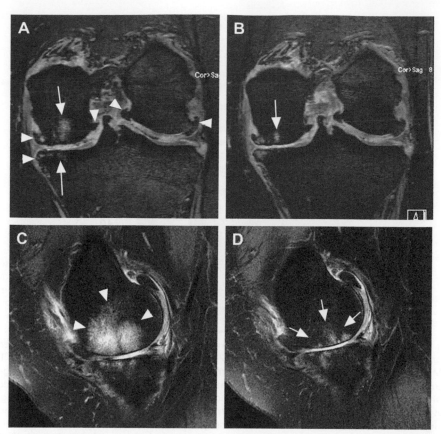

Fig. 12. Longitudinal SQ assessment of knee OA. (*A*) Baseline coronal dual-echo in the steady state image. Central OPs are scored for the medial and lateral compartment (*arrowheads*). Subchondral BMLs are shown (*arrows*). (*B*) 12-Month follow-up image shows increasing cartilage loss in the medial compartment but a decrease of the periarticular BMLs (*arrow*). Size of OPs has not changed. (*C*) Sagittal, proton density–weighted, fat-suppressed image. Large BML is seen in the central weight-bearing part of the medial femur (*arrowheads*). (*D*) 12-Month follow-up. Decrease in size and signal intensity of BML is shown (*arrows*). Note that BML is depicted superiorly on the spin-echo images (*C, D*) when compared with the gradient-echo images (*A, B*). Subchondral bone attrition, cartilage loss, meniscal damage, and posterior and anterior OPs are scored in same image. (*Courtesy of* the MOST study.)

however, demonstrate unchanged or decreased T2 with in vitro degeneration[78,84,85] and in clinical T2 images.[86]

A second parameter that has been investigated in depth for molecular imaging is T1rho. T1rho is similar to T2 in that it is sensitive to interactions of water with macromolecules. T1rho has been shown to correlate with the proteoglycan concentration in cartilage[87] and is sensitive to collagen.[78] T1rho initially was proposed as specific for glycosaminoglycan (GAG).[88] In support of that proposal, several studies have illustrated changes in T1rho in response to interventions that reduced tissue GAG.[85,89,90] T1rho, however, also is sensitive to many cartilage factors, in particular hydration, GAG, and collagen.[78] Furthermore, like T2, factors associated with cartilage degeneration may have differential and competing effects on T1rho.

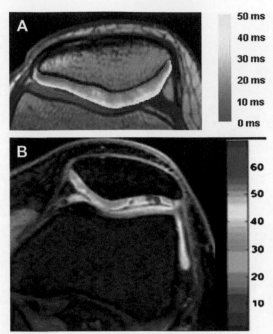

Fig. 13. (*A*) T2 map of patellar cartilage showing variation with cartilage depth. (*Reprinted from* Maier CF, Tan SG, Hariharan H, et al. T2 quantitation of articular cartilage at 1.5 T. J Magn Reson Imaging 2003:358–64; with permission.) (*B*) T1rho map of patellar cartilage demonstrating a lesion in cartilage that is morphologically thick and intact. (*Reprinted from* Borthakur A, Mellon E, Niyogi S, et al. Sodium and T1rho MRI for molecular and diagnostic imaging of articular cartilage. NMR Biomed 2006:781–821; with permission.) The variation and lesions apparent in maps of these parameters across morphologically intact cartilage enables one to potentially monitor biochemical changes in cartilage before morphologic changes become apparent.

Sodium MRI and the dGEMRIC technique are methods designed to measure fixed charge density in cartilage, adapting established biochemical and histologic approaches for measuring proteoglycan content.[91] The techniques are based on the premise that mobile ions distribute in cartilage in relation to the concentration of the charged proteoglycan molecules; in the MRI implementation of this principle, the mobile ions are the naturally abundant sodium or the proton MRI contrast agent, $Gd(DTPA)^{2-}$ (Magnevist) (Bayer HealthCare, Montville, New Jersey). Because the sodium ion is positively charged, sodium distributes in cartilage in proportion to the concentration of the negatively charged GAG molecules. The high concentration of sodium in cartilage initially was demonstrated by sodium MRI in 1988.[92] Sodium MRI later was shown to track GAG concentration[93] and sodium MRI has been shown clinically feasible.[94] This technique has the advantage that sodium is naturally present in cartilage yet is limited by low resolution and problematic for the thin and curved femoral cartilage, the very fast and variable T2, and the need for specialized hardware. In the dGEMRIC technique, $Gd(DTPA)^{2-}$ is injected intravenously and is given time (typically 90 minutes) to penetrate into cartilage before imaging. Because of the charge on the $Gd(DTPA)^{2-}$ molecule, it should distribute in cartilage in inverse relation to the negatively charged GAG molecular concentration (**Fig. 14**). Implementation of dGEMRIC has been limited. Although the method does not require any specialized equipment, the technique can be inconvenient (eg, it requires approximately a 2-hour delay between injection of the contrast agent and imaging), and the pulse sequences are not routinely available. Improved speed and ease of implementation of the pulse sequences are under development.[95] In addition, it may be possible to implement dGEMRIC at earlier times post injection, which has been shown to increase the separation between control and OA cartilage[96] and which also may enable the combination of dGEMRIC with first-pass contrast perfusion measurements of the synovium and bone and direct transport of molecules between bone and cartilage.[97]

Several other parameters for interrogating cartilage molecular composition, structure, and architecture have been evaluated, including diffusion and diffusion tensor imaging[98–101] and magnetization transfer.[102–106] In general they are limited by difficulties of in vivo implementation, poor spatial resolution, or limited sensitivity to degeneration and currently are not used in clinical trials.

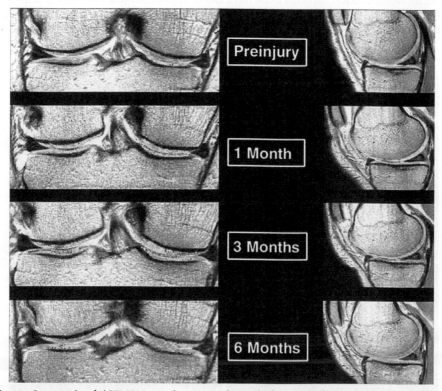

Fig. 14. Case study of dGEMRIC as a function of time before and after posterior cruciate ligament injury. A drop in the dGEMRIC Index is apparent at 1 month, with a further decrease at 3 months, and recovery at 6 months. These data illustrate the potential for biochemical monitoring of cartilage to demonstrate degeneration and recovery of the tissue from a traumatic injury. Similar studies might be used to monitor cartilage status improvement with other mechanical, surgical, or pharmaceutical interventions. (*Reprinted from* Young AA, Stanwell P, Williams A, et al. Glycosaminoglycan content of knee cartilage following posterior cruciate ligament rupture demonstrated by delayed gadolinium-enhanced magnetic resonance imaging of cartilage (dGEMRIC). A case report. J Bone Joint Surg Am 2005:2763–7; with permission.)

The ability of molecular MRI protocols to see OA as a regional and responsive (reversible) disease may lead to new paradigms for developing, circumstances for applying, and means of imaging the natural history of disease and therapeutic response to lifestyle, surgical, and disease-modifying drug interventions. In the long run, alterations in these molecular and physiologic metrics must be correlated with clinically meaningful endpoints, such as improvement in pain, function, or delay in the need for surgical intervention. Therefore, although the field is in its infancy, it has great potential for having an impact on the future understanding and development of disease-modifying therapies for OA.

Quantitative MRO (qMRI) of cartilage morphology has become of high interest over the past decade, because structural changes over time in OA generally are subtle and slow (see reviews by Eckstein and colleagues).[107–109] For quantitative measurement, the various cartilage plates in the joint are segmented by a trained user (**Fig. 15**), usually by tracing the bone-cartilage interface and the cartilage surface. Including appropriate quality control by an expert, this process may involve several hours per knee. After all slices of each cartilage plate have been segmented (**Fig. 16**), image analysis software can be used to compute a variety of morphologic parameters, such as the size of the subchondral bone area and cartilage surface, the denuded subchondral

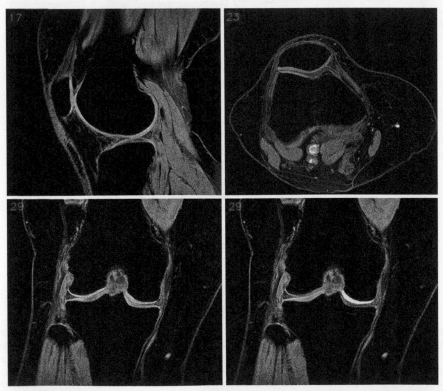

Fig. 15. MRI of the knee obtained with a SPGR sequences with water excitation: top left, sagittal image; top right, axial image of the same person; bottom left, coronal image of the same person; and bottom right, same coronal image with the medial tibial cartilage marked (segmented) blue; medial femoral cartilage, yellow; lateral tibial cartilage, green; and lateral femoral cartilage, red.

bone area, the cartilage thickness, volume, and others.[110] These quantitative MRI-based measures may reveal changes of small magnitude not immediately apparent to the human eye, in particular when extending over many slices. Small focal changes, in contrast, may be depicted more readily by expert scoring of MRI.

For quantifying cartilage morphology, water-excitation (or fat-suppressed), T1-weighted, spoiled gradient-echo (SPGR) sequences at 1.5 or 3 T represent the current gold standard.[107,111,112] 3-T qMRI has been shown slightly more precise (reproducible) than 1.5-T qMRI[113] and 3-T qMRI also recently was shown highly reproducible in multicenter (multivendor) trials.[114] A dedicated 1-T peripheral system recently was used successfully for quantitative assessment of cartilage morphology,[115] but systems operating at field strength of less than 1 T generally are not applicable to quantitative cartilage imaging.

There is great interest in identifying predictors of subsequent cartilage loss to understand the risk factors involved in disease progression. Also, detection of risk factors may enable selecting cohorts for pharmacologic intervention studies that can show protection from structural change in trials of short duration. Medial tibial cartilage loss was found associated with a lesser severity of baseline knee pain but was independent of age, body mass index (BMI), and other factors.[116] Raynauld and colleagues,[117] in contrast, observed that the rate of cartilage loss was associated with a high BMI and with meniscal extrusion, meniscal tears, and bone marrow edema. No association, however, was found with JSN (radiographs) or urine biomarker levels.[117] Another study confirmed the positive association of cartilage loss with BMI, meniscal changes, and BMLs and reported a significant association of cartilage loss with JSN.[118] Hunter and colleagues[119] recently investigated whether or not thin cartilage was a predisposing factor for OA: using a unilateral knee model in a large, community-based cohort, where one knee had radiographic change and one did not (the premorbid knee), the investigators observed that there was no difference of the mean cartilage thickness between premorbid knees and in knees of a non-OA subsample. Rather, the cartilage was normal or thicker with denuded areas, suggesting that the initial pathology in OA is focal cartilage loss and adjacent swelling rather than diffuse cartilage thinning.

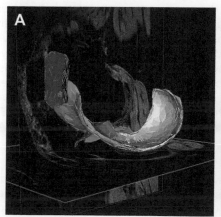
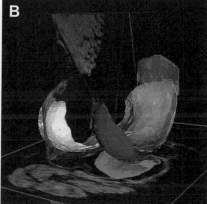

Fig. 16. 3-D reconstruction and visualization of knee cartilage plates from a sagittal MRI data set: medial tibial cartilage, blue; medial femoral cartilage, yellow; lateral tibial cartilage, green; lateral femoral cartilage, red; femoral trochlear cartilage, turquoise; and patellar cartilage, magenta.

When evaluating the effect of knee malalignment, Cicuttini and colleagues[120] reported significant femoral cartilage loss for increases in varus angulation, with less evidence for this relationship in tibial cartilage. In a cross-sectional study,[121] however, a higher correlation of tibial than femoral cartilage loss was reported with alignment in patients before knee arthroplasty. A recent study showed that varus malalignment increased the risk for cartilage loss in medial femorotibial compartment (tibia and femur) after adjusting for age, gender, BMI, medial meniscal damage and extrusion, and lateral laxity. The analysis by Sharma and colleagues[122] showed further that medial meniscal damage predicted cartilage loss in the medial femorotibial compartment and lateral meniscal damage cartilage loss in the lateral femorotibial compartment and that quantitative measures of cartilage morphology were superior in identifying these relationships to semiquantitative scores of cartilage pathology.

The OAI is an ongoing 4-year observational study of approximately 4800 participants, targeted at identifying the most reliable and sensitive biomarkers for evaluating the development and progression of symptomatic knee OA. First results from OAI pilot studies have been published[123–125] and the MRI data acquired at year 1 and baseline recently have been made publicly available for the first half of the cohort. In a subcohort of 160 participants (OAI public-use datasets 0.1.1, 0.B.1, and 1.B.1), cartilage changes observed over 1 year were small but significant; they were greater medially than laterally and greater in the medial weight-bearing femur than in the medial tibia.[126–129] Participants who had advanced radiographic disease and a high BMI tended to show faster progression than those who did not.[126] These and the upcoming data from the OAI should allow the research community to make rapid progress in understanding the risk factors involved in quantitative cartilage loss and eventually to investigate which imaging biomarkers best predict clinical outcomes, such as real or virtual total knee arthroplasty.

SUMMARY

Conventional radiography still is the first and most important imaging examination in a clinical setting when evaluating patients who have a known or suspected diagnosis of OA. In research and clinical trials it is a valuable tool for stratifying OA patients into different categories for inclusion criteria and eligibility. MRI has become crucial in understanding the natural history of the disease and in guiding future therapies because of its ability to image the knee as a whole organ and to assess, directly and 3-D, cartilage morphology and composition. Other modalities, discussed previously, are valuable additional techniques indicated on a case-by-case basis. US plays an important role for the diagnosis and follow-up of treatment of OA-related synovitis. CT arthrography is a modality that may precisely delineate most of the joint structures and especially the cartilage surface but it is invasive and conveys radiation. Other modalities, such as scintigraphy, single photon emission CT (SPECT), or FDG-PET currently are too nonspecific to have a relevant role in the diagnosis or follow-up of OA.

REFERENCES

1. Altman R, Asch E, Bloch D, et al. Development of criteria for the classification and reporting of osteoarthritis. Classification of osteoarthritis of the knee. Diagnostic and Therapeutic Criteria Committee of the American Rheumatism Association. Arthritis Rheum 1986;29:1039–49.
2. Altman R, Alarcon G, Appelrouth D, et al. The American College of Rheumatology criteria for the classification and reporting of osteoarthritis of the hip. Arthritis Rheum 1991;34:505–14.

3. Spector TD, Hart DJ, Doyle DV. Incidence and progression of osteoarthritis in women with unilateral knee disease in the general population: the effect of obesity. Ann Rheum Dis 1994;53:565–8.
4. Karachalios T, Zibis A, Papanagiotou P, et al. MR imaging findings in early osteoarthritis of the knee. Eur J Radiol 2004;50:225–30.
5. Raynauld JP, Martel-Pelletier J, Berthiaume MJ, et al. Quantitative magnetic resonance imaging evaluation of knee osteoarthritis progression over two years and correlation with clinical symptoms and radiologic changes. Arthritis Rheum 2004;50:476–87.
6. Buckland-Wright JC, Macfarlane DG, Lynch JA, et al. Joint space width measures cartilage thickness in osteoarthritis of the knee: high resolution plain film and double contrast macroradiographic investigation. Ann Rheum Dis 1995; 54:263–8.
7. Fife RS, Brandt KD, Braunstein EM, et al. Relationship between arthroscopic evidence of cartilage damage and radiographic evidence of joint space narrowing in early osteoarthritis of the knee. Arthritis Rheum 1991;34:377–82.
8. Jones G, Ding C, Scott F, et al. Early radiographic osteoarthritis is associated with substantial changes in cartilage volume and tibial bone surface area in both males and females. Osteoarthritis Cartilage 2004;12:169–74.
9. Cicuttini FM, Wluka AE, Forbes A, et al. Comparison of tibial cartilage volume and radiologic grade of the tibiofemoral joint. Arthritis Rheum 2003;48:682–8.
10. Altman RD, Hochberg M, Murphy WA Jr, et al. Atlas of individual radiographic features in osteoarthritis. Osteoarthritis Cartilage 1995;3(Suppl A):3–70.
11. Scott WW Jr, Lethbridge-Cejku M, Reichle R, et al. Reliability of grading scales for individual radiographic features of osteoarthritis of the knee. The Baltimore longitudinal study of aging atlas of knee osteoarthritis. Invest Radiol 1993;28: 497–501.
12. Duncan RC, Hay EM, Saklatvala J, et al. Prevalence of radiographic osteoarthritis—it all depends on your point of view. Rheumatology (Oxford) 2006;45: 757–60.
13. Merle-Vincent F, Vignon E, Brandt K, et al. Superiority of the Lyon schuss view over the standing anteroposterior view for detecting joint space narrowing, especially in the lateral tibiofemoral compartment, in early knee osteoarthritis. Ann Rheum Dis 2007;66:747–53.
14. Amin S, LaValley MP, Guermazi A, et al. The relationship between cartilage loss on magnetic resonance imaging and radiographic progression in men and women with knee osteoarthritis. Arthritis Rheum 2005;52:3152–9.
15. Ravaud P, Chastang C, Auleley GR, et al. Assessment of joint space width in patients with osteoarthritis of the knee: a comparison of 4 measuring instruments. J Rheumatol 1996;23:1749–55.
16. Buckland-Wright JC, Macfarlane DG, Jasani MK, et al. Quantitative microfocal radiographic assessment of osteoarthritis of the knee from weight bearing tunnel and semiflexed standing views. J Rheumatol 1994;21:1734–41.
17. Bruyere O, Henrotin YE, Honore A, et al. Impact of the joint space width measurement method on the design of knee osteoarthritis studies. Aging Clin Exp Res 2003;15:136–41.
18. Duryea J, Zaim S, Genant HK. New radiographic-based surrogate outcome measures for osteoarthritis of the knee. Osteoarthritis Cartilage 2003;11:102–10.
19. Duryea J, Li J, Peterfy CG, et al. Trainable rule-based algorithm for the measurement of joint space width in digital radiographic images of the knee. Med Phys 2000;27:580–91.

20. Peterfy C, Li J, Zaim S, et al. Comparison of fixed-flexion positioning with fluoro-scopic semi-flexed positioning for quantifying radiographic joint-space width in the knee: test-retest reproducibility. Skeletal Radiol 2003;32:128–32.

21. Conrozier T, Favret H, Mathieu P, et al. Influence of the quality of tibial plateau alignment on the reproducibility of computer joint space measurement from Lyon schuss radiographic views of the knee in patients with knee osteoarthritis. Osteoarthritis Cartilage 2004;12:765–70.

22. Buckland-Wright JC, Ward RJ, Peterfy C, et al. Reproducibility of the semiflexed (metatarsophalangeal) radiographic knee position and automated measure-ments of medial tibiofemoral joint space width in a multicenter clinical trial of knee osteoarthritis. J Rheumatol 2004;31:1588–97.

23. Kothari M, Guermazi A, von Ingersleben G, et al. Fixed-flexion radiography of the knee provides reproducible joint space width measurements in osteoarthri-tis. Eur Radiol 2004;14:1568–73.

24. Mazzuca SA, Hellio-Le Graverand MP, Vignon E, et al. Performance of a non-fluoroscopically assisted substitute for the Lyon-Schuss knee radiograph: qual-ity and reproducibility of positioning and sensitivity to joint space narrowing in osteoarthritic knees. Osteoarthritis Cartilage 2008 May 30 [Epub ahead of print].

25. Wakefield RJ, Gibbon WW, Emery P. The current status of ultrasonography in rheumatology. Rheumatology (Oxford) 1999;38:195–8.

26. Wakefield RJ, Gibbon WW, Conaghan PG, et al. The value of sonography in the detection of bone erosions in patients with rheumatoid arthritis: a comparison with conventional radiography. Arthritis Rheum 2000;43:2762–70.

27. Szkudlarek M, Narvestad E, Klarlund M, et al. Ultrasonography of the metatarso-phalangeal joints in rheumatoid arthritis: comparison with magnetic resonance imaging, conventional radiography, and clinical examination. Arthritis Rheum 2004;50:2103–12.

28. Hoving JL, Buchbinder R, Hall S, et al. A comparison of magnetic resonance imaging, sonography, and radiography of the hand in patients with early rheu-matoid arthritis. J Rheumatol 2004;31:663–75.

29. Keen HI, Wakefield RJ, Grainger AJ, et al. Can ultrasonography improve on radiographic assessment in osteoarthritis of the hands? A comparison between radiographic and ultrasonographic detected pathology. Ann Rheum Dis 2008; 67:1116–20.

30. Kim HR, So Y, Moon SG, et al. Clinical value of (99m)Tc-methylene di-phosphonate (MDP) bone single photon emission computed tomography (SPECT) in patients with knee osteoarthritis. Osteoarthritis Cartilage 2008;16: 212–8.

31. Aisen AM, McCune WJ, MacGuire A, et al. Sonographic evaluation of the carti-lage of the knee. Radiology 1984;153:781–4.

32. Monteforte P, Rovetta G. Sonographic assessment of soft tissue alterations in os-teoarthritis of the knee. Int J Tissue React 1999;21:19–23.

33. Martino F, Ettorre GC, Patella V, et al. Articular cartilage echography as a criterion of the evolution of osteoarthritis of the knee. Int J Clin Pharmacol Res 1993; 13(Suppl):35–42.

34. Tarhan S, Unlu Z. Magnetic resonance imaging and ultrasonographic evaluation of the patients with knee osteoarthritis: a comparative study. Clin Rheumatol 2003;22:181–8.

35. Jonsson K, Buckwalter K, Helvie M, et al. Precision of hyaline cartilage thickness measurements. Acta Radiol 1992;33:234–9.

36. Naredo E, Cabero F, Palop MJ, et al. Ultrasonographic findings in knee osteoarthritis: a comparative study with clinical and radiographic assessment. Osteoarthritis Cartilage 2005;13:568–74.
37. Karim Z, Wakefield RJ, Quinn M, et al. Validation and reproducibility of ultrasonography in the detection of synovitis in the knee: a comparison with arthroscopy and clinical examination. Arthritis Rheum 2004;50:387–94.
38. D'Agostino MA, Conaghan P, Le Bars M, et al. EULAR report on the use of ultrasonography in painful knee osteoarthritis. Part 1: prevalence of inflammation in osteoarthritis. Ann Rheum Dis 2005;64:1703–9.
39. Walther M, Harms H, Krenn V, et al. Synovial tissue of the hip at power Doppler US: correlation between vascularity and power Doppler US signal. Radiology 2002;225:225–31.
40. Walther M, Harms H, Krenn V, et al. Correlation of power Doppler sonography with vascularity of the synovial tissue of the knee joint in patients with osteoarthritis and rheumatoid arthritis. Arthritis Rheum 2001;44:331–8.
41. Schmidt WA, Volker L, Zacher J, et al. Colour Doppler ultrasonography to detect pannus in knee joint synovitis. Clin Exp Rheumatol 2000;18:439–44.
42. Ostergaard M, Court-Payen M, Gideon P, et al. Ultrasonography in arthritis of the knee. A comparison with MR imaging. Acta Radiol 1995;36:19–26.
43. Jan MH, Chai HM, Wang CL, et al. Effects of repetitive shortwave diathermy for reducing synovitis in patients with knee osteoarthritis: an ultrasonographic study. Phys Ther 2006;86:236–44.
44. de Miguel Mendieta E, Cobo Ibanez T, Uson Jaeger J, et al. Clinical and ultrasonographic findings related to knee pain in osteoarthritis. Osteoarthritis Cartilage 2006;14:540–4.
45. Qvistgaard E, Torp-Pedersen S, Christensen R, et al. Reproducibility and inter-reader agreement of a scoring system for ultrasound evaluation of hip osteoarthritis. Ann Rheum Dis 2006;65:1613–9.
46. Qvistgaard E, Kristoffersen H, Terslev L, et al. Guidance by ultrasound of intra-articular injections in the knee and hip joints. Osteoarthritis Cartilage 2001;9:512–7.
47. Hutton CW, Higgs ER, Jackson PC, et al. 99mTc HMDP bone scanning in generalised nodal osteoarthritis. II. The four hour bone scan image predicts radiographic change. Ann Rheum Dis 1986;45:622–6.
48. Boegard T, Rudling O, Dahlstrom J, et al. Bone scintigraphy in chronic knee pain: comparison with magnetic resonance imaging. Ann Rheum Dis 1999;58:20–6.
49. Dieppe P, Cushnaghan J, Young P, et al. Prediction of the progression of joint space narrowing in osteoarthritis of the knee by bone scintigraphy. Ann Rheum Dis 1993;52:557–63.
50. Mazzuca SA, Brandt KD, Schauwecker DS, et al. Severity of joint pain and Kellgren-Lawrence grade at baseline are better predictors of joint space narrowing than bone scintigraphy in obese women with knee osteoarthritis. J Rheumatol 2005;32:1540–6.
51. Mazzuca SA, Brandt KD, Schauwecker DS, et al. Bone scintigraphy is not a better predictor of progression of knee osteoarthritis than Kellgren and Lawrence grade. J Rheumatol 2004;31:329–32.
52. Nakamura H, Masuko K, Yudoh K, et al. Positron emission tomography with 18F-FDG in osteoarthritic knee. Osteoarthritis Cartilage 2007;15:673–81.
53. Thomas RH, Resnick D, Alazraki NP, et al. Compartmental evaluation of osteoarthritis of the knee. A comparative study of available diagnostic modalities. Radiology 1975;116:585–94.

54. Hechelhammer L, Pfirrmann CW, Zanetti M, et al. Imaging findings predicting the outcome of cervical facet joint blocks. Eur Radiol 2007;17:959–64.
55. Tuite MJ, Rubin D. CT and MR arthrography of the glenoid labroligamentous complex. Semin Musculoskelet Radiol 1998;2:363–76.
56. Vande Berg BC, Lecouvet FE, Poilvache P, et al. Assessment of knee cartilage in cadavers with dual-detector spiral CT arthrography and MR imaging. Radiology 2002;222:430–6.
57. Rand T, Brossmann J, Pedowitz R, et al. Analysis of patellar cartilage. Comparison of conventional MR imaging and MR and CT arthrography in cadavers. Acta Radiol 2000;41:492–7.
58. Daenen BR, Ferrara MA, Marcelis S, et al. Evaluation of patellar cartilage surface lesions: comparison of CT arthrography and fat-suppressed FLASH 3D MR imaging. Eur Radiol 1998;8:981–5.
59. Nishii T, Tanaka H, Sugano N, et al. Disorders of acetabular labrum and articular cartilage in hip dysplasia: evaluation using isotropic high-resolutional CT arthrography with sequential radial reformation. Osteoarthritis Cartilage 2007;15:251–7.
60. Gagliardi JA, Chung EM, Chandnani VP, et al. Detection and staging of chondromalacia patellae: relative efficacies of conventional MR imaging, MR arthrography, and CT arthrography. AJR Am J Roentgenol 1994;163:629–36.
61. Vande Berg BC, Lecouvet FE, Malghem J. Frequency and topography of lesions of the femoro-tibial cartilage at spiral CT arthrography of the knee: a study in patients with normal knee radiographs and without history of trauma. Skeletal Radiol 2002;31:643–9.
62. Guermazi A, Hunter DJ, Roemer FW, et al. MRI prevalence of different features of knee osteoarthritis in persons with normal knee X-rays. Arthritis Rheum 2007; 56:S128–9 [abstract].
63. Peterfy CG, Roberts T, Genant HK. Dedicated extremity MR imaging: an emerging technology. Magn Reson Imaging Clin N Am 1998;6:849–70.
64. Masciocchi C, Barile A, Satragno L, et al. Dedicated systems. Eur Radiol 2000;10: 250–5.
65. Englund M, Niu J, Guermazi A, et al. Effect of meniscal damage on the development of frequent knee pain, aching, or stiffness. Arthritis Rheum 2007;56: 4048–54.
66. Felson DT, Niu J, Guermazi A, et al. The development of knee pain correlates with enlarging bone marrow lesions on MRI. Arthritis Rheum 2007;56:2986–92.
67. Rhodes LA, Grainger AJ, Keenan AM, et al. The validation of simple scoring methods for evaluating compartment-specific synovitis detected by MRI in knee osteoarthritis. Rheumatology (Oxford) 2005;44:1569–73.
68. Grainger AJ, Rhodes LA, Keenan AM, et al. Quantifying peri-meniscal synovitis and its relationship to meniscal pathology in osteoarthritis of the knee. Eur Radiol 2007;17:119–24.
69. Peterfy CG, White D, Tirman P, et al. Whole-organ evaluation of the knee in osteoarthritis using MRI. Ann Rheum Dis 1999;38:342 [abstract].
70. Felson DT, Chaisson CE, Hill CL, et al. The association of bone marrow lesions with pain in knee osteoarthritis. Ann Intern Med 2001;134:541–9.
71. Hunter DJ, Zhang Y, Niu J, et al. Increase in bone marrow lesions associated with cartilage loss: a longitudinal magnetic resonance imaging study of knee osteoarthritis. Arthritis Rheum 2006;54:1529–35.
72. Roemer FW, Guermazi A, Javaid MK, et al. Change in MRI-Detected subchondral bone marrow lesions is associated with cartilage loss—the MOST study.

A longitudinal multicenter study of knee osteoarthritis. Ann Rheum Dis 2008; [Epub ahead of print].

73. Peterfy CG, Guermazi A, Zaim S, et al. Whole-organ magnetic resonance imaging score (WORMS) of the knee in osteoarthritis. Osteoarthritis Cartilage 2004; 12:177–90.

74. Kornaat PR, Ceulemans RY, Kroon HM, et al. MRI assessment of knee osteoarthritis: knee osteoarthritis scoring system (KOSS)—inter-observer and intra-observer reproducibility of a compartment-based scoring system. Skeletal Radiol 2005;34:95–102.

75. Hunter DJ, Lo GH, Gale D, et al. The development and reliability of a new scoring system for knee osteoarthritis MRI: BLOKS (Boston Leeds osteoarthritis knee score). Ann Rheum Dis 2008;67:206–11.

76. Roemer FW, Guermazi A, Lynch JA, et al. Short tau inversion recovery and proton density- weighted fat suppressed sequences for the evaluation of osteoarthritis of the knee with a 1.0 T dedicated extremity MRI: development of a time-efficient sequence protocol. Eur Radiol 2005;15:978–87.

77. Lehner KB, Rechl HP, Gmeinwieser JK, et al. Structure, function, and degeneration of bovine hyaline cartilage: assessment with MR imaging in vitro. Radiology 1989;170:495–9.

78. Menezes NM, Gray ML, Hartke JR, et al. T2 and T1rho MRI in articular cartilage systems. Magn Reson Med 2004;51:503–9.

79. David-Vaudey E, Ghosh S, Ries M, et al. T2 relaxation time measurements in osteoarthritis. Magn Reson Imaging 2004;22:673–82.

80. Watrin-Pinzano A, Ruaud JP, Olivier P, et al. Effect of proteoglycan depletion on T2 mapping in rat patellar cartilage. Radiology 2005;234:162–70.

81. Regatte RR, Akella SV, Lonner JH, et al. T1rho relaxation mapping in human osteoarthritis (OA) cartilage: comparison of T1rho with T2. J Magn Reson Imaging 2006;23:547–53.

82. Mosher TJ, Dardzinski BJ, Smith MB. Human articular cartilage: influence of aging and early symptomatic degeneration on the spatial variation of T2–preliminary findings at 3 T. Radiology 2000;214:259–66.

83. Dunn TC, Lu Y, Jin H, et al. T2 relaxation time of cartilage at MR imaging: comparison with severity of knee osteoarthritis. Radiology 2004;232:592–8.

84. Henkelman RM, Stanisz GJ, Menezes N, et al. Can MTR be used to assess cartilage in the presence of Gd-DTPA2-? Magn Reson Med 2002;48:1081–4.

85. Regatte RR, Akella SV, Borthakur A, et al. Proteoglycan depletion-induced changes in transverse relaxation maps of cartilage: comparison of T2 and T1rho. Acad Radiol 2002;9:1388–94.

86. Burstein D. MRI for development of disease-modifying osteoarthritis drugs. NMR Biomed 2006;19:669–80.

87. Borthakur A, Mellon E, Niyogi S, et al. Sodium and T1rho MRI for molecular and diagnostic imaging of articular cartilage. NMR Biomed 2006;19:781–821.

88. Duvvuri U, Reddy R, Patel SD, et al. T1rho-relaxation in articular cartilage: effects of enzymatic degradation. Magn Reson Med 1997;38:863–7.

89. Akella SV, Regatte RR, Gougoutas AJ, et al. Proteoglycan-induced changes in T1rho-relaxation of articular cartilage at 4T. Magn Reson Med 2001;46: 419–23.

90. Wheaton AJ, Dodge GR, Borthakur A, et al. Detection of changes in articular cartilage proteoglycan by T(1rho) magnetic resonance imaging. J Orthop Res 2005;23:102–8.

91. Gray ML, Burstein D, Kim YJ, et al. 2007 Elizabeth Winston Lanier Award Winner. Magnetic resonance imaging of cartilage glycosaminoglycan: basic principles, imaging technique, and clinical applications. J Orthop Res 2008;26:281–91.

92. Granot J. Sodium imaging of human body organs and extremities in vivo. Radiology 1988;167:547–50.

93. Lesperance LM, Gray ML, Burstein D. Determination of fixed charge density in cartilage using nuclear magnetic resonance. J Orthop Res 1992;10:1–13.

94. Shapiro EM, Borthakur A, Gougoutas A, et al. 23Na MRI accurately measures fixed charge density in articular cartilage. Magn Reson Med 2002;47:284–91.

95. Kimelman T, Vu A, Storey P, et al. Three-dimensional T1 mapping for dGEMRIC at 3.0 T using the look locker method. Invest Radiol 2006;41:198–203.

96. Tiderius CJ, Jessel R, Kim YJ, et al. Hip dGEMRIC in asymptomatic volunteers and patients with early osteoarthritis: the influence of timing after contrast injection. Magn Reson Med 2007;57:803–5.

97. Bashir A, Gray ML, Boutin RD, et al. Glycosaminoglycan in articular cartilage: in vivo assessment with delayed Gd(DTPA) (2-)-enhanced MR imaging. Radiology 1997;205:551–8.

98. Burstein D, Gray ML, Hartman AL, et al. Diffusion of small solutes in cartilage as measured by nuclear magnetic resonance (NMR) spectroscopy and imaging. J Orthop Res 1993;11:465–78.

99. Mlynarik V, Sulzbacher I, Bittsansky M, et al. Investigation of apparent diffusion constant as an indicator of early degenerative disease in articular cartilage. J Magn Reson Imaging 2003;17:440–4.

100. Filidoro L, Dietrich O, Weber J, et al. High-resolution diffusion tensor imaging of human patellar cartilage: feasibility and preliminary findings. Magn Reson Med 2005;53:993–8.

101. Deng X, Farley M, Nieminen MT, et al. Diffusion tensor imaging of native and degenerated human articular cartilage. Magn Reson Imaging 2007;25: 168–71.

102. Wolff SD, Chesnick S, Frank JA, et al. Magnetization transfer contrast: MR imaging of the knee. Radiology 1991;179:623–8.

103. Gray ML, Burstein D, Lesperance LM, et al. Magnetization transfer in cartilage and its constituent macromolecules. Magn Reson Med 1995;34:319–25.

104. Seo GS, Aoki J, Moriya H, et al. Hyaline cartilage: in vivo and in vitro assessment with magnetization transfer imaging. Radiology 1996;201:525–30.

105. Wachsmuth L, Juretschke HP, Raiss RX. Can magnetization transfer magnetic resonance imaging follow proteoglycan depletion in articular cartilage? MAGMA 1997;5:71–8.

106. Regatte RR, Akella SV, Reddy R. Depth-dependent proton magnetization transfer in articular cartilage. J Magn Reson Imaging 2005;22:318–23.

107. Eckstein F, Cicuttini F, Raynauld JP, et al. Magnetic resonance imaging (MRI) of articular cartilage in knee osteoarthritis (OA): morphological assessment. Osteoarthritis Cartilage 2006;14(Suppl A):A46–75.

108. Eckstein F, Burstein D, Link TM. Quantitative MRI of cartilage and bone: degenerative changes in osteoarthritis. NMR Biomed 2006;19:822–54.

109. Eckstein F, Mosher T, Hunter D. Imaging of knee osteoarthritis: data beyond the beauty. Curr Opin Rheumatol 2007;19:435–43.

110. Eckstein F, Ateshian G, Burgkart R, et al. Proposal for a nomenclature for magnetic resonance imaging based measures of articular cartilage in osteoarthritis. Osteoarthritis Cartilage 2006;14:974–83.

111. Gold GE, Burstein D, Dardzinski B, et al. MRI of articular cartilage in OA: novel pulse sequences and compositional/functional markers. Osteoarthritis Cartilage 2006;14(Suppl A):A76–86.
112. Peterfy CG, Gold G, Eckstein F, et al. MRI protocols for whole-organ assessment of the knee in osteoarthritis. Osteoarthritis Cartilage 2006;14(Suppl A):A95–111.
113. Eckstein F, Charles HC, Buck RJ, et al. Accuracy and precision of quantitative assessment of cartilage morphology by magnetic resonance imaging at 3.0T. Arthritis Rheum 2005;52:3132–6.
114. Eckstein F, Buck RJ, Burstein D, et al. Precision of 3.0 Tesla quantitative magnetic resonance imaging of cartilage morphology in a multi center clinical trial. Ann Rheum Dis 2008 Feb 18 [Epub ahead of print].
115. Inglis D, Pui M, Ioannidis G, et al. Accuracy and test-retest precision of quantitative cartilage morphology on a 1.0 T peripheral magnetic resonance imaging system. Osteoarthritis Cartilage 2007;15:110–5.
116. Wluka AE, Forbes A, Wang Y, et al. Knee cartilage loss in symptomatic knee osteoarthritis over 4.5 years. Arthritis Res Ther 2006;8:R90.
117. Raynauld JP, Martel-Pelletier J, Berthiaume MJ, et al. Long term evaluation of disease progression through the quantitative magnetic resonance imaging of symptomatic knee osteoarthritis patients: correlation with clinical symptoms and radiographic changes. Arthritis Res Ther 2006;8:R21.
118. Pelletier JP, Raynauld JP, Berthiaume MJ, et al. Risk factors associated with the loss of cartilage volume on weight-bearing areas in knee osteoarthritis patients assessed by quantitative magnetic resonance imaging: a longitudinal study. Arthritis Res Ther 2007;9:R74.
119. Hunter DJ, Niu J, Zhang Y, et al. Premorbid knee OA is not characterized by diffuse thinness: The Framingham Study. Ann Rheum Dis 2008 Jan 24 [Epub ahead of print].
120. Cicuttini F, Wluka A, Hankin J, et al. Longitudinal study of the relationship between knee angle and tibiofemoral cartilage volume in subjects with knee osteoarthritis. Rheumatology (Oxford) 2004;43:321–4.
121. von Eisenhart-Rothe R, Graichen H, Hudelmaier M, et al. Femorotibial and patellar cartilage loss in patients prior to total knee arthroplasty, heterogeneity, and correlation with alignment of the knee. Ann Rheum Dis 2006;65:69–73.
122. Sharma L, Eckstein F, Song J, et al. The relationship of meniscal damage, meniscal extrusion, malalignment, and joint laxity to subsequent cartilage loss in osteoarthritic knees. Arthritis Rheum 2008;58(6):1716–26.
123. Eckstein F, Hudelmaier M, Wirth W, et al. Double echo steady state magnetic resonance imaging of knee articular cartilage at 3 Tesla: a pilot study for the osteoarthritis initiative. Ann Rheum Dis 2006;65:433–41.
124. Eckstein F, Kunz M, Hudelmaier M, et al. Impact of coil design on the contrast-to-noise ratio, precision, and consistency of quantitative cartilage morphometry at 3 Tesla: a pilot study for the osteoarthritis initiative. Magn Reson Med 2007;57:448–54.
125. Eckstein F, Kunz M, Schutzer M, et al. Two year longitudinal change and test-re-test-precision of knee cartilage morphology in a pilot study for the osteoarthritis initiative. Osteoarthritis Cartilage 2007;15:1326–32.
126. Eckstein F, Maschek S, Wirth W, et al. One year change of knee cartilage morphology in the first release of participants from the osteoarthritis initiative progression subcohort—association with sex, body mass index, symptoms, and radiographic OA status. Ann Rheum Dis 2008 Jul 7 [Epub ahead of print].

127. Hunter DJ, Niu J, Zhang Y, et al. Change in cartilage morphometry: a sample of the progression cohort of the osteoarthritis initiative. Ann Rheum Dis 2008 Apr 13 [Epub ahead of print].
128. Maier CF, Tan SG, Hariharan H, et al. T2 quantitation of articular cartilage at 1.5 T. J Magn Reson Imaging 2003;17:358–64.
129. Young AA, Stanwell P, Williams A, et al. Glycosaminoglycan content of knee cartilage following posterior cruciate ligament rupture demonstrated by delayed gadolinium-enhanced magnetic resonance imaging of cartilage (dGEMRIC). A case report. J Bone Joint Surg Am 2005;87:2763–7.

The Management of Osteoarthritis: An Overview and Call to Appropriate Conservative Treatment

David J. Hunter, MBBS, MSc, PhD[a],*, Grace H. Lo, MD, MSc[b]

KEYWORDS

• Osteoarthritis • Diagnosis • Treatment

Osteoarthritis (OA) is a rising epidemic. In 2000, OA was present in 25 million north Americans (United States and Canada).[1,2] By 2020, the number of people with OA will have doubled, in large part owing to the exploding prevalence of obesity and the graying of the "baby boomer" generation. The largest increase will occur among older adults, for whom OA also has the greatest functional impact. When OA becomes symptomatic in the knee, as it does in about 13% of adults aged more than 55 years,[3] the impact can be debilitating. OA of the knee is the single most prevalent cause of mobility dependency and disability.[4] Despite growing concern, OA remains a poorly understood disease, and recent doubts about the safety of several commonly prescribed OA medications have served to highlight deficiencies in the traditional medical approach to management. Current clinical management of OA is often limited to analgesic medication and cautious waiting[5] for the sometimes eventual referral for total joint replacement. With few conservative options offered by physicians, increasing numbers of patients are turning to untested folk remedies and aggressively

A version of this article originally appeared in the 34:3 issue of the *Rheumatic Disease Clinics of North America*.

The corresponding author (DJH) had full access to all of the data in this study and had final responsibility for the decision to submit for publication. Dr. Hunter receives research or institutional support from AstraZeneca, DonJoy, Lilly, Merck, NIH, Pfizer, Stryker, and Wyeth.

[a] Division of Research, New England Baptist Hospital, 125 Parker Hill Avenue, Boston, MA 02120, USA

[b] Tufts Medical Center, Divison of Rheumatology, 800 Washington Street, Box #406, Boston, MA 02111, USA

* Corresponding author. Division of Research, New England Baptist Hospital, 125 Parker Hill Avenue, Boston, MA 02120.

E-mail address: djhunter@caregroup.harvard.edu (D.J. Hunter).

Med Clin N Am 93 (2009) 127–143

doi:10.1016/j.mcna.2008.07.009

marketed dietary supplements with little substantive evidence to support their efficacy. There is a great demand for nonpharmacologic therapies and a pressing need for physicians to revisit the current clinical management of OA.

This article presents a general outline for the management of the patient with OA in the form of a narrative review considering diagnosis, investigation, and treatment. It is not a comprehensive discussion (subsequent articles on imaging, weight management, exercise, braces and orthotics, pharmacologic intervention, and surgery provide more detail); rather, it provides the clinician with an overview of what is available. For the interested clinician, further references are provided that can facilitate additional reading and, it is hoped, practice change.[6–11] Inevitably, there is much the interested clinician can do rather than practice nihilistic waiting. The authors encourage active clinician involvement and instilling self-management strategies in patients to further promote effective long-term treatment of this pervasive disease.

DIAGNOSIS OF OSTEOARTHRITIS

In clinical practice, the diagnosis of OA should be made on the basis of history and physical examination. The role of radiography is to confirm this clinical suspicion and rule out other conditions.[12] The cardinal features that suggest a diagnosis of OA include pain, stiffness, reduced movement, swelling, and crepitus in typically involved joints (eg, hand distal interphalangeals and proximal interphalangeals, hips, knees, and metatarsophalangeals) in individuals who are older (eg, the occurrence of OA is unusual before age 40 years unless there is a history of predisposing factors such as prior trauma) and in the absence of systemic features (eg, fever).

Typically, the patient who has OA presents to the clinician with joint pain. Peat and colleagues[13] presented research demonstrating that, during a 1-year period, 25% of persons aged more than 55 years have a persistent episode of knee pain, of whom about one in six consult their general practitioner about it in the same time period. Approximately 50% of these persons have radiographic knee OA. Many of the remainder also likely have knee OA (although not detectable as yet on a plain radiograph) or an alternate source of knee pain such as pes anserine bursitis or iliotibial band syndrome.[14]

The joint pain of OA is typically described as mechanical. It is exacerbated by activity, especially weight-bearing activity, and relieved by rest. In more advanced disease OA can cause rest and night pain. The source of pain is not particularly well understood and is best framed in a biopsychosocial framework.[15] This framework includes complex interactions among what a person is doing in his or her everyday life, local events in the joint, pain sensitization, and the cortical experience of pain.

Although a great deal of attention has been directed at the articular cartilage in this disease, there is little evidence to suggest that articular cartilage loss contributes directly to pain because this structure is aneural.[16–18] In contrast, the subchondral bone, periosteum, synovium, and joint capsule are all richly innervated and contain nerve endings[16,19,20] that could be the source of nociceptive stimuli in OA.

Physical examination should include an assessment of body mass index (BMI) to assess for a status of being "overweight" (BMI ≥25) or "obese" (BMI ≥30), joint range of motion, point tenderness, muscle strength, and ligament stability. The features on physical examination that suggest a diagnosis of OA include the following:

- Tenderness, usually located over the joint line
- Crepitus with movement of the joint (eg, in the knee, which can involve the patellofemoral or the tibiofemoral compartments)

- Bony enlargement of the joint (eg, Heberden's and Bouchard's nodes, squaring of the first carpal metacarpal, typically along the affected joint line in the knee)
- Restricted joint range of motion
- Pain on passive range of motion
- Deformity (eg, angulation of the distal interphalangeal and proximal interphalangeal joints in the hands, varus [bowed legs] or valgus [knock kneed] alignment in the knees)
- Instability of the joint
- Weakness of the periarticular muscles, especially the quadriceps muscles related to knee OA

INVESTIGATION OF OSTEOARTHRITIS

Imaging can assist in making a diagnosis, predominantly by assessing the constellation of presenting clinical features. When disease is advanced, it is visible on plain radiographs, which show narrowing of joint space (in most joints due to loss of hyaline articular cartilage and, in the knee, also due to damage to the meniscus,[21] osteophytes, and sometimes changes in the subchondral bone). In light of the lack of therapy that can modify the disease course and measurement imprecision, there is no rationale for obtaining serial radiographs if the clinical state is unchanged.

When making the diagnosis of OA, one should consider using the criteria of the American College of Rheumatology (ACR) for diagnostic purposes and classification of OA of the hip, knee, and hands in patients with pain in these joints.[12,22] The ACR clinical and radiographic criteria for classification of knee OA have a sensitivity of 91% and specificity of 86% and include knee pain, osteophytes on radiographs of the knee, and at least one of the following: age greater than 50 years, stiffness lasting less than 30 minutes, and crepitus.

As is true for most diagnostic criteria, these factors are used primarily for inclusion into research studies. Although they can be helpful in informing the diagnosis of OA, individuals are not required to meet all criteria to receive a clinical diagnosis of OA or to receive treatment for this condition. Information gathering should not be limited to these criteria, particularly considering the wealth of other information that patients with OA may provide that can help to confirm or refute a diagnosis of OA.

Bearing in mind that radiographs are notoriously insensitive to the earliest pathologic features of knee OA, the absence of positive radiographic findings should not be interpreted as confirming the complete absence of symptomatic disease. Conversely, the presence of positive radiographic findings does not guarantee that an OA joint is also the active source of the patient's current knee symptoms.[23] Asymptomatic knee OA is common, especially among older patients with a contralateral knee with symptomatic radiographic OA and in those with OA in neighboring hip or low back joints.

MRI should be used in infrequent circumstances to facilitate the diagnosis of other causes of knee pain that can be confused with OA (eg, osteochondritis dissecans, avascular necrosis). The presence of a meniscal tear on MRI in a person with knee OA is almost uniform and is not necessarily a cause of increased symptoms.[24] The penchant to remove menisci should be avoided unless there are symptoms of locking or extension blockade,[25] because there are strong data to support that meniscectomy, even partial meniscectomy, increases the risk for progression of OA.[26]

To date, no reliable laboratory tests can establish the diagnosis of OA. Because OA is considered to be a non-inflammatory arthritis, laboratory testing is expected to be normal; however, because the prevalence of OA is high in the general population, especially in elderly patients, laboratory abnormalities such as an elevated erythrocyte sedimentation rate and anemia will be detected frequently. One should consider testing for a full blood count, creatinine level, and liver function before initiating nonsteroidal anti-inflammatory drugs (NSAIDs) for OA, especially in elderly patients or in patients with other chronic illnesses. Biochemical markers at present are a research tool. One should consider aspirating a joint if a diagnosis other than OA (ie, septic arthritis, gout, pseudogout) is suspected. Synovial fluid from OA joints tends to be non-inflammatory (ie, leukocyte count <2000/mm^3, clear, viscous).

POTENTIAL DIFFERENTIAL DIAGNOSES

Other forms of arthritis may present with hand, knee, or hip pain, including rheumatoid arthritis, psoriatic arthritis, other seronegative spondyloarthropathies (ankylosing spondylitis, arthritis associated with inflammatory bowel disease (IBD), reactive arthritis), and sarcoidosis. Several other diseases may also predispose to the development of OA and should be treated, including metabolic diseases (hemachromatosis, Wilson's disease, ochronosis), endocrine disease (acromegaly, hyperparathyroidism), hypermobility (Ehlers-Danlos), crystal arthropathy (gout, calcium pyrophosphate dihydrate deposition [CPPD]), neuropathic joints, and chondrodysplasias.

In addition, patients may present with other sources of regional pain. Common reasons for local pain in the regions commonly affected by OA include the following:

Hip pain, including trochanteric bursitis, iliopsoas tendonitis, referred pain from the lumbosacral spine, avascular necrosis, inguinal hernia, and hip fracture[27]

Knee pain, including pes anserine bursitis, iliotibial band friction syndrome (runner's knee), patella tendonitis, patellofemoral pain syndrome, prepatellar bursitis, and semimembranous bursitis[28]

Hand pain, including De Quervain's tenosynovitis, carpal tunnel syndrome (median nerve compression), flexor tenosynovitis (trigger finger), and ulnar nerve compression

In the first instance, the clinician should consider these diagnoses in the differential when a patient complains of pain in these areas and should tailor the history and physical examination to exclude them.

TREATMENT

The aims of management of OA are (1) patient education about the disease and its management, (2) pain control, (3) improved function and decreased disability, and (4) altering the disease process and its consequences.

The management of OA should be individualized and will likely consist of a combination of treatment options. Unfortunately, the overwhelming preponderance of treatments tested and used for OA are currently drugs or surgery. In a recent meta-analysis of trials in OA, 60% assessed the effect of drug treatment and 26% evaluated surgical procedures.[29] The toxicity and adverse event profiles of the most commonly used existing therapies (eg, NSAIDs, cyclooxygenase-2 [COX-2] inhibitors, and total joint replacement) are unfavorable when compared with conservative interventions such as exercise, weight loss, braces, and orthotics.[6] Options for the conservative care of patients with knee OA are often overlooked.[5] In the authors' opinion, only when conservative efforts fail to improve function should pharmaceuticals be offered, and, certainly, surgical interventions should be a last resort.

In the absence of a cure, current therapy primarily attempts to reduce pain and improve joint function by employing modalities targeted toward symptom relief that do not facilitate any improvement in joint structure. The management of OA should be individualized so that it conforms to the specific findings of the clinical examination, especially when the findings include obesity, malalignment, and muscle weakness. Comprehensive management always includes a combination of treatment options that are directed toward the common goal of improving the patient's pain and tolerance for functional activity. Treatment plans should never be defined rigidly according to the radiographic appearance of the joint but should instead remain flexible so that they can be altered according to the functional and symptomatic responses obtained.

The recommended hierarchy of management should consist of nonpharmacologic modalities first, followed by drugs and then surgery. Too frequently, the first step is forgotten or not emphasized sufficiently to the patient's detriment. In addition, combinations of treatments are frequently used in clinical practice and may have additional synergistic benefits (**Fig. 1**).

Several well-written guidelines describe the management of OA that are based on evidence from trials and expert consensus.[6–9] The ACR released expert-guided consensus guidelines for the management of the hip and knee in 2000.[8] These guidelines are now somewhat outdated, and the Osteoarthritis Research Society International (OARSI) or European League Against Rheumatism (EULAR) guidelines and recommendations should be used in preference to these.

The EULAR final set of ten recommendations for management of OA of the knee (**Table 1**), published in 2003, were developed using an evidence-based medicine and expert opinion approach.[6] These updated recommendations support some of the previous propositions for the large number of treatment options available for knee OA but also include modified statements and new propositions. Further consensus guidelines agreed upon after three anonymous Delphi rounds were developed for management of OA of the hip in 2005 (**Table 2**).[7] Ten key recommendations for the treatment of hip OA were developed based on research evidence and expert consensus. The effectiveness and cost-effectiveness of these recommendations were evaluated, and the strength of recommendation was scored.

Updated evidence-based, international consensus recommendations for the management of OA of the hip and knee have been developed by the OARSI Treatment Guidelines Committee.[9] This committee undertook a critical appraisal of published guidelines, and a systematic review of more recent evidence for relevant therapies was completed and published in two parts in late 2007 and early 2008. The first part of the work of this committee was to undertake a critical appraisal of all existing evidence-based and consensus guidelines for the treatment of OA of the knee or hip

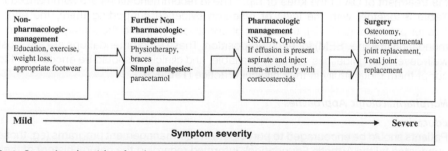

Fig. 1. Stepwise algorithm for the management of OA. This suggested treatment algorithm is modified according to the patient's response and the clinician's preference. It highlights the encompassing need to consider nonpharmacologic management as the first-line treatment for all patients. (*From* Hunter D, Felson D. Osteoarthritis [review]. BMJ 2006;332(7542): 639–42; with permission.)

Table 1
EULAR 2003 management recommendations for osteoarthritis of the knee

Number	Proposition
1	The optimal management of knee OA requires a combination of nonpharmacologic and pharmacologic treatment modalities.
2	The treatment of knee OA should be tailored according to (a) knee risk factors (obesity, adverse mechanical factors, physical activity), (b) general risk factors (age, comorbidity, polypharmacy), (c) the level of pain intensity and disability, (d) signs of inflammation (eg, effusion), and (e) the location and degree of structural damage.
3	Nonpharmacologic treatment of knee OA should include regular education, exercise, appliances (sticks, insoles, knee bracing), and weight reduction.
4	Paracetamol is the oral analgesic to try first and, if successful, the preferred long-term oral analgesic.
5	Topical applications (NSAIDs, capsaicin) have clinical efficacy and are safe.
6	NSAIDs should be considered in patients unresponsive to paracetamol. In patients with an increased gastrointestinal risk, nonselective NSAIDs and effective gastroprotective agents or selective COX-2 inhibitors should be used.
7	Opioid analgesics, with or without paracetamol, are useful alternatives in patients in whom NSAIDs, including COX-2 selective inhibitors, are contraindicated, ineffective, or poorly tolerated.
8	SYSADOA (glucosamine sulfate, chondroitin sulfate, ASU, diacerein, hyaluronic acid) have symptomatic effects and may modify structure.
9	Intra-articular injection of long-acting corticosteroids is indicated for flare of knee pain, especially if accompanied by effusion.
10	Joint replacement has to be considered in patients with radiographic evidence of knee OA who have refractory pain and disability.

Abbreviations: ASU, avocado soybean unsaponifiable; SYSADOA, symptomatic slow-acting drugs for osteoarthritis.
From Jordan KM, Arden NK, Doherty M, et al. EULAR recommendations 2003: an evidence based approach to the management of knee osteoarthritis. Report of a Task Force of the Standing Committee for International Clinical Studies Including Therapeutic Trials (ESCISIT) [review]. Ann Rheum Dis 2003;62(12):1145–55; with permission.

and a systematic review of the recent research evidence. The second part of the report contains the current OARSI evidence-based, expert consensus recommendations for the treatment of OA of the knee or hip.[9] These recommendations are summarized in **Table 3** together with the level of research evidence supporting them, the effect size for pain relief (95% CI), the extent of consensus (%), and the strength of recommendation (mean ± SEM) for each proposition. These recommendations are the most well-developed guidelines currently available, and clinicians should be encouraged to adopt them thoughtfully in their clinical practice (**Table 3**).

Nonpharmacologic Approaches

Education
Patients should be encouraged to participate in self-management programs (eg, those conducted by the Arthritis Foundation), informed regarding the natural history of their disease (the Arthritis Foundation provides reliable information for patients at their Web site www.arthritis.org under the topic of "Diseases" and the subheading "Disease Center"), and provided resources for social support and instruction on coping skills.[30,31]

Table 2
Experts' propositions developed through three Delphi rounds ordered according to topic (general, nonpharmacologic, pharmacologic, invasive, and surgical)

Number	Proposition
1	The optimal management of hip OA requires a combination of nonpharmacologic and pharmacologic treatment modalities.
2	The treatment of hip OA should be tailored according to (a) hip risk factors (obesity, adverse mechanical factors, physical activity, dysplasia); (b) general risk factors (age, sex, comorbidity, comedication); (c) the level of pain intensity, disability, and handicap; (d) the location and degree of structural damage; and (e) the wishes and expectations of the patient.
3	Nonpharmacologic treatment of hip OA should include regular education, exercise, appliances (sticks, insoles), and weight reduction if the patient is obese or overweight.
4	Because of its efficacy and safety, paracetamol (up to 4 g/d) is the oral analgesic of first choice for mild-to-moderate pain and, if successful, is the preferred long-term oral analgesic.
5	NSAIDs at the lowest effective dose should be added or substituted in patients who respond inadequately to paracetamol. In patients with increased gastrointestinal risk, nonselective NSAIDs plus a gastroprotective agent or selective COX-2 inhibitors should be used.
6	Opioid analgesics, with or without paracetamol, are useful alternatives in patients in whom NSAIDs, including COX-2 selective inhibitors (coxibs), are contraindicated, ineffective, or poorly tolerated.
7	SYSADOA (glucosamine sulfate, chondroitin sulfate, diacerein, avocado soybean unsaponifiable, and hyaluronic acid) have symptomatic effects and low toxicity, but effect sizes are small, suitable patients are not well defined, and clinically relevant structure modification and pharmacoeconomic aspects are not well established.
8	Intra-articular steroid injections (guided by ultrasound or radiography) may be considered in patients with a flare that is unresponsive to analgesic and NSAIDs.
9	Osteotomy and joint-preserving surgical procedures should be considered in young adults with symptomatic hip OA, especially in the presence of dysplasia or varus/valgus deformity.
10	Joint replacement has to be considered in patients with radiographic evidence of hip OA who have refractory pain and disability.

Abbreviation: SYSADOA, symptomatic slow-acting drugs for osteoarthritis.
From Zhang W, Doherty M, Arden N, et al. EULAR evidence based recommendations for the management of hip osteoarthritis: report of a task force of the EULAR Standing Committee for International Clinical Studies Including Therapeutics (ESCISIT)[see comment] [review]. Ann Rheum Dis 2005;64(5):669–81; with permission.

Weight loss

Clinicians should encourage overweight and obese patients with hip and knee OA to lose weight through a combination of diet and exercise. Weight loss facilitates load reduction experienced by the weight-bearing hips and knees. The Arthritis, Diet, and Activity Promotion trial showed that diet and exercise leads to overall improvements in self-reported measures of pain and function in older overweight and obese adults with knee OA,[32] even with loss of just 5% of their total weight over 18 months.

Exercise

Exercise increases aerobic capacity, muscle strength, and endurance and also facilitates weight loss.[32,33] All persons capable of exercise should be encouraged to

Table 3
OARSI recommendations and research evidence for the management of osteoarthritis of the hip and knee

Proposition	Level of Evidence[a]	Effect Size for Pain (95% CI)[b]	Frequency Recommended in Existing Guidelines	Level of Consensus (%)	Strength of Recommendation (%) (95% CI)
General					
1. Optimal management of OA requires a combination of nonpharmacologic and pharmacologic modalities.	IV	—	12/12	100	96 (93–99)
Nonpharmacologic modalities of treatment					
2. All patients with hip and knee OA should be given information, access to, and education about the objectives of treatment and the importance of changes in lifestyle, exercise, pacing of activities, weight reduction, and other measures to unload the damaged joint(s). The initial focus should be on self-help and patient-driven treatments rather than on passive therapies delivered by health professionals. Subsequently, emphasis should be placed on encouraging adherence to the regimen of nonpharmacologic therapy.	Ia (education) IV (adherence)	0.06 (0.02, 0.10)	8/8	92	97 (95–99)
3. The clinical status of patients with hip or knee OA can be improved if patients are contacted regularly by phone.	Ia	0.12 (0.00, 0.24)	2/2	77	66 (57–75)
4. Patients with symptomatic hip and knee OA may benefit from referral to a physical therapist for evaluation and instruction in appropriate exercises to reduce pain and improve functional capacity. This evaluation may result in provision of assistive devices such as canes and walkers, as appropriate.	IV	—	5/5	100	89 (82–96)
5. Patients with hip and knee OA should be encouraged to undertake, and continue to undertake, regular aerobic, muscle-strengthening, and range of motion exercises. For patients with symptomatic hip OA, exercises in water can be effective.	Ia (knee) IV(hip) Ib (hip, water-based)	Aerobic, 0.52 (0.34, 0.70) Strength, 0.32 (0.23, 0.42) Water-based, 0.25 (0.02, 0.47)	21/21 21/21 8/8	85	96 (93–99)

Recommendation					
6. Patients with hip and knee OA who are overweight should be encouraged to lose weight and maintain their weight at a lower level.	Ia	0.13 (−0.12, 0.38)	13/14	100	96 (92–100)
7. Walking aids can reduce pain in patients with hip and knee OA. Patients should be given instruction in the optimal use of a cane or crutch in the contralateral hand. Frames or wheeled walkers are often preferable for those with bilateral disease.	IV	—	11/11	100	90 (84–96)
8. In patients with knee OA and mild-to-moderate varus or valgus instability, a knee brace can reduce pain, improve stability, and diminish the risk of falling.	Ia		8/9	92	76 (69–83)
9. Every patient with hip or knee OA should receive advice concerning appropriate footwear. In patients with knee OA, insoles can reduce pain and improve ambulation. Lateral wedged insoles can be of symptomatic benefit for some patients with medial tibiofemoral compartment OA.	IV (footwear) Ia (insole)	—	12/13	92	77 (66–88)
10. Some thermal modalities may be effective for relieving symptoms in hip and knee OA.	Ia	0.69 (−0.07, 1.45)	7/10	77	64 (60–68)
11. Transcutaneous electrical nerve stimulation can help with short-term pain control in some patients with hip or knee OA.	Ia	—	8/10	69	58 (45–72)
12. Acupuncture may be of symptomatic benefit in patients with knee OA.	Ia	0.51 (0.23, 0.79)	5/8	69	59 (47–71)
Pharmacologic modalities of treatment					
13. Acetaminophen (up to 4 g/d) can be an effective initial oral analgesic for treatment of mild-to-moderate pain in patients with knee or hip OA. In the absence of an adequate response, or in the presence of severe pain or inflammation, alternative pharmacologic therapy should be considered based on relative efficacy and safety, as well as concomitant medications and comorbidities.	Ia (knee) IV (hip)	0.21 (0.02, 0.41)	16/16	77	92 (88–99)

(continued on next page)

Table 3
(continued)

Proposition	Level of Evidence[a]	Effect Size for Pain (95% CI)[b]	Frequency Recommended in Existing Guidelines	Level of Consensus (%)	Strength of Recommendation (%) (95% CI)
14. In patients with symptomatic hip or knee OA, NSAIDs should be used at the lowest effective dose, but their long-term use should be avoided if possible. In patients with increased gastrointestinal risk, either a COX-2 selective agent or a nonselective NSAID with co-prescription of a proton pump inhibitor or misoprostol for gastroprotection may be considered, but NSAIDs, including both nonselective and COX-2 selective agents, should be used with caution in patients with cardiovascular risk factors.	Ia (knee) Ia (hip)	0.32 (0.24, 0.39)	NSAID + PPi, 8/8 NSAID + misoprostol, 8/8 COX-2 inhibitors, 11/11	100	93 (88–99)
15. Topical NSAIDs and capsaicin can be effective as adjunctives and alternatives to oral analgesic/anti-inflammatory agents in knee OA.	Ia (NSAIDs) Ia (capsaicin)	0.41 (0.22, 0.59)	7/9 8/9	100	85 (75–95)
16. Intra-articular injections with corticosteroids can be used in the treatment of hip or knee OA and should be considered particularly when patients have moderate-to-severe pain not responding satisfactorily to oral analgesic/anti-inflammatory agents and in patients with symptomatic knee OA with effusions or other physical signs of local inflammation.	Ib (hip) Ia (knee)	0.72 (0.42, 1.02)	11/13	69	78 (61–95)
17. Injections of intra-articular hyaluronate may be useful in patients with knee or hip OA. They are characterized by delayed onset but prolonged duration of symptomatic benefit when compared with intra-articular injections of corticosteroids.	Ia (knee) Ia (hip)	0.32 (0.17, 0.47)	8/9	85	64 (43–85)
18. Treatment with glucosamine and/or chondroitin sulfate may provide symptomatic benefit in patients with knee OA. If no response is apparent within 6 months, treatment should be discontinued.	Ia (glucosamine) Ia (chondroitin)	0.45 (0.04, 0.86) 0.30 (−0.10, 0.70)	6/10 2/7	92	63 (44–82)

Recommendation	Strength of recommendation			
19. In patients with symptomatic knee OA, glucosamine sulfate and chondroitin sulfate may have structure-modifying effects, whereas diacerein may have structure-modifying effects in patients with symptomatic OA of the hip.	Ib (knee) Ib (hip)	—	69	41 (20–62)
20. The use of weak opioids and narcotic analgesics can be considered for the treatment of refractory pain in patients with hip or knee OA when other pharmacologic agents have been ineffective or are contraindicated. Stronger opioids should only be used for the management of severe pain in exceptional circumstances. Nonpharmacologic therapies should be continued in such patients and surgical treatments considered.	Ia (week opioids) IV (strong opioids) IV (others)	9/9	92	82 (74–90)
Surgical modalities of treatment				
21. Patients with hip or knee OA who are not obtaining adequate pain relief and functional improvement from a combination of nonpharmacologic and pharmacologic treatment should be considered for joint replacement surgery. Replacement arthroplasties are effective and cost-effective interventions for patients with significant symptoms or functional limitations associated with a reduced health-related quality of life despite conservative therapy.	III	14/14	92	96 (94–98)
22. Unicompartmental knee replacement is effective in patients with knee OA restricted to a single compartment.	IIb	—	100	76 (64–88)
23. Osteotomy and joint-preserving surgical procedures should be considered in young adults with symptomatic hip OA, especially in the presence of dysplasia. For the young and physically active patient with significant symptoms from unicompartmental knee OA, high tibial osteotomy may offer an alternative intervention that delays the need for joint replacement some 10 years.	IIb	10/10	100	75 (64–86)

(continued on next page)

Table 3
(continued)

Proposition	Level of Evidence[a]	Effect Size for Pain (95% CI)[b]	Frequency Recommended in Existing Guidelines	Level of Consensus (%)	Strength of Recommendation (%) (95% CI)
24. The role of joint lavage and arthroscopic debridement in knee OA is controversial. Although some studies have demonstrated short-term symptom relief, others suggest that improvement in symptoms could be attributable to a placebo effect.	Ib (lavage) Ib (debridement)	0.09 (−0.27, 0.44) −0.01 (−0.37, 0.35)	3/3 5/6	100	60 (47–82)
25. In patients with OA of the knee, joint fusion can be considered as a salvage procedure when joint replacement has failed.	IV	—	2/2	100	69 (57–82)

[a] Level of evidence: Ia, meta-analysis of randomized controlled trials; Ib, randomized controlled trial; IIa, controlled study without randomization; IIb, quasi-experimental study (eg, uncontrolled trial, one arm dose-response trial); III, observational studies (eg, case-control, cohort, cross-sectional studies); IV, expert opinion.

[b] Effect size (ES) is the standard mean difference, that is, the mean difference between a treatment and a control group divided by the standard deviation of the difference. ES = 0.2 is considered small, ES = 0.5 is moderate, and ES >0.8 is large.

From Zhang W, Moskovitz R, Nuki G, et al. OARSI recommendations for the management of hip and knee osteoarthritis. Part II. OARSI evidence-based, expert consensus guidelines. Osteoarthritis Cartilage 2008;16(2):137–62; with permission.

partake in a low impact aerobic exercise program (walking, biking, swimming, or other aquatic exercise). Quadriceps strengthening exercises have been demonstrated to lead to improvements in pain and function.[34–36]

Physical therapy
Physical therapy consists of several strategies to facilitate symptom resolution and improve functional deficits, including range of motion exercise, muscle strengthening, muscle stretching, and soft tissue mobilization. Although the results of a recent randomized, double blind, placebo-controlled trial found that regular contact with a therapist (sham ultrasound therapy) provided an equivalent effect in reducing pain and disability, the effects in both groups in symptom improvement were substantial.[37] It is possible that the sham ultrasound therapy may have provided some treatment (eg, massage). Another randomized controlled trial focused more on quadriceps strengthening did show a benefit of physical therapy in OA of the knee.[38] A recent randomized controlled trial also found that application of taping was efficacious in the management of pain and disability in persons with OA of the knee.[39]

Knee braces and orthotics
Because involvement of the medial tibiofemoral compartment is especially frequent, interventions whose goal is to realign the knee so as to reduce transarticular loading on the medial compartment, such as valgus bracing, are sometimes used clinically. Despite knowing for many years that altering loads in patients with OA of the knee is a safe, inexpensive, and effective modality of treatment, few studies have evaluated these therapies.[40–43] For persons with instability of the knee, evidence suggests that valgus bracing and orthotics shift the load away from the medial compartment and, in doing so, may provide considerable relief of pain and improvement in function.[42–44] To the authors' knowledge, only two randomized trials of the effectiveness of unloader braces for the treatment of varus knee OA have been reported.[41,42] These studies demonstrated that wearing a valgus brace results in a clinically significant and immediate improvement in the pain and function of patients with medial OA of the knee. In both studies there was an approximately 50% improvement in pain and function, which is much more than seen with typical NSAID prescription.[45,46]

With regard to orthotics, observational studies suggest that lateral heel wedges could reduce medial compartmental loading; however, two randomized controlled trials of lateral heel wedges in medial knee OA have not demonstrated an improvement in symptoms.[47,48] Conceptually, there may still be merit to using orthotics to restore normal foot anatomy in patients with foot pathology (ie, hallicus valgus or planovalgus deformities), particularly because all forces that go through the knee and hip pass through the foot first.

Use of a cane in the hand contralateral to the painful joint should be considered in patients with persistent ambulatory pain from OA of the hip or knee. A cane reduces loading force on the joint and is associated with a decrease in pain in patients with hip and knee OA.[49] Appropriate footwear advice should be given to all patients with OA of the knee and hip.

Pharmacologic Approaches

Structure-modifying efficacy has not been convincingly demonstrated for any of the existing pharmacologic agents. Furthermore, current drug treatment paradigms reduce the symptoms of OA, but their efficacy is limited, leaving the patients with a substantial pain burden. The difference between placebo and active treatment for many widely used current therapies including hyaluronic acid and glucosamine is exceedingly difficult to detect.[50,51] This observation is further compounded by the fact that many of these agents have side-effect profiles that are raising a number of legitimate concerns about their long- term safety, especially COX-2 inhibitors.[52] Judicious use of topical NSAIDs has been demonstrated to be effective in relieving pain in OA when compared with placebo for both hand and knee OA.[53,54] This route possibly reduces gastrointestinal adverse reactions by maximizing local delivery and minimizing systemic toxicity.

Surgical Approaches

Surgery should be resisted when symptoms can be managed by other treatment modalities. The typical indications for surgery are debilitating pain and major limitation of function such as walking, working, or sleeping. Although this treatment for knee OA has a large effect size,[55–57] it is an invasive modality that has attendant risks. If surgical intervention is to be pursued, recent evidence has shown that patients operated on in low-volume hospitals or by low-volume surgeons have worse functional outcomes 2 years post total knee replacement than those operated on in high-volume hospitals by high-volume surgeons.[58]

SUMMARY

Despite the increasing prevalence of OA, many uncertainties exist pertaining to its management. Many putative risk factors are characterized by excessive loading of vulnerable joint structures. Clinical examination should include an assessment of joint function and the influence of modifiable risks such as malalignment, muscle strength, and obesity. Braces, footwear, exercises, and dieting are prescribed for the purpose of improving the distribution of loads on the joints and reducing the likelihood that OA and its symptoms will worsen. In this conservative approach, pharmaceuticals of low toxicity are preferred and given only when other methods fail to achieve functional improvement. Attention to these factors in managing the patient with OA is critical if we are to impact the increasing burden of this disease among older adults.

REFERENCES

1. Lawrence RC, Helmick CG, Arnett FC, et al. Estimates of the prevalence of arthritis and selected musculoskeletal disorders in the United States [see comments]. Arthritis Rheum 1998;41(5):778–99.
2. Badley E, DesMeules M. Arthritis in Canada: an ongoing challenge. Ottawa (ON): Canada; 2003. Ref Type: Report.
3. Felson DT. An update on the pathogenesis and epidemiology of osteoarthritis [review]. Radiol Clin North Am 2004;42(1):1–9.
4. Guccione AA, Felson DT, Anderson JJ, et al. The effects of specific medical conditions on the functional limitations of elders in the Framingham study. Am J Public Health 1994;84(3):351–8.
5. Glazier RH, Dalby DM, Badley EM, et al. Management of common musculoskeletal problems: a survey of Ontario primary care physicians [see comment]. CMAJ 1998;158(8):1037–40.
6. Jordan KM, Arden NK, Doherty M, et al. EULAR recommendations 2003: an evidence based approach to the management of knee osteoarthritis. Report of a Task Force of the Standing Committee for International Clinical Studies Including Therapeutic Trials (ESCISIT) [review]. Ann Rheum Dis 2003;62(12):1145–55.
7. Zhang W, Doherty M, Arden N, et al. EULAR evidence based recommendations for the management of hip osteoarthritis: report of a task force of the EULAR

Standing Committee for International Clinical Studies Including Therapeutics (ESCISIT) [see comment] [review]. Ann Rheum Dis 2005;64(5):669–81.

8. Anonymous. Recommendations for the medical management of osteoarthritis of the hip and knee: 2000 update. American College of Rheumatology Subcommittee on Osteoarthritis Guidelines. Arthritis Rheum 2000;43(9):1905–15.

9. Zhang W, Moskovitz R, Nuki G, et al. OARSI recommendations for the management of hip and knee osteoarthritis. Part II. OARSI evidence-based, expert consensus guidelines. Osteoarthritis Cartilage 2008;16(2):137–62.

10. Hunter D. In the clinic: osteoarthritis [review]. Ann Intern Med 2007;147(3): ITC8-1-6.

11. Hunter D, Felson D. Osteoarthritis [review]. BMJ 2006;332(7542):639–42.

12. Altman R, Asch E, Bloch D, et al. Development of criteria for the classification and reporting of osteoarthritis: classification of osteoarthritis of the knee. Diagnostic and Therapeutic Criteria Committee of the American Rheumatism Association. Arthritis Rheum 1986;29(8):1039–49.

13. Peat G, McCarney R, Croft P. Knee pain and osteoarthritis in older adults: a review of community burden and current use of primary health care [see comments] [review]. Ann Rheum Dis 2001;60(2):91–7.

14. Hill CL, Gale DG, Chaisson CE, et al. Knee effusions, popliteal cysts, and synovial thickening: association with knee pain in osteoarthritis. J Rheumatol 2001;28(6): 1330–7.

15. Dieppe PA, Lohmander LS. Pathogenesis and management of pain in osteoarthritis [review]. Lancet 2005;365(9463):965–73.

16. Witonski D, Wagrowska-Danilewicz M, Raczynska-Witonska G, et al. Distribution of substance P nerve fibers in osteoarthritis knee joint. Pol J Pathol 2005;56(4): 203–6.

17. Wojtys EM, Beaman DN, Glover RA, et al. Innervation of the human knee joint by substance P fibers. Arthroscopy 1990;6(4):254–63.

18. Benedek TG, Benedek TG. A history of the understanding of cartilage [review]. Osteoarthritis & Cartilage 2006;14(3):203–9.

19. Freeman MA, Wyke B. The innervation of the knee joint: an anatomical and histological study in the cat. J Anat 1967;101(Pt 3):505–32.

20. Marshall KW, Theriault E, Homonko DA, et al. Distribution of substance P and calcitonin gene related peptide immunoreactivity in the normal feline knee. J Rheumatol 1994;21(5):883–9.

21. Hunter DJ, Zhang YQ, Tu X, et al. Change in joint space width: hyaline articular cartilage loss or alteration in meniscus? Arthritis Rheum 2006;54(8):2488–95.

22. Altman RD. Classification of disease: osteoarthritis [review]. Semin Arthritis Rheum 1991;20(6 Suppl 2):40–7.

23. Hannan MT, Felson DT, Pincus T. Analysis of the discordance between radiographic changes and knee pain in osteoarthritis of the knee. J Rheumatol 2000;27(6):1513–7.

24. Bhattacharyya T, Gale D, Dewire P, et al. The clinical importance of meniscal tears demonstrated by magnetic resonance imaging in osteoarthritis of the knee [comment]. J Bone Joint Surg Am 2003;85(1):4–9.

25. Englund M, Lohmander LS. Risk factors for symptomatic knee osteoarthritis fifteen to twenty-two years after meniscectomy. Arthritis Rheum 2004;50(9):2811–9.

26. Roos EM, Ostenberg A, Roos H, et al. Long-term outcome of meniscectomy: symptoms, function, and performance tests in patients with or without radiographic osteoarthritis compared to matched controls. Osteoarthritis & Cartilage 2001;9(4):316–24.

27. Zacher J, Gursche A. Regional musculoskeletal conditions: 'hip' pain [review]. Best Pract Res Clin Rheumatol 2003;17(1):71–85.
28. Calmbach WL, Hutchens M. Evaluation of patients presenting with knee pain. Part II. Differential diagnosis [review]. Am Fam Physician 2003;68(5):917–22.
29. Tallon D, Chard J, Dieppe P. Relation between agendas of the research community and the research consumer. Lancet 2000;355(9220):2037–40.
30. Superio-Cabuslay E, Ward MM, Lorig KR. Patient education interventions in osteoarthritis and rheumatoid arthritis: a meta-analytic comparison with non-steroidal anti-inflammatory drug treatment. Arthritis Care Res 1996;9(4):292–301.
31. Marks R, Allegrante JP, Lorig K. A review and synthesis of research evidence for self-efficacy–enhancing interventions for reducing chronic disability: implications for health education practice (part I) [review]. Health Promot Pract 2005;6(1):37–43.
32. Messier SP, Loeser RF, Miller GD, et al. Exercise and dietary weight loss in overweight and obese older adults with knee osteoarthritis: the Arthritis, Diet, and Activity Promotion Trial [see comment]. Arthritis Rheum 2004;50(5):1501–10.
33. Ettinger WHJ, Burns R, Messier SP, et al. A randomized trial comparing aerobic exercise and resistance exercise with a health education program in older adults with knee osteoarthritis: the Fitness Arthritis and Seniors Trial (FAST) [see comment]. JAMA 1997;277(1):25–31.
34. Roddy E, Zhang W, Doherty M, et al. Aerobic walking or strengthening exercise for osteoarthritis of the knee? A systematic review [see comment] [review]. Ann Rheum Dis 2005;64(4):544–8.
35. Roddy E, Zhang W, Doherty M, et al. Evidence-based recommendations for the role of exercise in the management of osteoarthritis of the hip or knee—the MOVE consensus [see comment] [review]. Rheumatology 2005;44(1):67–73.
36. Schattner A. Review: both aerobic and home-based quadriceps strengthening exercises reduce pain and disability in knee osteoarthritis. ACP J Club 2005; 143(3):71.
37. Bennell KL, Hinman RS, Metcalf BR, et al. Efficacy of physiotherapy management of knee joint osteoarthritis: a randomised, double blind, placebo controlled trial. Ann Rheum Dis 2005;64(6):906–12.
38. Deyle GD, Henderson NE, Matekel RL, et al. Effectiveness of manual physical therapy and exercise in osteoarthritis of the knee: a randomized, controlled trial [see comment]. Ann Intern Med 2000;132(3):173–81.
39. Hinman RS, Crossley KM, McConnell J, et al. Efficacy of knee tape in the management of osteoarthritis of the knee: blinded randomised controlled trial [see comment]. BMJ 2003;327(7407):135.
40. Hillstrom H, Mcguire J, Whitney K, et al. Immediate effects of conservative realignment therapies of varus knee osteoarthritis [abstract]. Arthritis Rheum 1998;1556.
41. Horlick S, Loomer R. Valgus knee bracing for medial gonarthrosis. Clin J Sport Med 1993;3:251–5.
42. Kirkley A, Webster-Bogaert S, Litchfield R, et al. The effect of bracing on varus gonarthrosis. J Bone Joint Surg 1999;81(4):539–48.
43. Draper ER, Cable JM, Sanchez-Ballester J, et al. Improvement in function after valgus bracing of the knee: an analysis of gait symmetry. J Bone Joint Surg Br 2000;82(7):1001–5.
44. Pollo FE, Otis JC, Backus SI, et al. Reduction of medial compartment loads with valgus bracing of the osteoarthritic knee. Am J Sports Med 2002;30(3):414–21.
45. Brouwer R, Jakma T, Verhagen A, et al. Braces and orthoses for treating osteoarthritis of the knee. Cochrane Database Syst Rev 2005;2:CD004020.

46. Todd PA, Clissold SP. Naproxen: a reappraisal of its pharmacology and therapeutic use in rheumatic diseases and pain states [review]. Drugs 1990; 40(1):91–137.
47. Maillefert JF, Hudry C, Baron G, et al. Laterally elevated wedged insoles in the treatment of medial knee osteoarthritis: a prospective randomized controlled study. Osteoarthritis & Cartilage 2001;9(8):738–45.
48. Baker K, Goggins J, Xie H, et al. A randomized crossover trial of a wedged insole for treatment of knee osteoarthritis. Arthritis Rheum 2007;56(4):1198–203.
49. Neumann DA, Neumann DA. Biomechanical analysis of selected principles of hip joint protection [review]. Arthritis Care Res 1989;2(4):146–55.
50. Lo GH, LaValley M, McAlindon T, et al. Intra-articular hyaluronic acid in treatment of knee osteoarthritis: a meta-analysis [see comment]. JAMA 2003;290(23): 3115–21.
51. Clegg DO, Reda DJ, Harris CL, et al. Glucosamine, chondroitin sulfate, and the two in combination for painful knee osteoarthritis [see comment]. N Engl J Med 2006;354(8):795–808.
52. Ortiz E. Market withdrawal of Vioxx: is it time to rethink the use of COX-2 inhibitors? J Bone Joint Surg Br 2004;10(6):551–4.
53. Bookman AA, Williams KS, Shainhouse JZ, et al. Effect of a topical diclofenac solution for relieving symptoms of primary osteoarthritis of the knee: a randomized controlled trial [see comment]. CMAJ 2004;171(4):333–8.
54. Lin J, Zhang W, Jones A, et al. Efficacy of topical non-steroidal anti-inflammatory drugs in the treatment of osteoarthritis: meta-analysis of randomised controlled trials [see comment]. BMJ 2004;329(7461):324.
55. Liang MH, Larson MG, Cullen KE, et al. Comparative measurement efficiency and sensitivity of five health status instruments for arthritis research. Arthritis Rheum 1985;28(5):542–7.
56. Roos E, Nilsdotter A, Toksvig-Larsen S. Patient expectations suggest additional outcomes in total knee replacement [abstract]. Arthritis Rheum 2002;46(Suppl 9):199.
57. Cohen J. Statistical power analysis for the behavioral sciences. New York: Academic Press; 1977.
58. Katz JN, Mahomed NN, Baron JA, et al. Association of hospital and surgeon procedure volume with patient-centered outcomes of total knee replacement in a population-based cohort of patients age 65 years and older. Arthritis Rheum 2007;56(2):568–74.

Obesity and Osteoarthritis: Disease Genesis and Nonpharmacologic Weight Management

Stephen P. Messier, PhD

KEYWORDS

• Function • Gait • Inflammation • Exercise • Weight loss

OBESITY AND RISK FOR OSTEOARTHRITIS DEVELOPMENT

First documented in 1945,[1] the strong association between obesity and knee osteoarthritis (OA) has been widely verified. Leach and colleagues[2] found that 83% of their female subjects who had knee OA were obese compared with 42% of the control group. In a case-controlled study of 675 matched pairs, Coggon and colleagues[3] determined that the risk for knee OA in people who had a body mass index (BMI) of 30 kg/m^2 or greater was 6.8 times that of normal-weight controls. Felson and colleagues[4] showed that a 5.1-kg loss in body mass over a 10-year period reduced the odds of developing OA by more than 50%. Ettinger and colleagues[5] examined the effects of comorbid diseases on disability and found that people who had a BMI greater than 30 kg/m^2 were 4.2 times more likely to have knee OA than leaner people. Knee OA and obesity were each significantly associated with poorer physical function, with odds ratios of 4.3 and 1.7, respectively; when obesity was combined with knee OA, the odds ratio increased to 9.8. Taken together, these studies indicate that obesity is a major risk factor for knee OA and associated functional impairment. A high BMI is also associated with faster disease progression.[6]

OA is most commonly located in the small joints of the hand. Unlike knee OA, the association between obesity and hand OA is not strong. Doherty and colleagues[7] reviewed the literature on hand OA and concluded that BMI and waist circumference were not risk factors, especially in older adults. Similarly, Kalichman and Kobyliansky[8] used an observational, cross-sectional design to study 745 women who had hand OA

A version of this article originally appeared in the 34:3 issue of the *Rheumatic Disease Clinics of North America.*
Supported by NIH grants 1R01AR052528-01 and M01-RR-0021.
J.B. Snow Biomechanics Laboratory, Department of Health and Exercise Science, Wake Forest University, Winston-Salem, NC 27109, USA
E-mail address: messier@wfu.edu

Med Clin N Am 93 (2009) 145–159
doi:10.1016/j.mcna.2008.09.011
0025-7125/08/$ – see front matter

and saw no relationship with BMI or waist circumference. The authors suggested that obesity might be a mechanical rather than a systemic risk factor for OA, which would explain its strong association with OA in weight-bearing joints relative to the small joints of the hand.

IMPACT OF OBESITY ON FUNCTION AND GAIT

The National Health and Nutrition Examination Survey I and Epidemiologic Follow-up studies revealed that obesity at baseline increased upper and lower body disability across 20 years.[5,9] More recently, Jenkins[10] found that functional impairment in older adults increased with BMI. In the Cardiovascular Health Study, an adjusted odds ratio of 2.94 for self-reported mobility-related disability was found for those in the highest versus the lowest quintile of fat mass.[11]

As body weight increases, fat mass and fat-free mass increase.[12] The relationship between fat-free mass and BMI is stronger in men, suggesting that increased BMI in women is attributable predominantly to an increase in fat mass. Although these data seem to imply that obese people are stronger than their nonobese counterparts, the opposite is true. Specifically, when strength is represented as a function of body weight, obese men and women are weaker, irrespective of age.[13] In obese men aged 60 to 80, mean knee strength is 65% of body weight, as compared with 77% for controls; for their female counterparts, mean knee strength is 50% of body weight, compared with 62% for nonobese women.

Muscle weakness in older adults can have dire consequences. It is the second leading cause of falls in the elderly, accounting for 17%.[14] Falls are the leading cause of death by injury in older adults, and 75% of deaths attributable to falls occur in adults older than 65 years of age. Only one half of older adults hospitalized because of falls are alive after 1 year. By 2030, 280,000 Americans will die annually from falls.[15]

Loss of balance causes falls, so balance measures are used to identify people who are more susceptible. Kejonen and colleagues[16] found significant correlations between poor balance and high BMI in women but not men, once again suggesting that muscle weakness is a mediator of poor balance and falls. Jadelis and colleagues[17] found that for older adults who had a BMI greater than 30 kg/m^2 and a given amount of knee strength, the more obese, the worse the balance, suggesting that obesity, independent of strength, is a risk factor for poor balance and falls.

Not without reason, then, obesity is related to a fear of falling and injury risk.[18,19] Austin and colleagues[18] followed 1282 community-dwelling women aged 70 to 85 years for 3 years and found that obesity was independently associated with fear of falling at baseline and with the onset of this fear in women who were symptom-free at baseline. In a sample of more than 42,000 adults, the odds of sustaining an injury were greater among those who had excess weight. As BMI category increased from overweight ($25.0 \ kg/m^2 \leq BMI \leq 29.9 \ kg/m^2$) to class III obesity ($BMI \geq 40.0 \ kg/m^2$), the odds of sustaining an injury, including those related to falls, increased from 15% to 48%.[19]

Obese adults make adjustments to help stabilize their larger mass and reduce fall risk. DeVita and Hortobagyi[20] compared obese and lean adults and noted that the obese group increased ankle torque during walking but showed no difference in knee or hip torque. Specifically, the ankle plantar flexors act eccentrically to control the forward motion of the leg throughout stance to stabilize body mass and at toe-off to assist in propulsion. Their greater mass requires more ankle plantar flexor torque to perform these tasks.

Obese people try to reduce the load on their knees by shortening their stride and reducing knee extensor torque. In an obese cohort, the greater the BMI, the shorter the stride and the lower the knee-joint extensor/flexor torque, actually shifting from an overall extensor torque to a dominant flexor torque at high BMIs. This switch results in the hamstrings, rather than the quadriceps, providing knee stability. In lean subjects, no relationship exists among BMI, stride length, and knee torques, indicating that lower BMI values have little effect on gait.[20]

Liu and Nigg[21] examined the effects of rigid and soft tissue mass on impact forces during running. They termed the soft tissue mass "wobbling mass." Their spring-damper-mass model consisted of upper- and lower-body rigid and wobbling masses. A computer simulation found that upper-body wobbling mass had no effect on impact forces but strongly influenced the propulsive peak. As upper-body wobbling mass increased, vertical force propulsive peaks increased, suggesting that obese individuals exert greater forces during gait because of their greater wobbling mass.

Empiric data support Liu and Nigg's model. Messier and colleagues[22] found a strong positive association between BMI and peak ground reaction forces ($r = 0.76, P = .0001$) in older adults who had knee OA. A study by Browning and Kram[23] found that obese people exerted 60% greater vertical ground reaction forces compared with normal-weight people (**Fig. 1**).

Abnormal gait is characteristic of obese people. Messier and colleagues[24] found that a severely overweight population walked with bilaterally abducted forefeet, or a stance that was 276% more toed-out than that of a normal-weight group. Chodera and Levell[25] suggested that the feet have different functions, with the more abducted forefoot responsible for balance and the less abducted foot responsible for direction. In severely obese people, the amount of abduction is significantly greater in the feet relative to a normal weight control group, suggesting that balance is more important than direction.[24]

In addition to greater forefoot angles, severely obese people have more rearfoot motion: typically, greater touchdown angle, more pronation range of motion, and

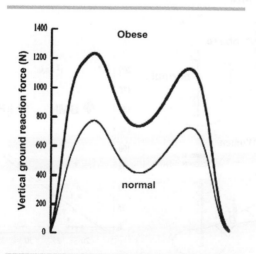

Fig. 1. Obese individuals exert 60% more force than normal-weight individuals. (*From* Browning RC, Kram R. Effects of obesity on the biomechanics of walking at different speeds. Med Sci Sports Exerc 2007;39(9):1635; with permission.)

faster pronation. This excessive rearfoot motion may cause injury and discomfort and negatively affect mobility.

Plantar fasciitis and heel pain are commonly associated with obesity. In a case-controlled study, obese subjects were five times more likely to have heel pain than their nonobese counterparts, with an odds ratio of 5.6.[26] Similarly, obese men and women exert greater plantar pressure while standing and walking.[27-31] Hills and colleagues[28] found a significant correlation (r = 0.81) between midfoot peak pressure and BMI (**Fig. 2**A, B). Gravante and colleagues[32] found greater midfoot weight-bearing area in obese men and women versus a control. The additional pressure on the medial longitudinal arch could have a detrimental effect on the plantar ligaments, causing them to collapse. Considering that the medial longitudinal arch is critical in distributing loads to the rearfoot and forefoot, it is not surprising that foot ailments are common among the obese.

In summary, obese adults exert greater forces than normal-weight adults during gait. As obesity worsens they try to minimize these loads by shortening their stride. Adjusting gait mechanics without reducing body weight does not eliminate obesity's detrimental effects on the lower extremities, however.

What role obesity plays in the degenerative process is unclear. The multiphasic nature of articular cartilage permits it to withstand compressive stresses as high as 20 MPa, or 3000 lb/in^2.[33] A densely woven collagen fibrillar network, water (normally <80% by wet weight), and ionic species of Na^+, Ca^{++}, and Cl^- provide a unique combination of material properties that prevents such high loads from crushing the tissue. Cartilage has little permeability, resulting in large interstitial fluid pressures inside the tissue during compression. This pressurized fluid accounts for most of the load-bearing capability and protects proteoglycans and chondrocytes from dangerously high stresses and strains. Moderate running increases cartilage matrix synthesis and

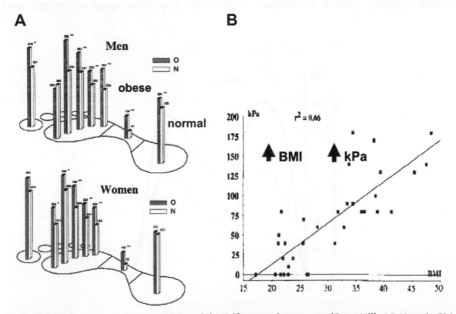

Fig. 2. (A) Peak pressure during walking. (B) Midfoot peak pressure. (*From* Hills AP, Hennig EM, McDonald M, et al. Plantar pressure differences between obese and non-obese adults: a biomechanical analysis. Int J Obes Relat Metab Disord 2001;25(11):1677; with permission.)

may have a protective effect on the joint.[34,35] Peak knee-joint compressive forces in humans during long-distance running range between 10 to 14 times body weight.[36] Despite these high forces, most studies have shown no relationship between running and OA.[37] Compressive loads during walking are less than half those found during running.[38] The cumulative effect of obesity on knee-joint loads during daily activities must therefore play the critical role in the disease process.

OBESITY AND INFLAMMATION

Obesity is typified by nutrient excess and insulin resistance, which are closely related to the excessive proinflammatory cytokine production seen in chronic inflammation.[39] Nutrient excess produces reactive oxygen species, resulting in oxidative stress that damages cells and triggers an inflammatory response. The increased inflammation blocks the protective action of insulin, which normally stimulates target cells to take up nutrients. Unfortunately, as excessive nutrients are consumed, neighboring cells and tissues that remain insulin sensitive are placed at risk. As insulin resistance progresses, inflammation is exacerbated, initiating a cycle of excessive nutrient intake/insulin resistance/inflammation.[40] In some cells, nutrient excess impairs endoplasmic reticulum function and accelerates the accumulation of fatty acid derivatives that also promote inflammation.[39]

The broad inflammatory response characteristic of obesity was first demonstrated by Hotamisligil and colleagues[41] in 1993. They showed that the inflammatory cytokine tumor necrosis factor alpha (TNF-α) was overexpressed 5 to 10 fold in obese compared with lean mice. TNF-α activates signal transduction cascades that result in insulin resistance. The inflammatory response seems to be triggered and to reside predominantly in adipose tissue, which secretes various hormones known collectively as adipokines. Deregulation of these proteins is associated with excessive weight gain, an inflammatory state, and various chronic diseases, including knee OA.[42]

INFLAMMATION AND OSTEOARTHRITIS

Because obese individuals have higher concentrations of inflammatory markers, inflammation may contribute to functional limitation and disease progression in those who have OA. Besides direct effects on the joint, inflammatory mediators can affect muscle function and lower the pain threshold. Recent studies confirm that low-grade inflammation plays a pathophysiologic role in OA. One of our earlier studies showed that the inflammatory cytokine interleukin-1 beta, believed to mediate joint inflammation and cartilage degradation in OA, was present in the joint fluids of patients who had OA.[43] Likewise, an inflammatory component associated with OA can be detected in the circulation because serum concentrations of inflammatory markers, such as cytokines (interleukin-6, TNF-α) and the acute-phase reactant C-reactive protein (CRP), are higher in people who have knee or hip OA.[44–46] Longitudinal studies demonstrate that high serum levels of CRP and TNF-α predict increased radiographic progression of knee OA as long as 5 years later.[45,47,48] A few studies, including one by our group,[49] associate OA severity and the resulting impaired physical function with higher inflammatory markers in the blood.[50,51] Severity, mobility, pain, stiffness, and radiographic progression are at least partly mediated by the level of chronic inflammation in a patient who has OA. Diffusion of cytokines from the synovial fluid into the cartilage could contribute to the cartilage matrix loss observed in OA by stimulating chondrocyte catabolic activity and inhibiting anabolic activity. The adipokine leptin increases TGF-β synthesis within the joint; TGF-β is a known stimulator of osteophyte formation.[52]

Weight loss lowers serum leptin levels in subjects who have OA and is related to improved function.[53]

No experimental studies in humans show that weight loss prevents knee OA. Felson and colleagues[4] demonstrated that a 5.1-kg loss over 10 years decreased the odds of developing knee OA by more than 50% in an observational study, however. Hartz and colleagues[54] suggested that the strong link between obesity and knee OA is related to the additional mechanical stress on the knees. It follows that weight loss should relieve this mechanical stress, improving function and reducing pain in the affected knee. In a case-controlled study, the odds ratio for knee OA prevalence with a BMI 30 kg/m^2 or greater was 6.8 compared with a reference group with a BMI between 20.0 and 24.9 kg/m^2. The authors predicted that 24% of surgical procedures for knee OA could be avoided by controlling obesity.[3] Inflammation and joint loads are important mechanisms in osteoarthritis disease pathogenesis; however, their exact roles in the process and their association with obesity remain unclear.

MANAGING BODY WEIGHT

Given the important influence obesity has in OA pathogenesis, intervening on this modifiable risk is a critically important public health goal. Wadden and colleagues[55,56] noted that obese individuals have difficulty achieving permanent weight loss. Successful weight loss and maintenance programs involve attention to several factors, including behavioral change strategies, extended treatment, increased hours of intervention contact, adherence to a rigorous diet, exercise, and inclusion of significant others.[57,58] Wing improved weight loss with increased treatment duration and intensity.[59] Although maintaining weight loss is challenging, individual attention to coping strategies and increased intervention efforts during the maintenance phase have produced success. Approximately 80% of clients on moderate calorie restriction remain in treatment for 20 weeks, and approximately 50% lose 9.1 kg or more. An average weekly loss of 0.4 to 0.5 kg, with an average 33% regained 1 year after treatment, is expected.

Maintaining weight loss seems to require rigorous follow-up contacts. Perri and colleagues[60] showed that participants in a 20-week behavioral therapy program, followed by an 18-week maintenance program with biweekly contact, maintained a 13.15-kg loss. Esposito and colleagues[61] produced a 14.7% loss over a 2-year period in women following a moderate energy-restricted diet of 1300 kcal/d for year 1 and 1500 kcal/d for year 2. This intervention used education, individualized goal setting, self-monitoring, and a structured exercise program. In the longest (3 years) and largest (n = 1032) study to date, Svetkey and colleagues[62] found that participants randomized to a personal contact intervention regained less weight during the 30-month maintenance phase that followed the 6-month loss period than participants in an interactive technology intervention or a self-directed control group. Personal contact seems to be a vital component of successful, long-term dietary weight-loss programs.

The long-term effectiveness of low-fat and low-carbohydrate diets is currently under debate. Meta-analyses have found them no more effective than a low-calorie diet in reducing weight and improving cardiovascular risk factors.[63,64] Increasingly popular meal-replacement diet drinks have been studied as a complement to reduced-calorie diets. Heymsfield and colleagues[65] performed meta- and pooled analyses of six clinical trials that compared partial meal replacement to reduced-calorie diet plans and found greater weight loss, reduced risk factors, and a lower drop-out rate with the partial meal replacement plan, but the small number of trials limited conclusions.

Weight loss reduces risk factors for symptomatic knee OA and lowers proinflammatory cytokines and adipokines believed to play a role in cartilage degradation. Our Arthritis, Diet, and Activity Promotion Trial (ADAPT)[66] diet groups achieved 5% weight loss over 18 months using a reduced-calorie diet with behavioral strategies, and the Physical Activity, Inflammation, and Body Composition Trial (PACT) pilot study achieved a 9% weight loss over 6 months in obese older adults who had knee OA by combining a partial meal replacement plan with accepted behavioral strategies.[67] Using a similar cohort and an intensive low-energy diet that achieved an 11% weight loss, Christensen and colleagues[68] found a threefold improvement in Western Ontario and McMaster Osteoarthritis Index (WOMAC) function over an 8-week period compared with a control diet group who lost 4% of their body weight. Cognitive strategies were used to promote behavior change. A recent meta-analysis of 35 potential trials identified only 4 that met the authors' inclusion criteria. From these 4 studies, they concluded that weight loss in patients who had knee OA significantly reduces disability and that a weight loss of at least 10% would result in a moderate to large clinical effect.[69] Christensen and colleagues[68] concluded that weight loss should be the first-choice therapy for obese adults who have knee OA.

Randomized clinical trials (RCTs) that examined weight loss in adults older than 65 years reported no difference in mortality compared with groups that did not lose weight.[70,71] Diehr and colleagues[72] suggested that for the aged population, quality of life and years of healthy life may be more appropriate outcomes. These measures have important public health implications for morbidity and daily living activities. Moreover, for older adults who have knee OA, pain reduction and improved mobility are important outcomes.

Loss of bone and muscle mass is a problem in weight-loss programs for older adults. Weight loss is associated with decreased bone mineral density,[73,74] increased bone turnover,[74] and increased fracture rates.[75,76] Fiatarone Singh[77] noted that combining hypocaloric diets with aerobic exercise in older adults resulted in loss of lean mass, which resistance training tended to offset. Janssen and colleagues[78] found no lean tissue loss when diet was combined with resistance or aerobic training in premenopausal women. In contrast, Wang and colleagues[79] found that a 6-month weight-loss intervention that incorporated partial meal replacements and aerobic and resistance exercises for older obese adults who had knee OA resulted in an 8.1% weight loss of which 19.9% was lean mass. The exercise training improved knee extensor strength 37% compared with a 1% loss of strength in a weight-stable control group, however. These results show that intentional weight loss, when combined with aerobic and resistance exercise training, improves knee extensor strength despite loss of lean body mass.

EXERCISE INTERVENTIONS

Although patients who have OA commonly avoid activity, physical exercise is an effective nonpharmacologic treatment. Several studies have shown that pain, physical function, and walking distance improve an average of 26%, 31%, and 15%, respectively, with short-term exercise.[80,81] Furthermore, long-term walking and resistance training programs have made significant, if modest, improvements in self-reported function (1%–11%), slowing the decline in physical function commonly seen in this disabled population (**Fig. 3**).[82–84] Participants in the Fitness Arthritis in Seniors Trial (FAST) who were randomized to either 18-month aerobic or resistance-training interventions showed a dose response to exercise, with higher compliance yielding better function, less pain, and longer 6-minute walking distance and similar gains being

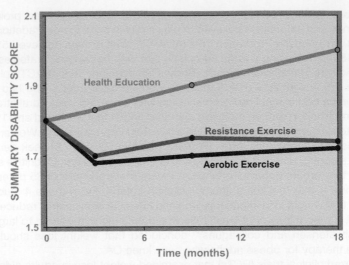

Fig. 3. Disability versus time with lower values, indicating less disability. (*From* Ettinger WH Jr, Burns R, Messier SP, et al. A randomized trial comparing aerobic exercise and resistance exercise with a health education program in older adults with knee osteoarthritis. The Fitness Arthritis and Seniors Trial (FAST). JAMA 1997;277(1):29; with permission.)

found in both groups compared with an attention control group.[82] Recently, the exercise group in our ADAPT trial showed statistically significant and clinically relevant (16%) long-term gains in mobility, effectively slowing the impairment common in the older OA population.[66]

Exercise interventions in older adults who have knee OA, however, tend to help them to maintain their weight more than to lose it. The exercise-only group in ADAPT lost 3.5 kg, or 3.7% of their baseline body weight, after 18 months of intervention compared with 5.2 kg (5.7%) and 4.6 kg (4.9%) for the diet-plus-exercise and diet-only groups, respectively.[66] In the ADAPT pilot study, a 6-month exercise program resulted in a 1.8-kg weight loss, whereas the exercise-and-diet group lost 8.5 kg.[43] In summary, long-term exercise programs in this disabled population improve mobility and pain and are effective in maintaining body weight.

CONCEPTUAL BASIS AND DELIVERY OF THE LIFESTYLE INTERVENTION

The reciprocal interaction of personal factors (eg, beliefs and values), social influence (eg, support and strain), and physical environment (eg, structure and access to resources) can improve weight loss and fitness by modifying eating and physical activity behaviors.[85] Our clinical trial protocols (FAST, ADAPT, and, currently, Intensive Diet and Exercise for Arthritis [IDEA]) evolved from social cognitive theory, group dynamics literature, and more than 15 years' experience in clinical trial research.

Social cognitive theory is based on three constructs: self-efficacy expectations, outcome expectations, and incentives. Self-efficacy expectations arise from individuals' beliefs that they can act to satisfy the demands of a situation. Such beliefs are determined by prior behavior, physical symptoms (eg, pain, fatigue), appetite, affect, and social/environmental factors.[85] The physical activity literature studies them to predict the ability to perform functional tasks or physical challenges of varying difficulty,[86–88] and the physical activity and eating behavior literatures have examined them under various environmental, social, and emotional stressors. Because self-regulation is important to successful behavior change, our clinical trials use goal setting and self-monitoring.[89,90]

Outcome expectations refer to the anticipated costs and benefits of a behavior. People are more likely to try a behavior if the perceived consequences have a favorable cost/benefit ratio.[89] Some people simply do not know the negative health effects of being overweight/obese and sedentary or are unduly optimistic about their own fate. They often become discouraged when lifestyle interventions (1) do not meet their unrealistic expectations about how much weight they can lose, (2) cause pain and fatigue, or (3) prohibit a valued food.

Incentives refer to the value that people associate with outcomes.[89] In our weight-loss clinical trials, the nutrition interventionist personalizes the protocol by learning how much participants value controlling their physical disability or reducing their weight; the dissatisfaction differential between the goal and the current weight; and the commitment to competing behaviors, such as responsibilities to families or friends. In the IDEA trial, we train our diet and exercise interventionists in social cognitive behavioral strategies, reinforced by discussion of success stories. They review participant programs with our health psychologist biweekly, developing strategies to use with participants who are finding it difficult to adhere.

THE FUTURE OF BEHAVIORAL WEIGHT-LOSS INTERVENTIONS

Osteoarthritis Research Society International (OARSI) guidelines recommend a combination of nonpharmacologic and pharmacologic interventions for the treatment of knee OA.[91] In addition to the challenges presented by any weight-loss intervention, the knee OA population's typical age and chronic pain create barriers. Dietary weight-loss trials nevertheless demonstrate significant improvements in pain and function with only a 5% loss, especially if exercise is included as part of the intervention. Weight loss reduces inflammation and joint loads, but no evidence indicates that it alters disease progression. A meta-analysis of previous weight-loss interventions suggests that at least 10% loss is necessary for a large clinical effect, but such results lasting longer than 1 year are rare. The ongoing IDEA clinical trial will determine if a 10% to 15% weight loss over 18 months either slows or stops OA disease progression. We hypothesize that a weight loss of this magnitude—two to three times that achieved in previous long-term OA weight-loss trials—will reduce inflammation and knee-joint loads sufficiently to retard joint destruction and to improve function and pain far beyond what has previously been attained.

TRANSLATING TRIAL RESULTS TO CLINICAL PRACTICE

The National Institutes of Health (NIH) have identified research on intervention approaches that incorporate primary care practice as a high priority.[92] Patients generally believe that their primary care physician should have a role in weight management.[93] A recent study found that only 42% of obese adults who had visited their health care professional during a 12-month span were advised to lose weight.[94] More disturbing, when either diet or exercise was discussed, a median of 0.7 minutes (42 seconds) was spent on this pressing and pervasive public health concern.[95]

Integrating the primary care physician and nurse into weight-loss intervention trials has met with modest success. Ashley and colleagues[96] enrolled 113 overweight, premenopausal women in a 1-year weight-loss program. A primary care office intervention (meeting with the primary care physician or nurse) combined with partial meal replacement was compared with traditional dietitian-led groups with and without meal replacement. Over the course of 52 weeks, the dietitian-led group with meal replacement produced greater weight loss (9.1%) than the traditional dietitian group (4.1%) and the primary-care-plus-meal-replacement group (4.3%). All three groups were successful in achieving and maintaining weight loss, however.

An evidence-based weight management model was implemented in 47 clinical practices involving 1256 obese patients.[97] It involved four phases: setting priorities, setting guidelines, measuring performance, and improving performance. General practice physicians and practice nurses were recruited at each clinical site. The weight-loss target was 5% to 10% of baseline weight. Preliminary results indicated that one third of all patients had a clinically relevant loss of more than 5% of baseline body weight at 12-month follow-up. Of the 58 general practices that began the trial, 15 dropped out, primarily because of lack of resources and time. The authors concluded that a primary care weight-management model can be used as part of a multistrategic approach to manage obesity in the community.

Clinical trial results can only be integrated into clinical practice if it is financially viable. We recommend that primary care physicians and rheumatologists urge their obese patients to enroll in a comprehensive weight-loss and exercise program run by a nurse, dietitian, or physician assistant in collaboration with an American College of Sports Medicine (ACSM)-certified exercise specialist. For such a program to be successful, however, several barriers must be addressed, including lack of reimbursement, lack of training, time constraints during normal office hours, and physicians' perceptions that these behavioral interventions are generally unsuccessful.[94]

SUMMARY

Obesity plays an important role through mechanical forces and inflammation in predisposing to OA development. Interventions designed to promote dietary weight loss and exercise in obese people who have OA have demonstrated clinically significant improvements in symptoms and disease risk factors. Dissemination of these pivotal research findings into clinical practice is facing several obstacles that health care practitioners can become more involved in removing to facilitate addressing this pervasive but modifiable public health problem.

ACKNOWLEDGMENTS

The assistance of my colleague Dr. Shannon Mihalko in completing the section entitled Conceptual Basis and Delivery of the Lifestyle Intervention is gratefully acknowledged.

REFERENCES

1. Fletcher E, Lewis-Faning E. Chronic rheumatic diseases: statistical study of 1000 cases of chronic rheumatism. Postgrad Med J 1945;21:137–76.
2. Leach RE, Baumgard S, Broom J. Obesity: its relationship to osteoarthritis of the knee. Clin Orthop 1973;93:271–3.
3. Coggon D, Reading I, Croft P, et al. Knee osteoarthritis and obesity. Int J Obes Relat Metab Disord 2001;25(5):622–7.
4. Felson DT, Zhang Y, Anthony JM, et al. Weight loss reduces the risk for symptomatic knee osteoarthritis in women. The Framingham Study. Ann Intern Med 1992; 116(7):535–9.

5. Ettinger WH, Davis MA, Neuhaus JM, et al. Long-term physical functioning in persons with knee osteoarthritis from NHANES. I: Effects of comorbid medical conditions. J Clin Epidemiol 1994;47(7):809–15.

6. Raynauld JP, Martel-Pelletier J, Berthiaume MJ, et al. Long term evaluation of disease progression through the quantitative magnetic resonance imaging of symptomatic knee osteoarthritis patients: correlation with clinical symptoms and radiographic changes. Arthritis Res Ther 2006;8(1).

7. Doherty M, Spector TD, Serni U. Session 1: epidemiology and genetics of hand osteoarthritis. Osteoarthr Cartil 2000;8(Suppl A):S14–5.

8. Kalichman L, Kobyliansky E. Age, body composition, and reproductive indices as predictors of radiographic hand osteoarthritis in Chuvashian women. Scand J Rheumatol 2007;36(1):53–7.

9. Davis MA, Ettinger WH, Neuhaus JM. Obesity and osteoarthritis of the knee: evidence from the National Health and Nutrition Examination Survey (NHANES I). Semin Arthritis Rheum 1990;20(3 Suppl 1):34–41.

10. Jenkins KR. Obesity's effects on the onset of functional impairment among older adults. Gerontologist 2004;44(2):206–16.

11. Ettinger WH Jr, Fried LP, Harris T, et al. Self-reported causes of physical disability in older people: the Cardiovascular Health Study. CHS Collaborative Research Group. J Am Geriatr Soc 1994;42(10):1035–44.

12. Sartorio A, Proietti M, Marinone PG, et al. Influence of gender, age and BMI on lower limb muscular power output in a large population of obese men and women. Int J Obes Relat Metab Disord 2004;28(1):91–8.

13. Miyatake N, Fujii M, Nishikawa H, et al. Clinical evaluation of muscle strength in 20-79-years-old obese Japanese. Diabetes Res Clin Pract 2000;48(1):15–21.

14. Rubenstein LZ. Falls in older people: epidemiology, risk factors and strategies for prevention. Age Ageing 2006;35(Suppl 2):ii37–41.

15. Center for disease control and prevention. State-specific prevalence of obesity among adults—Unites States, 2005. MMWR Morb Mortal Wkly Rep 2006; 55(36):985–8.

16. Kejonen P, Kauranen K, Vanharanta H. The relationship between anthropometric factors and body-balancing movements in postural balance. Arch Phys Med Rehabil 2003;84(1):17–22.

17. Jadelis K, Miller ME, Ettinger WH Jr, et al. Strength, balance, and the modifying effects of obesity and knee pain: results from the Observational Arthritis Study in Seniors (OASIS). J Am Geriatr Soc 2001;49(7):884–91.

18. Austin N, Devine A, Dick I, et al. Fear of falling in older women: a longitudinal study of incidence, persistence, and predictors. J Am Geriatr Soc 2007;55(10): 1598–603.

19. Finkelstein EA, Chen H, Prabhu M, et al. The relationship between obesity and injuries among U.S. adults. Am J Health Promot 2007;21(5):460–8.

20. DeVita P, Hortobagyi T. Obesity is not associated with increased knee joint torque and power during level walking. J Biomech 2003;36(9):1355–62.

21. Liu W, Nigg BM. A mechanical model to determine the influence of masses and mass distribution on the impact force during running. J Biomech 2000;33(2):219–24.

22. Messier SP, Ettinger WH, Doyle TE, et al. Obesity: effects on gait in an osteoarthritic population. J Appl Biomech 1996;12:161–72.

23. Browning RC, Kram R. Effects of obesity on the biomechanics of walking at different speeds. Med Sci Sports Exerc 2007;39(9):1632–41.

24. Messier SP, Davies AB, Moore DT, et al. Severe obesity: effects on foot mechanics during walking. Foot Ankle Int 1994;15(1):29–34.

25. Chodera JD, Levell RW. Footprint patterns during walking. In: Kenedi RM, editor. Perspectives in biomedical engineering. Baltimore (MD): University Park Press; 1973. p. 81–90.
26. Riddle DL, Pulisic M, Pidcoe P, et al. Risk factors for plantar fasciitis: a matched case-control study. J Bone Joint Surg Am 2003;85(5):872–7.
27. Hills AP, Hennig EM, Byrne NM, et al. The biomechanics of adiposity—structural and functional limitations of obesity and implications for movement. Obes Rev 2002;3(1):35–43.
28. Hills AP, Hennig EM, McDonald M, et al. Plantar pressure differences between obese and non-obese adults: a biomechanical analysis. Int J Obes Relat Metab Disord 2001;25(11):1674–9.
29. Wearing SC, Hennig EM, Byrne NM, et al. Musculoskeletal disorders associated with obesity: a biomechanical perspective. Obes Rev 2006;7(3):239–50.
30. Wearing SC, Hennig EM, Byrne NM, et al. The biomechanics of restricted movement in adult obesity. Obes Rev 2006;7(1):13–24.
31. Wearing SC, Hennig EM, Byrne NM, et al. The impact of childhood obesity on musculoskeletal form. Obes Rev 2006;7(2):209–18.
32. Gravante G, Russo G, Pomara F, et al. Comparison of ground reaction forces between obese and control young adults during quiet standing on a baropodometric platform. Clin Biomech (Bristol, Avon) 2003;18(8):780–2.
33. Lu XL, Mow VC. Biomechanics of articular cartilage and determination of material properties. Med Sci Sports Exerc 2008;40(2):193–9.
34. Kiviranta I, Tammi M, Jurvelin J, et al. Moderate running exercise augments glycosaminoglycans and thickness of articular cartilage in the knee joint of young beagle dogs. J Orthop Res 1988;6(2):188–95.
35. Palmoski MJ, Colyer RA, Brandt KD. Joint motion in the absence of normal loading does not maintain normal articular cartilage. Arthritis Rheum 1980;23(3):325–34.
36. Nigg BM. Biomechanical aspects of running. In: Nigg BM, editor. Biomechanics of running shoes. Champaign (IL): Human Kinetics Publishers, Inc; 1986. p. 1–25.
37. Paty JG Jr. Running injuries. Curr Opin Rheumatol 1994;6(2):203–9.
38. Messier SP, Devita P, Cowan RE, et al. Do older adults with knee osteoarthritis place greater loads on the knee during gait? A preliminary study. Arch Phys Med Rehabil 2005;86(4):703–9.
39. Hotamisligil GS. Inflammation and metabolic disorders. Nature 2006;444(7121): 860–7.
40. Wisse BE, Kim F, Schwartz MW. An integrative view of obesity. Science 2007; 318(5852):928–9.
41. Hotamisligil GS, Shargill NS, Spiegelman BM. Adipose expression of tumor necrosis factor-alpha: direct role in obesity-linked insulin resistance. Science 1993;259(5091):87–91.
42. Behre CJ. Adiponectin, obesity and atherosclerosis. Scand J Clin Lab Invest 2007;67(5):449–58.
43. Messier SP, Loeser RF, Mitchell MN, et al. Exercise and weight loss in obese older adults with knee osteoarthritis: a preliminary study. J Am Geriatr Soc 2000;48(9): 1062–72.
44. Otterness IG, Swindell AC, Zimmerer RO, et al. An analysis of 14 molecular markers for monitoring osteoarthritis: segregation of the markers into clusters and distinguishing osteoarthritis at baseline. Osteoarthr Cartil 2000;8(3):180–5.
45. Spector TD, Hart DJ, Nandra D, et al. Low-level increases in serum C-reactive protein are present in early osteoarthritis of the knee and predict progressive disease. Arthritis Rheum 1997;40(4):723–7.

46. Van Loan MD, Johnson HL, Barbieri TF. Effect of weight loss on bone mineral content and bone mineral density in obese women. Am J Clin Nutr 1998;67(4): 734–8.
47. Goldring MB. Osteoarthritis and cartilage: the role of cytokines. Curr Rheumatol Rep 2000;2(6):459–65.
48. Sharif M, Shepstone L, Elson CJ, et al. Increased serum C reactive protein may reflect events that precede radiographic progression in osteoarthritis of the knee. Ann Rheum Dis 2000;59(1):71–4.
49. Penninx BW, Messier SP, Rejeski WJ, et al. Physical exercise and the prevention of disability in activities of daily living in older persons with osteoarthritis. Arch Intern Med 2001;161(19):2309–16.
50. Otterness IG, Weiner E, Swindell AC, et al. An analysis of 14 molecular markers for monitoring osteoarthritis. Relationship of the markers to clinical end-points. Osteoarthr Cartil 2001;9(3):224–31.
51. Wolfe F. The C-reactive protein but not erythrocyte sedimentation rate is associated with clinical severity in patients with osteoarthritis of the knee or hip. J Rheumatol 1997;24(8):1486–8.
52. Scharstuhl A, Glansbeek HL, van Beuningen HM, et al. Inhibition of endogenous TGF-beta during experimental osteoarthritis prevents osteophyte formation and impairs cartilage repair. J Immunol 2002;169(1):507–14.
53. Miller GD, Nicklas B, Ambrosius W, et al. Is serum leptin related to physical function and is it modifiable through weight loss and exercise in older adults with knee osteoarthritis? Int J Obes 2004;28:1383–90.
54. Hartz AJ, Fischer ME, Bril G, et al. The association of obesity with joint pain and osteoarthritis in the HANES data. J Chronic Dis 1986;39(4):311–9.
55. Wadden TA, Vogt RA, Andersen RE, et al. Exercise in the treatment of obesity: effects of four interventions on body composition, resting energy expenditure, appetite, and mood. J Consult Clin Psychol 1997;65(2):269–77.
56. Wadden TA, Berkowitz RI, Sarwer DB, et al. Benefits of lifestyle modification in the pharmacologic treatment of obesity: a randomized trial. Arch Intern Med 2001; 161(2):218–27.
57. Kayman S, Bruvold W, Stern JS. Maintenance and relapse after weight loss in women: behavioral aspects. Am J Clin Nutr 1990;52(5):800–7.
58. Perri MG, Martin AD, Leermakers EA, et al. Effects of group- versus home-based exercise in the treatment of obesity. J Consult Clin Psychol 1997;65(2):278–85.
59. Wing RR, Epstein LH, Paternostro-Bayles M, et al. Exercise in a behavioural weight control programme for obese patients with Type 2 (non-insulin-dependent) diabetes. Diabetologia 1988;31(12):902–9.
60. Perri MG, McAllister DA, Gange JJ, et al. Effects of four maintenance programs on the long-term management of obesity. J Consult Clin Psychol 1988;56(4): 529–34.
61. Esposito K, Pontillo A, Di Palo C, et al. Effect of weight loss and lifestyle changes on vascular inflammatory markers in obese women: a randomized trial. JAMA 2003;289(14):1799–804.
62. Svetkey LP, Stevens VJ, Brantley PJ, et al. Comparison of strategies for sustaining weight loss: the weight loss maintenance randomized controlled trial. JAMA 2008;299(10):1139–48.
63. Pirozzo S, Summerbell C, Cameron C, et al. Advice on low-fat diets for obesity. Cochrane Database Syst Rev 2002;(2):CD003640.
64. Bravata DM, Sanders L, Huang J, et al. Efficacy and safety of low-carbohydrate diets: a systematic review. JAMA 2003;289(14):1837–50.

65. Heymsfield SB, van Mierlo CA, van der Knaap HC, et al. Weight management using a meal replacement strategy: meta and pooling analysis from six studies. Int J Obe Relat Metab Disord 2003;27(5):537–49.
66. Messier SP, Loeser RF, Miller GD, et al. Exercise and dietary weight loss in overweight and obese older adults with knee osteoarthritis: the arthritis, diet, and activity promotion trial. Arthritis Rheum 2004;50(5):1501–10.
67. Miller GD, Nicklas BJ, Davis C, et al. Intensive weight loss program improves physical function in older obese adults with knee osteoarthritis. Obesity (Silver Spring) 2006;14(7):1219–30.
68. Christensen R, Astrup A, Bliddal H. Weight loss: the treatment of choice for knee osteoarthritis? A randomized trial. Osteoarthr Cartil 2005;13(1):20–7.
69. Christensen R, Bartels EM, Astrup A, et al. Effect of weight reduction in obese patients diagnosed with knee osteoarthritis: a systematic review and meta-analysis. Ann Rheum Dis 2007;66(4):433–9.
70. Wedick NM, Barrett-Connor E, Knoke JD, et al. The relationship between weight loss and all-cause mortality in older men and women with and without diabetes mellitus: the Rancho Bernardo study. J Am Geriatr Soc 2002;50(11): 1810–5.
71. Newman AB, Yanez D, Harris T, et al. Weight change in old age and its association with mortality. J Am Geriatr Soc 2001;49(10):1309–18.
72. Diehr P, Newman AB, Jackson SA, et al. Weight-modification trials in older adults: what should the outcome measure be? Curr Control Trials Cardiovasc Med 2002;3(1):1.
73. Andersen RE, Wadden TA, Herzog RJ. Changes in bone mineral content in obese dieting women. Metabolism 1997;46(8):857–61.
74. Hyldstrup L, Andersen T, McNair P, et al. Bone metabolism in obesity: changes related to severe overweight and dietary weight reduction. Acta Endocrinol (Copenh) 1993;129(5):393–8.
75. Andersen RE, Wadden TA, Bartlett SJ, et al. Relation of weight loss to changes in serum lipids and lipoproteins in obese women. Am J Clin Nutr 1995;62(8): 350–7.
76. Ensrud KE, Cauley J, Lipschutz R, et al. Weight change and fractures in older women. Study of Osteoporotic Fractures Research Group. Arch Intern Med 1997;157(8):857–63.
77. Fiatarone Singh MA. Combined exercise and dietary intervention to optimize body composition in aging. Ann N Y Acad Sci 1998;854:378–93.
78. Janssen I, Fortier A, Hudson R, et al. Effects of an energy-restrictive diet with or without exercise on abdominal fat, intermuscular fat, and metabolic risk factors in obese women. Diabetes Care 2002;25(3):431–8.
79. Wang X, Miller GD, Messier SP, et al. Knee strength maintained despite loss of lean body mass during weight loss in older obese adults with knee osteoarthritis. J Gerontol A Biol Sci Med Sci 2007;62(8):866–71.
80. Kovar PA, Allegrante JP, MacKenzie CR, et al. Supervised fitness walking in patients with osteoarthritis of the knee. A randomized, controlled trial. Ann Intern Med 1992;116(7):529–34.
81. Minor MA, Hewett JE, Webel RR, et al. Efficacy of physical conditioning exercise in patients with rheumatoid arthritis and osteoarthritis. Arthritis Rheum 1989; 32(11):1396–405.
82. Ettinger WH Jr, Burns R, Messier SP, et al. A randomized trial comparing aerobic exercise and resistance exercise with a health education program in older adults with knee osteoarthritis. The Fitness Arthritis and Seniors Trial (FAST). JAMA 1997;277(1):25–31.

83. Thomas KS, Muir KR, Doherty M, et al. Home based exercise programme for knee pain and knee osteoarthritis: randomised controlled trial. BMJ 2002; 325(7367):752–6.
84. van Baar ME, Assendelft WJ, Dekker J, et al. Effectiveness of exercise therapy in patients with osteoarthritis of the hip or knee: a systematic review of randomized clinical trials. Arthritis Rheum 1999;42(7):1361–9.
85. Bandura A. Self-efficacy: the exercise of control. New York: W.H. Freeman and Co.; 1997.
86. McAuley E, Blissmer B. Self-efficacy determinants and consequences of physical activity. Exerc Sport Sci Rev 2000;28(2):85–8.
87. McAuley E, Blissmer B, Katula J, et al. Physical activity, self-esteem, and self-efficacy relationships in older adults: a randomized controlled trial. Ann Behav Med 2000;22(2):131–9.
88. McAuley E, Blissmer B, Katula J, et al. Exercise environment, self-efficacy, and affective responses to acute exercise in older adults. Psychol Health 2000; 15(3):341–55.
89. McAuley E, Mihalko SL. Measuring exercise-related self-efficacy. In: Duda JL, editor. Advances in sport and exercise psychology measurement. Morgantown (WV): Fitness Information Technology, Inc.; 1998. p. 371–89.
90. Rejeski WJ, Mihalko SL. Physical activity and quality of life in older adults. J Gerontol A Biol Sci Med Sci 2001;56:23–35.
91. Zhang W, Moskowitz RW, Nuki G, et al. OARSI recommendations for the management of hip and knee osteoarthritis, Part II: OARSI evidence-based, expert consensus guidelines. Osteoarthr Cartil 2008;16(2):137–62.
92. Blair SN, Applegate WB, Dunn AL, et al. Activity Counseling Trial (ACT): rationale, design, and methods. Activity Counseling Trial Research Group. Med Sci Sports Exerc 1998;30(7):1097–106.
93. Tan D, Zwar NA, Dennis SM, et al. Weight management in general practice: what do patients want? Med J Aust 2006;185(2):73–5.
94. Galuska DA, Will JC, Serdula MK, et al. Are health care professionals advising obese patients to lose weight? JAMA 1999;282(16):1576–8.
95. Flocke SA, Stange KC. Direct observation and patient recall of health behavior advice. Prev Med 2004;38(3):343–9.
96. Ashley JM, St Jeor ST, Schrage JP, et al. Weight control in the physician's office. Arch Intern Med 2001;161(13):1599–604.
97. The Counterweight Project Team. A new evidence-based model for weight management in primary care: the counterweight programme. J Hum Nutr Diet 2004;17:191–208.

Muscle and Exercise in the Prevention and Management of Knee Osteoarthritis: an Internal Medicine Specialist's Guide

Kim L. Bennell, PhD[a],*, Michael A. Hunt, PhD[a], Tim V. Wrigley, MSc[a],
Boon-Whatt Lim, MSc[b], Rana S. Hinman, PhD[a]

KEYWORDS

• Knee osteoarthritis • Muscle • Rehabilitation • Strengthening

Despite overwhelming evidence supporting the benefits of exercise in osteoarthritis and clinical guidelines recommending the inclusion of exercise in intervention strategies,[1] getting patients with knee osteoarthritis to exercise remains a challenge. Whilst there are many barriers to the uptake of exercise in the osteoarthritis population, there are two of particular importance: (1) failure on the part of medical practitioners to properly recommend exercise to patients and make appropriate referrals to exercise professionals and (2) failure of patients to comply with prescribed exercise programs.

Exercise is underused by medical practitioners as a treatment strategy for osteoarthritis.[2] In a survey of 3000 French general practitioners, less than 15% reported that they would prescribe exercise for knee osteoarthritis as a first-line therapeutic approach. Additionally, a survey of patients with osteoarthritis in Canada revealed that only one third had been advised to exercise for their condition.[3] However, 73% reported that they had tried exercise in the past. Given the large number of patients who chose to exercise independently, it is possible that many failed to consult a professional regarding the most appropriate exercise. Thus, it is important to understand the reasons for prescribing exercise to these patients and the potential benefits such exercise offers. Much of the evidence supporting the utility of exercise interventions

A version of this article originally appeared in the 34:3 issue of the *Rheumatic Disease Clinics of North America*.
[a] Centre for Health, Exercise and Sports Medicine, School of Physiotherapy, The University of Melbourne, 200 Berkeley Street, Carlton, Victoria 3010, Australia
[b] School of Sport, Health and Leisure, Republic Polytechnic, Singapore
* Corresponding author.
E-mail address: k.bennell@unimelb.edu.au (K.L. Bennell).

Med Clin N Am 93 (2009) 161–177
doi:10.1016/j.mcna.2008.08.006
0025-7125/08/$ – see front matter © 2008 Elsevier Inc. All rights reserved.

medical.theclinics.com

for patients with knee osteoarthritis points to the important role of lower-limb muscle function in the genesis and management of this health condition.

At the knee, muscles function to produce movement but also to absorb limb loading and provide dynamic joint stability. Muscle weakness has been identified as a potential risk factor for disease development due to increased joint loading. Additionally, the presence of osteoarthritis undermines the integrity of the structure and function of muscles, potentially further affecting the disease process.

Recent research has provided a rationale for the use of muscle rehabilitation as part of the overall treatment regimen for knee osteoarthritis to improve joint integrity, reduce symptoms, increase function, and possibly protect against disease progression. A detailed understanding of the role of muscle in knee osteoarthritis can, therefore, aid in the implementation of effective rehabilitation strategies and may also form the basis of primary prevention strategies against disease development.

This review outlines the influence of muscle activity on knee-joint loading, describes the deficits in muscle function observed in people with knee osteoarthritis, and summarizes available evidence pertaining to the role of muscle in the development and progression of knee osteoarthritis. The review focuses on whether muscle deficits can be modified in knee osteoarthritis and whether improvements in muscle function lead to improved symptoms and joint structure. This review concludes with a discussion of exercise prescription for muscle rehabilitation in knee osteoarthritis.

INFLUENCE OF MUSCLE ACTIVITY ON KNEE-JOINT LOADING

Because knee osteoarthritis is thought to be due to joint loading acting within the context of systemic and local susceptibility, the influence of muscle activity on knee-joint load is important to understand. To achieve equilibrium of motion and joint stability, all external forces acting on a joint must be counteracted by internal forces equal in magnitude, but opposite in direction. External knee-joint loading experienced during human movement is primarily derived from the ground reaction forces and inertial properties of the lower limb, resulting in a total tibiofemoral joint force approaching three times body weight[4,5] during gait. The medial compartment is loaded to a greater extent than the lateral compartment.[6] Partly because of this higher level of loading, the medial compartment has a higher prevalence of osteoarthritis.

Of particular interest to the pathogenesis of medial knee osteoarthritis is the ability to counteract the external adduction moment (torque) applied about the knee in the frontal plane during stance phase as this moment is suggested to influence disease initiation,[7] disease severity[8] and disease progression,[9] and is believed to be an indirect measure of medial tibiofemoral joint load.[6,10] Dynamic stability of the knee depends upon the load-sharing characteristics of many passive soft tissues and active muscle forces.[6] Although no in vivo data exist to quantify the relative contributions of knee-joint structures in generating internal forces, many biomechanical modeling studies provide estimations of these forces.

Schipplein and Andriacchi[6] were among the first to evaluate passive soft tissue and active muscle contributions to dynamic knee stability during walking. They found that activation of the quadriceps muscles in isolation was insufficient to balance the external adduction moment and that cocontraction from the hamstrings or tension in lateral soft tissues was required to produce an internal abduction moment to maintain dynamic equilibrium in the frontal plane. They also found that increased coactivation of the quadriceps and hamstrings could support larger external adduction moments while reducing the amount of soft tissue tension or medial compartment joint compression. This apparent off-loading suggests a potentially protective role of muscles against large medial compartment contact forces and likely subsequent articular cartilage degeneration.

The requirement of active muscle contributions to internal abduction moment generation has been supported by subsequent studies examining isometric loading.[11,12] Buchanan and Lloyd[12] reported individual activation patterns of many lower-limb muscles during static loads in the frontal plane. Muscles active during the production of internal abduction forces include sartorius, gracilis, quadriceps (primarily rectus femoris), long head of biceps femoris, and lateral gastrocnemius. Shelburne and colleagues[4] recently showed in a biomechanical modeling study that, although these muscles are capable of producing internal abduction moments isometrically, much of the contribution to the total abduction moment during normal gait came from the quadriceps (early stance) and gastrocnemius (late stance).

Taken together, these findings indicate that, for a given external load, muscles are capable of generating enough force to produce the majority of the internal balancing load. However, other soft tissue structures, such as bone and articular cartilage, still must sustain loads. Clearly, muscle force generation is of particular interest to clinicians given that the individual can consciously control it and improve it with training. Improving the load-bearing capacities of lower-limb muscles—in particular, the quadriceps—through strength-training and muscle-rehabilitation programs may protect against soft tissue damage resulting from excessive load.

It is unclear, however, if the increase in the total joint reaction force occurring with muscle contraction may actually *accelerate* the degeneration of articular cartilage, rather than prevent it. Indeed, while muscle activity—in particular, cocontraction of the quadriceps and hamstrings—may balance the external adduction moment and improve the dynamic stability of the knee joint during walking, axial compression due to the muscles' line of pull may place the cartilage in an environment of excessive and prolonged load. Alterations in muscle activation in association with osteoarthritis are discussed in detail in the following section, but it is apparent that further research into the effects of muscle cocontraction on the health of articular cartilage in the tibiofemoral joint is needed.

DEFICITS IN MUSCLE FUNCTION IN KNEE OSTEOARTHRITIS

Given the role of muscles in influencing knee-joint load and knee stability, an understanding of deficits in muscle function associated with knee osteoarthritis is important. Most studies of muscle function in knee osteoarthritis have concerned muscle strength. However, other aspects of muscle function are also affected by the osteoarthritis disease process, including activation patterns and proprioceptive acuity. Understanding how muscle function is impaired will assist clinicians in prescribing more effective rehabilitation programs and improving clinical outcome.

Strength

Muscle weakness is a well-accepted impairment in knee osteoarthritis. However, measurement of strength is not straightforward and has not always been well conducted in osteoarthritis studies. The ability to generate muscle force is a function of muscle cross-sectional area and the ability to recruit and fire descending alpha motor neurons to muscle fibers at appropriate frequencies.[13,14] That force then acts in conjunction with the muscle's moment arm to generate a torque or moment about a particular joint.[13,14]

Results of the relatively few studies that have correctly reported strength (torque normalized for body mass differences [Nm/kg]) show that patients with knee osteoarthritis are 20% to 40% weaker in relative quadriceps strength than healthy controls.[15–17] The strength of other lower-limb muscles in knee osteoarthritis has received less attention. Further work is particularly necessary on the strength of the hip muscles, although these muscle groups are harder to measure.

There are several contributors to muscle weakness in individuals with knee osteoarthritis. The assessment of strength typically requires a maximal contraction, something that most patients would not have attempted for some time. Pain, anxiety, motivation, effusion, muscle atrophy, and aberrant joint mechanics can all contribute to a loss of measurable strength. Some of the weakness in relation to body size seen in osteoarthritis is likely due to the obesity that is also commonly present, as the proportion of total body mass made up of force-generating muscle is by definition reduced. Primary deficits in muscle strength may be associated with muscle fiber atrophy (ie, loss of muscle cross-sectional area), reduced ability to activate muscle fibers, or both.

Few studies have investigated muscle atrophy in osteoarthritis. Ikeda and colleagues[18] recently found that quadriceps cross-sectional area was significantly reduced by an average of 12% in women with incident radiological osteoarthritis without symptoms, compared to age- and body mass–matched women with no signs of osteoarthritis. In later-stage disease, more obvious signs of muscle fiber atrophy have been reported.[19,20] Thus, it appears likely that at least some strength loss in osteoarthritis is due to loss of muscle cross-sectional area.

Where muscle atrophy cannot explain the full extent of muscle weakness, inhibition in the ability to activate muscle is implicated. Overall, there is a large variation in the results of studies assessing the extent of maximal voluntary muscle activation typically possible in osteoarthritis. However, the literature consistently shows that patients with osteoarthritis commonly exhibit impaired activation compared to healthy controls.[21–25] Pain is commonly presumed to be a major source of inhibition in the ability to voluntarily activate muscle surrounding arthritic joints.[26] Joint effusion has also been found to be a potent inhibitor of maximal muscle activation, even at low levels that might otherwise not be deemed clinically important.[27] While effusion is often associated with osteoarthritis,[28] it is not clear if it plays an important role in the reduced activation associated with knee osteoarthritis.

The source of muscle weakness is important because it determines how restoration of muscle strength might be approached therapeutically. If the deficit is primarily due to atrophy, then a pure muscle-strengthening approach should be taken. Alternatively, if the deficit is primarily in the ability to activate an essentially normal muscle, then attention might be directed towards removing the inhibitory sources that prevent sufficient activation (such as pain and effusion) and retraining the patient to activate his or her muscles fully.

Muscle Activation Patterns

In recent years, there has been increasing interest in the patterns of muscle activation associated with knee osteoarthritis. It appears that some patients are able to activate their knee muscles in a way that is most efficient for counter-balancing the external knee adduction moment during gait whilst satisfying the other requirements for weight support and propulsion. However, other patients adopt a less efficient strategy that involves activating many muscles in a less specific fashion, which may increase overall joint loading.[25,29] It appears that, as disease progresses, a less specific and efficient activation of a greater number of knee muscles may become more apparent.

Whether these differences reflect the increasing difficulty in activating muscles efficiently for ambulation in the face of pain and deteriorating joint mechanics, or are in fact involved in disease progression itself, needs to be clarified. There is also little current evidence showing that such patterns can be altered; nor is it entirely clear what would constitute a desirable alteration.

Proprioception

Knee-joint proprioception is essential to the coordinated activity of surrounding muscles. Proprioceptive afferent information from mechanoreceptors, particularly in muscles, but also in ligaments, capsule, menisci, and skin, contribute at the spinal level to arthrokinetic and muscular reflexes, which play a large part in dynamic joint stability.[30] The information is also conveyed to supraspinal centers where it is integral to motor learning and the on-going programming of complex movements. Abnormal proprioception could predispose to musculoskeletal pathology by altering the control of movement leading to abnormal stresses on tissues.[31] Alternatively, pathology and pain may alter proprioceptive information, further compounding functional deficits.[32,33]

Compared to similarly aged asymptomatic individuals, deficits in knee-joint proprioception have been found in patients with knee osteoarthritis.[34–38] However, the link between impaired proprioception and function is less clear. While some studies have found a relationship between proprioceptive impairment and either physical function[38–41] or pain[38] in individuals with osteoarthritis, others have failed to do so.[41–43]

EVIDENCE FOR THE ROLE OF MUSCLE IN OSTEOARTHRITIS DEVELOPMENT AND PROGRESSION

This section discusses the limited cross-sectional and cohort studies and randomized controlled trials that link impaired muscle function to the development and progression of knee osteoarthritis. These have focused primarily on muscle strength with few studies evaluating links with other aspects of muscle function.

Some evidence suggests that quadriceps weakness precedes the onset of knee osteoarthritis and hence could increase the risk of disease development, particularly in women. In a large community-based cross-sectional study involving 462 volunteers, Slemenda and colleagues[17] demonstrated that absolute quadriceps strength was lower in women with radiographic knee osteoarthritis but without any history of knee pain. In a follow-up study on 280 volunteers over a mean period of 31 months,[44] the same investigators demonstrated that baseline absolute quadriceps strength (statistically adjusted for body mass) was 18% lower in women who developed incident radiographic osteoarthritis, compared to women who did not develop osteoarthritis. These results were confirmed in another longitudinal cohort study involving 3081 adults without osteoarthritis where higher isokinetic quadriceps strength relative to body mass was associated with a 55% reduced risk of developing knee osteoarthritis in women, with similar, but nonsignificant, results found in men.[45] Thus, there may be a potential role for quadriceps-strengthening exercises in women in the prevention of osteoarthritis development.

There is presently limited evidence to suggest stronger muscles can protect against osteoarthritis progression in those with established disease. A longitudinal study on 79 women with radiographic knee osteoarthritis[46] reported peak absolute and relative isokinetic quadriceps strength and radiographic disease severity at baseline. The investigators found that the mean absolute quadriceps strength of women with progressive osteoarthritis (defined as worsening of the Kellgren and Lawrence grade over 2.5 years) was about 9% lower than those with radiographically stable osteoarthritis, but this was not significant.

In another longitudinal cohort study, Sharma and colleagues[47] measured absolute quadriceps strength at baseline and prevalence of disease progression (defined as an increase in the grade of joint space narrowing in the medial or lateral compartment) 18 months later. After adjusting for age, body mass index, disease severity, and physical activity, *greater* absolute quadriceps strength at baseline increased the risk of disease progression in people with malaligned knees (defined as >5° deviation from the mechanical axis) but not in those with neutral alignment. The investigators suggested that the inability of malaligned knees to evenly distribute muscle forces could result in focal stress while the increase in muscle contraction to stabilize lax knees could lead to higher joint-reaction forces.

This study generated a substantial amount of publicity and its findings were generalized to muscle strengthening. However, this was an observational study, not an intervention. It highlights the need for further work in this area.

Recently, Amin and colleagues[48] have briefly reported a longitudinal study investigating the association between isokinetic quadriceps strength (absolute or relative to body mass not specified) and cartilage loss over 30 months. MRI was used to quantify cartilage volume in the tibiofemoral and patellofemoral joints in 265 elderly individuals with symptomatic knee osteoarthritis, including stratification for alignment. They found no relationship between quadriceps strength and cartilage loss over 15 and 30 months anywhere except the lateral compartment of the patellofemoral joint, where increased quadriceps strength was protective against cartilage degeneration.

Though the role of muscle function on *structural* disease development and progression has received most of the attention in the literature, its effects on *functional* progression are less well known. Sharma and colleagues[49] conducted a 3-year longitudinal cohort study investigating factors contributing to poor physical functioning in 257 patients with knee osteoarthritis. They found that, in addition to such factors as age, reduced absolute quadriceps and hamstrings strength and poor proprioceptive acuity increased the likelihood of poor physical functioning as measured by the time to perform five repetitions of rising and sitting in a chair. Taken together, these findings suggest strong interrelationships between muscle function, physical functioning, and joint integrity over time in those with knee osteoarthritis.

CAN MUSCLE DEFICITS BE MODIFIED IN KNEE OSTEOARTHRITIS?

Whilst it is important to understand the muscle function deficits associated with knee osteoarthritis, it is also imperative to appreciate which deficits are amenable to change with intervention. This allows the clinician to tailor treatment to the nature of the presenting muscle deficit.

Muscle Strength

Ample research indicates that muscle strength can be improved with an appropriately targeted strengthening program in people with knee osteoarthritis.[50] Whilst the majority of research has focused on the quadriceps muscle,[51–54] strength gains have also been observed in the hamstrings and the hip musculature with exercise.[55–58] Strength gains have been observed both with supervised programs[52,55–57] and home exercise regimes.[51,53,54] The magnitude of strength gain achieved with resistance training varies according to the intensity of training (resistance applied as well as frequency), patient compliance, and the specificity of training, which probably explains why strength increases in knee osteoarthritis vary from 5% to 71% (from pre-exercise levels) in the literature.[51,52,54,57]

Muscle Atrophy and Activation

Despite atrophy being implicated in the weakness associated with osteoarthritis, work is still required to determine if the increasing strength found with training in osteoarthritis is associated with reversal of any previous loss of muscle cross-sectional area. Similarly, few studies have evaluated whether changes in muscle activation are possible with treatment. Some studies have demonstrated improvements in voluntary activation of the quadriceps following an exercise regime, usually including quadriceps strengthening exercises.[51,52] Mean within-group increases in activation ranging from 5% to 14% have been reported.[51,52] Another study has demonstrated that pain relief via local anesthetic injection resulted in an 11% to 12% increase in percentage activation of the quadriceps,[59] confirming that at least some of the reduced voluntary activation observed in knee osteoarthritis is due to the inhibition of pain. No study to date has evaluated whether exercise can alter muscle activation timing or patterns of recruitment in knee osteoarthritis.

Proprioception

There is some evidence that impairments in proprioceptive acuity in knee osteoarthritis can be enhanced. One nonrandomized study reported significant improvements in proprioception following a multifaceted exercise program,[52] while another randomized study demonstrated that the addition of kinesthesia and balance exercises to a strengthening program did not offer any additional improvement in proprioceptive acuity beyond that offered by a strengthening program alone.[60] Because a nonexercising control group was not included, it is unclear whether a true change in proprioception occurred with either exercise intervention. Another study compared proprioceptive function following computerized proprioception facilitation exercise and closed kinetic chain exercise in knee osteoarthritis[61] and found that both programs were more effective in improving proprioception than a no-exercise program for the control group. Also, some evidence suggests that knee bandaging or bracing can improve proprioception in knee osteoarthritis.[35,62] However, findings are inconsistent across the literature.[63] Thus, it appears that some treatments show some promise for enhancing proprioceptive acuity in knee osteoarthritis. However, reported mean changes are generally quite small and it is unclear if such changes are clinically relevant or merely within the realm of measurement error.

DO IMPROVEMENTS IN MUSCLE FUNCTION LEAD TO IMPROVED SYMPTOMS AND JOINT STRUCTURE IN KNEE OSTEOARTHRITIS?

Ample evidence demonstrates that muscle-strengthening exercises result in improvements in pain, physical function, and quality of life in people with knee osteoarthritis.[50,64] Again, the majority of research has focused on quadriceps-strengthening programs. A recent systematic review noted small to moderate effect sizes for both pain and physical function following quadriceps strengthening.[64]

While the improvements observed in pain and physical function following strengthening programs are often attributed to improvements in muscle strength, studies generally do not correlate changes in muscle function with clinical improvements following intervention. Indeed, many clinical trials involving exercise do not include measures of muscle function in their test battery. Thus, it is not clear if an increase in muscle strength is directly responsible for the improvements in pain or function, or whether a general increase in physical activity is a more important factor. For example, a randomized controlled trial investigating the efficacy of a 6-month home-based quadriceps-strengthening program in a large group of older adults with knee pain found that pain at follow-up was reduced by 23% in the exercise group, compared to only 6% in the control group, which did not exercise.[51] Physical function scores improved by 17% in the exercise group and were unchanged in the control group. In this study, significant gains in quadriceps strength were evident in the exercise group compared to the controls, with small increases in quadriceps activation also noted. However, correlations between muscle function parameters and clinical outcome were not performed. While it is likely that improvements in muscle function contributed to the improvements in pain and function noted in this study, definitive conclusions regarding the mechanistic effects of quadriceps strengthening cannot be drawn.

Improvements in clinical state with strengthening exercise are generally not maintained once the patient ceases exercising. A study by van Baar and colleagues[65] evaluated the long-term effectiveness of a multifaceted exercise program, which included muscle strengthening, in hip and knee osteoarthritis. Participants were evaluated 6 months after completion of the 3-month exercise program. Although exercise was associated with reductions in pain and observed disability at 3 months,[55] these improvements had disappeared 6 months later.[65] This study showed that the beneficial effects of exercise decline over time and eventually disappear in the absence of ongoing exercise. This decline may partially be due to the gradual loss of improvement in muscle function once exercise has ceased. Muscle strength had essentially returned to baseline levels 3 months after completion of the exercise program. Thus, for ongoing improvements in pain and function, and to maintain increases in muscle strength, long-term involvement in exercise is necessary.

Only one study has specifically evaluated whether improvements in muscle function have any discernable impact on joint structure in knee osteoarthritis. A recent randomized controlled trial evaluated the effects of muscle strength training on incidence and progression of knee osteoarthritis in older adults.[66] Older adults with and without knee pain were randomly allocated to either a strength-training or range-of-motion exercise group. Exercise was initially supervised for 12 weeks and thereafter increasingly performed at home up until 30 months. Strength training was directed to both the upper and lower limbs but with an emphasis on quadriceps and hamstrings. To evaluate joint structural change over time, measurements from radiographs were taken of joint space width in the medial tibiofemoral compartment. Whilst participants in both exercise groups actually *lost* lower-extremity muscle strength over 30 months, the rate of loss was slower with strength training compared to range-of-motion exercises. In participants with established knee osteoarthritis at baseline, the mean loss of joint space width in the strengthening group was 37% less than that in the range-of-motion group. However, this difference was not statistically significant. Semiquantitative ratings of loss of joint space width revealed that joint space narrowing occurred less frequently in the strengthening group compared to range-of-motion exercise. Trends in data from this study suggest that lower-limb strength training may have a role in slowing deterioration over time in established knee osteoarthritis, but further large-scale studies using more sensitive imaging techniques (such as magnetic resonance) are needed before conclusions can be drawn.

EXERCISE PRESCRIPTION FOR MUSCLE REHABILITATION

Given the deficits in muscle function present in those with knee osteoarthritis, muscle rehabilitation plays an important role in disease management, particularly for management aimed at reducing symptoms and improving function. This section discusses practical aspects related to prescribing exercise for patients and reviews current evidence about the best mode of delivery, type of exercise, and dosage (**Box 1**).

> **Box 1**
> **Summary of exercise prescription for muscle rehabilitation**
>
> - Refer to health professional for appropriate exercise prescription.
> - Recommend supervised group or individual treatments, which are superior to independent home exercise for pain reduction.
> - Supplement home exercise with initial group exercise.
> - Do not depend entirely on exercise handouts or audiovisual material, which alone are ineffective.
> - Target quadriceps, hamstrings, and hip abductors for strengthening.
> - Minimize compressive joint forces.
> - Remember that the type of strengthening exercise does not influence clinical outcome.
> - Use a combined program of strengthening, flexibility, and functional exercises.
> - Employ strategies to maximize long-term patient compliance to exercise.

Mode of Delivery

Exercise may be delivered via individual treatments, supervised group classes, or performed at home. Advantages of group-based exercise programs include the social aspects of group therapy and the ability to minimize resources and cost. Disadvantages include greater difficulty in tailoring exercise to individual patients and the need for patients to attend a specific location at a set time. Home exercise entails little financial outlay and provides the patient with greater flexibility regarding timing of the exercise session. However, there is a lack of supervision and often a lack of suitable equipment.

A Cochrane Review compared the effect sizes of different exercise delivery modes in knee osteoarthritis.[67] For pain, comparable medium effect sizes were observed with individual treatments and group classes, whilst a small effect size was evident for home exercise. For physical function, small effect sizes were reported for all modes of delivery. This suggests that supervised group or individual treatments are superior to independent home exercise for reduction of pain whilst all exercise modes produce similar results for physical function. However, it appears that supplementing home exercises with an initial physiotherapist-supervised class-based program can lead to greater improvements in pain and locomotor function with home exercises in the longer term.[68] Economic analyses demonstrate that the additional cost of the group exercise classes can be offset by reductions in resource use elsewhere in the health care system.[69] Thus, exercise class supplementation represents a more cost-effective method of maximizing the benefits of a home exercise program, which would otherwise result in only small benefits.

One mode of exercise delivery that has been shown to be ineffective is a "minimalist" approach whereby patients are simply given a pamphlet or audiovisual material outlining a standardized exercise program. In a large study, this exercise approach delivered by rheumatologists yielded similar clinical outcomes to usual care after 6 months.[70] Numerous factors likely contributed to the ineffectiveness of exercise in this study. Patients were poorly compliant and an unsupervised standardized exercise program and dosage was used, which may have been ineffective for such a heterogeneous patient group. Whilst a videotape demonstration of the exercises was provided, it would appear that technology is no substitute for personal demonstration and tuition in correct exercise technique. As a result, it is possible that many patients were performing the exercises incorrectly, further reducing their effectiveness.

Type of Program

Quadriceps strengthening has formed the cornerstone of traditional osteoarthritis exercise therapy. Quadriceps-strengthening exercises may be performed in a variety of modes, including isometric, isotonic, or isokinetic, the latter two of which may be concentric, eccentric, or both concentric and eccentric. A meta-analysis published in 2004 identified 22 trials of strengthening exercise on individuals with knee osteoarthritis employing a variety of modes.[50] The results of this meta-analysis found no evidence that the type of strengthening exercise (ie, isometric, isotonic, or isokinetic) influences outcome, although more work is needed in this area. However, it is likely that the magnitude of the load and pattern of loading throughout the range-of-motion exercise and overall volume of exercise performed are more important for increasing strength than the resistance apparatus on which exercise is performed. Exercises may also be performed in an open kinetic or closed kinetic chain manner. Open kinetic chain exercises at the knee are non–weight bearing whilst closed kinetic chain exercises are typically weight bearing, involving multiple joints, and are thought to be more functional. However, the important issue for osteoarthritis is keeping compressive joint forces as low as possible while still achieving an adequate muscle-strengthening stimulus. Load magnitude and range of motion may be more important in determining compressive forces than whether the exercise is performed in an open or closed kinetic chain fashion. Findings also suggest that the effectiveness of joint-specific strengthening is maximized when combined with general strength, flexibility, and functional exercises.[50]

A factor that may influence choice of treatment is the degree to which a reduction in muscle strength is due to disuse muscle atrophy or to muscle inhibition. The latter may be due to effusion or pain and, as such, may require targeted interventions such as ice, compression bandaging, anti-inflammatory medication, and other pain-relieving modalities to remove the source of the inhibition. However, it is generally not possible to measure muscle inhibition in the clinical setting, although large discrepancies between apparent muscle mass and measured muscle strength (ie, a low strength score in relation to body mass) could indicate its presence. These other interventions may be reserved for cases when traditional strengthening does not seem to provide the expected increases in muscle strength.

Other factors that may influence the type of exercise prescribed are the coexistence of symptoms arising from the patellofemoral joint, the presence of obesity, and greater disease severity. In these cases, strengthening may need to be performed in positions that minimize patellofemoral contact forces and knee loading. Such positions include, for example, non–weight bearing positions and those involving lesser degrees of knee flexion. Exercise prescription may need to emphasize lower loads and a greater number of repetitions. Hydrotherapy may also be a useful way to strengthen muscles whilst minimizing joint loading, particularly in the obese or in those with more advanced disease or with greater abnormalities in the local mechanical environment. A recent clinical trial comparing 18 weeks of hydrotherapy or land-based exercise in 64 people with knee osteoarthritis found similar improvements in pain and function.[71] This suggests that, when prescribing exercise, hydrotherapy can be considered a suitable and effective alternative to land-based exercise. Obesity alone results in reduced strength relative to the increased body mass. So strategies to reduce obesity also yield improvements in relative strength that should lead to improved function.

Muscle rehabilitation for knee osteoarthritis has largely focused on strengthening lower-limb muscles. However, neuromuscular retraining exercise may be important in people with knee osteoarthritis who report instability, buckling, slipping, or giving way of the knee during functional activities.[72] Furthermore, research showing differences in the muscular strategies employed by the central nervous system in people with knee osteoarthritis compared to those in healthy individuals (see earlier discussion of muscle activation patterns) also highlights a potential role for muscle rehabilitation that emphasizes neuromuscular retraining. One option may be to train patients to activate appropriate selective muscles through specific exercises[73] and through real-time biofeedback and motor control relearning. In this, the movement is broken down into smaller components and the person is made aware of the muscle activity required. Repetition and feedback are key components. Whether such techniques are effective in reducing knee loading or influencing disease progression has not been formally tested.

Dosage

The frequency, duration, and intensity of the exercise program may affect clinical outcomes. However, the possible relationship between outcomes and exercise frequency, duration, and intensity has not been well studied in people with knee osteoarthritis. Although a definitive dose-based response to exercise has been reported, there may be issues with maintaining high compliance in programs with long durations. Most exercise guidelines would suggest a physiological response can be attained with as little as three exercise sessions per week, and research into the effectiveness of exercise programs in individuals with knee osteoarthritis have shown improvements after 8- or 12-week programs.[74–76]

The optimal intensity of a strengthening program for osteoarthritis is unclear. High-intensity training (high resistance/load) might be expected to result in greater strength gains than low-intensity training but could potentially overload the joint and exacerbate such symptoms as pain, inflammation, and swelling. A recent study compared the effects of 8 weeks of high- and low-intensity closed kinetic chain knee-strengthening exercise performed thrice weekly in 102 people with knee osteoarthritis.[77] High-intensity training was defined as three sets of eight repetitions with an exercise weight set initially at 60% of one repetition maximum whilst low-intensity training was defined as 10 sets of 15 repetitions with an initial exercise weight of 10% of one repetition maximum. This ensured that both groups were performing a similar overall volume of mechanical work. The results showed that both strengthening programs were beneficial for pain, function, walking time, and muscle strength. However, although not significantly different, the effect sizes were larger for high-resistance strength training. From a practical perspective, the high-intensity program took 20 minutes less to perform per session than the low-intensity program, which could facilitate patient compliance.

Enhancing Uptake of Exercise and Patient Compliance

Patient compliance is a key factor in determining outcome from exercise therapy in patients with knee osteoarthritis. Many studies have reported significant differences in outcome response after an exercise intervention based on the number of completed sessions,[51,53,56,78–80] with those individuals exhibiting higher adherence to the program achieving more beneficial results. A number of factors can contribute to compliance rates for exercise programs in individuals with knee osteoarthritis. Compliance is improved when patients receive attention from health professionals rather than without such attention in an exercise program based primarily at home.[69] Psychosocial attributes of the individual also influence compliance. Better compliance with therapy has been found to be related to the perception of more severe knee symptoms, belief in the effectiveness of the intervention, and understanding of the pathogenesis of knee osteoarthritis (those who are less compliant tend to believe that osteoarthritis is part of the natural ageing process or that it is simply a "wear and tear" disease).[81] Self-efficacy, or one's belief in his or her own ability to perform tasks, is also associated with higher compliance and better outcome.[82]

Many strategies have been suggested to improve patient compliance when prescribing exercise interventions for those with knee osteoarthritis. Tailoring the exercise program to the unique requirements of the patient as well as ensuring availability of resources can be effective in maximizing compliance. Other methods suggested to improve compliance include monitoring via telephone contact[83] or self-reported diary,[84–86] graphic feedback on exercise goals and progress,[87] and lifestyle retraining.[84] While monitoring from a health care professional is the preferred method of contact, patients can rely on their own social support network when an appropriate health care professional is unavailable.[84,88,89] Additionally, self-monitoring via positive feedback loops based on level of physical function and attainment of goals may be useful for some patients.

SUMMARY

Lower-limb muscles, particularly the quadriceps, influence knee-joint load, a major contributor to knee osteoarthritis. Impairments in muscle function, including weakness, altered activation patterns, and proprioceptive deficits, are commonly found in association with knee osteoarthritis. Furthermore, there is some evidence that muscle weakness may predispose to the onset of knee osteoarthritis. Exercise is a key component of conservative management of knee osteoarthritis and has been found to be effective in symptom reduction. Further research is needed to determine whether exercise influences disease development and progression.

REFERENCES

1. Zhang W, Moskowitz R, Nuki G, et al. OARSI recommendations for the management of hip and knee osteoarthritis, part II: OARSI evidence-based, expert consensus guidelines. Osteoarthritis Cartilage 2008;16:137–62.
2. DeHaan MN, Guzman J, Bayley MT, et al. Knee osteoarthritis clinical practice guidelines—how are we doing? J Rheumatol 2007;34(10):2099–105.
3. Li L, Maetzel A, Pencharz J, et al. Use of mainstream nonpharmacologic treatment by patients with arthritis. Arthritis Rheum (Arthritis Care & Research) 2004;51(2):203–9.
4. Shelburne K, Torry M, Pandy M. Contributions of muscles, ligaments, and the ground-reaction force to tibiofemoral joint loading during normal gait. J Orthop Res 2006;24:1983–90.
5. Taylor W, Heller M, Bergmann G, et al. Tibio-femoral loading during human gait and stair climbing. J Orthop Res 2004;22:625–32.
6. Schipplein OD, Andriacchi TP. Interaction between active and passive knee stabilizers during level walking. J Orthop Res 1991;9:113–9.
7. Amin S, Luepongsak N, McGibbon C, et al. Knee adduction moment and development of chronic knee pain in elders. Artritis Care Res 2004;51:371–6.
8. Sharma L, Hurwitz DE, Thonar E, et al. Knee adduction moment, serum hyaluronan level, and disease severity in medial tibiofemoral osteoarthritis. Arthritis Rheum 1998;41:1233–40.

9. Miyazaki T, Wada M, Kawahara H, et al. Dynamic load at baseline can predict radiographic disease progression in medial compartment knee osteoarthritis. Ann Rheum Dis 2002;61:617–22.

10. Zhao D, Banks S, Mitchell K, et al. Correlation between the knee adduction torque and medial contact force for a variety of gait patterns. J Orthop Res 2007;25: 789–97.

11. Lloyd D, Buchanan T. A model of load sharing between muscles and soft tissues at the human knee during static tasks. J Biomech Eng 1996;118:367–76.

12. Buchanan T, Lloyd D. Muscle activation at the human knee during isometric flexion-extension and varus-valgus loads. J Orthop Res 1997;15:11–7.

13. Lieber R. Skeletal muscle structure, function & plasticity: the physiological basis of rehabilitation. Philadelphia: Lippincott Williams & Wilkins; 2002.

14. Enoka R. Neuromechanics of human movement. Champaign (IL): Human Kinetics; 2002.

15. Messier SP, Loeser RF, Hoover JL, et al. Osteoarthritis of the knee: effects on gait, strength, and flexibility. Arch Phys Med Rehabil 1992;73:29–36.

16. Jan MH, Lai JS, Tsauo JY, et al. Isokinetic study of muscle strength in osteoarthritic knees of females. J Formos Med Assoc 1990;89:873–9.

17. Slemenda C, Brandt KD, Heilman DK, et al. Quadriceps weakness and osteoarthritis of the knee. Ann Intern Med 1997;127:97–104.

18. Ikeda S, Tsumura H, Torisu T. Age-related quadriceps-dominant muscle atrophy and incident radiographic knee osteoarthritis. J Orthop Sci 2005;10:121 6.

19. Fink B, Egl M, Singer J, et al. Morphologic changes in the vastus medialis muscle in patients with osteoarthritis of the knee. Arthritis Rheum 2007;56:3626–33.

20. Glasberg MR, Glasberg JR, Jones RE. Muscle pathology in total knee replacement for severe osteoarthritis: a histochemical and morphometric study. Henry Ford Hosp Med J 1986;34:37–40.

21. Stevens JE, Mizner RL, Snyder-Mackler L. Quadriceps strength and volitional activation before and after total knee arthroplasty for osteoarthritis. J Orthop Res 2003;21:775–9.

22. O'Reilly SC, Jones A, Muir KR, et al. Quadriceps weakness in knee osteoarthritis: the effect on pain and disability. Ann Rheum Dis 1998;57:588–94.

23. Berth A, Urbach D, Awiszus F. Improvement of voluntary quadriceps muscle activation after total knee arthroplasty. Arch Phys Med Rehabil 2002;83: 1432–6.

24. Lewek MD, Rudolph KS, Snyder-Mackler L. Control of frontal plane knee laxity during gait in patients with medial compartment knee osteoarthritis. Osteoarthritis Cartilage 2004;12:745–51.

25. Childs JD, Sparto PJ, Fitzgerald GK, et al. Alterations in lower extremity movement and muscle activation patterns in individuals with knee osteoarthritis. Clin Biomech 2004;19:44–9.

26. Moskowitz R, Howell D, Goldberg V, et al. Osteoarthritis diagnosis and medical/ surgical management. Philadelphia: WB Saunders Co; 1992.

27. Wrigley T. Physiological responses to injury: muscle. In: Zuluaga M, Briggs C, Carlisle J, et al, editors. Sports physiotherapy: applied science & practice. Edinburgh (UK): Churchill Livingstone; 1995. p. 17–42.

28. Ledingham J, Regan M, Jones A, et al. Factors affecting radiographic progression of knee osteoarthritis. Ann Rheum Dis 1995;54:53–8.

29. Astephen JL, Deluzio KJ, Caldwell GE, et al. Gait and neuromuscular pattern changes are associated with differences in knee osteoarthritis severity levels. J Biomech 2008;41:868–76.

30. Jerosch J, Prymka M. Proprioception and joint stability. Knee Surg Sports Traumatol Arthrosc 1996;4:171–9.
31. Sharma L, Pai Y. Impaired proprioception and osteoarthritis. Curr Opin Rheumatol 1997;9:253–8.
32. Lephart SM, Pincivero DM, Giraldo JL, et al. The role of proprioception in the management and rehabilitation of athletic injuries. Am J Sports Med 1997;25:130–7.
33. Fischer-Rasmussen T, Jensen P. Proprioceptive sensitivity and performance in anterior cruciate ligament-deficient knee joints. Scand J Med Sci Sports 2000;10:85–9.
34. Barrack RL, Skinner HB, Cook SD, et al. Effect of articular disease and total knee arthroplasty on knee joint-position sense. J Neurophysiol 1983;50:684–7.
35. Barrett DS, Cobb AG, Bentley G. Joint proprioception in normal, osteoarthritic and replaced knees. J Bone Joint Surg [Br] 1991;73:53–6.
36. Hassan BS, Mockett S, Doherty M. Static postural sway, proprioception, and maximal voluntary quadriceps contraction in patients with knee osteoarthritis and normal control subjects. Ann Rheum Dis 2001;60:612–8.
37. Koralewicz LM, Engh GA. Comparison of proprioception in arthritic and age-matched normal knees. J Bone Joinit Surg [Am] 2000;82:1582–8.
38. Pai YC, Rymer WZ, Chang RW, et al. Effect of age and osteoarthritis on knee proprioception. Arthritis Rheum 1997;40:2260–5.
39. Marks R. An investigation of the influence of age, clinical status, pain and position sense on stair walking in women with osteoarthrosis. Int J Rehabil Res 1994;17:151–8.
40. Marks R. Correlations between measurements of the sense of knee position and the severity of joint lesions in knee osteoarthritis. Rev Rhum Ed Fr 1994;61:423–30.
41. Skinner HB, Barrack RL, Cook SD, et al. Joint position sense in total knee arthroplasty. J Orthop Res 1984;1:276–83.
42. Bennell KL, Hinman RS, Metcalf BR, et al. Relationship of knee joint proprioception to pain and disability in individuals with knee osteoarthritis. J Orthop Res 2003;21:792–7.
43. Hurley MV, Scott DL, Rees J, et al. Sensorimotor changes and functional performance in patients with knee osteoarthritis. Ann Rheum Dis 1997;56(11):641–8.
44. Slemenda C, Heilman D, Brandt K, et al. Reduced quadriceps strength relative to body weight: a risk factor for knee osteoarthritis in women? Arthritis Rheum 1998;41:1951–9.
45. Hootman J, Fitzgerald S, Macera C, et al. Lower extremity muscle strength and risk of self-reported hip or knee osteoarthritis. J Phys Act Health 2004;1:321–30.
46. Brandt KD, Heilman DK, Slemenda C, et al. Quadriceps strength in women with radiographically progressive osteoarthritis of the knee and those with stable radiographic changes. J Rheumatol 1999;26:2431–7.
47. Sharma L, Dunlop DD, Song J, et al. Quadriceps strength and osteoarthritis progression in maligned and lax knees. Ann Intern Med 2003;138(8):613–9.
48. Amin S, Baker K, Niu J, et al. Quadriceps strength and its relation to cartilage loss in knee osteoarthritis. Paper presented at: American College of Rheumatology, Washington, DC; 2006.
49. Sharma L, Cahue S, Song J, et al. Physical functioning over three years in knee osteoarthritis. Role of psychosocial, local mechanical, and neuromusculsr factors. Arthritis Rheum 2003;48:3359–70.

50. Pelland L, Brosseau L, Wells G, et al. Efficacy of strengthening exercises for osteoarthritis (part I): a meta-analysis. Phys Ther Rev 2004;9:77–108.
51. O'Reilly SC, Muir KR, Doherty M. Effectiveness of home exercise on pain and disability from osteoarthritis of the knee: a randomised controlled trial. Ann Rheum Dis 1999;58:15–9.
52. Hurley MV, Scott DL. Improvements in quadriceps sensorimotor function and disability of patients with knee osteoarthritis following a clinically practicable exercise regime. Br J Rheumatol 1998;37:1181–7.
53. Thomas K, Muir K, Doherty M, et al. Home based exercise programme for knee pain and knee osteoarthritis: randomised controlled trial. BMJ 2002; 325:752–6.
54. Baker K, Nelson M, Felson D, et al. The efficacy of home based progressive strength training in older adults with knee osteoarthritis: a randomized controlled trial. J Rheumatol 2001;28:1655–65.
55. Van Baar ME, Dekker J, Oostendorp RAB, et al. The effectiveness of exercise therapy in patients with osteoarthritis of the hip or knee: a randomized clinical trial. J Rheumatol 1998;25:2432–9.
56. Ettinger WH, Burns R, Messier SP, et al. A randomized trial comparing aerobic exercise and resistance exercise with a health education program in older adults with knee osteoarthritis. JAMA 1997;277:25–31.
57. Fisher NM, Gresham G, Pendergast DR. Effects of a quantitative progressive rehabilitation program applied unilaterally to the osteoarthritic knee. Arch Phys Med Rehabil 1993;74:1319–26.
58. Hinman R, Heywood S, Day A. Aquatic physical therapy for hip and knee osteoarthritis: results of a single-blind randomized controlled trial. Phys Ther 2007;87: 32–43.
59. Hassan B, Doherty S, Mockett S, et al. Effect of pain reduction on postural sway, proprioception, and quadriceps strength in subjects with knee osteoarthritis. Ann Rheum Dis 2002;61:422–8.
60. Diracoglu D, Aydin R, Baskent A, et al. Effects of kinesthesia and balance exercises in knee osteoarthritis. J Clin Rheumatol 2005;11(6):303–10.
61. Lin D, Lin Y, Chai H, et al. Comparison of proprioceptive functions between computerized proprioception facilitation exercise and closed kinetic chain exercise in patients with knee osteoarthritis. Clin Rheumatol 2007;26(4):520–8.
62. Birmingham T, Kramer J, Kirkley A, et al. Knee bracing for medial compartment osteoarthritis: effects on proprioception and postural control. Rheumatology 2001;40:285–9.
63. Hassan B, Mockett S, Doherty M. Influence of elastic bandage on knee pain, proprioception, and postural sway in subjects with knee osteoarthritis. Ann Rheum Dis 2002;61:24–8.
64. Roddy E, Zhang W, Doherty M. Aerobic walking or strengthening exercise for osteoarthritis of the knee? A systematic review. Ann Rheum Dis 2005;64:544–8.
65. van Baar M, Dekker J, Oostendorp R, et al. Effectiveness of exercise in patients with osteoarthritis of the hip or knee: nine months' follow up. Ann Rheum Dis 2001; 60:1123–30.
66. Mikesky A, Mazzuca S, Brandt K, et al. Effects of strength training on the incidence and progression of knee osteoarthritis. Arthritis Rheum 2006;55:690–9.
67. Fransen M, McConnell S, Bell M. Exercise for osteoarthritis of the hip or knee (cochrane review). In: The Cochrane library, vol. 4. Chichester (UK): John Wiley & Sons, Ltd; 2003.

68. McCarthy C, Mills P, Pullen R, et al. Supplementing a home exercise programme with a class-based exercise programme is more effective than home exercise alone in the treatment of knee osteoarthritis. Rheumatology 2004;43:880–6.
69. McCarthy C, Mills P, Pullen R, et al. Supplementation of a home-based exercise programme with a class-based programme for people with osteoarthritis of the knees: a randomised controlled trial and health economic analysis. Health Technol Assess 2004;46:1–61.
70. Ravaud P, Giraudeau B, Logeart I, et al. Management of osteoarthritis (OA) with an unsupervised home based exercise programme and/or patient administered tools. A cluster randomised controlled trial with a 2×2 factorial design. Ann Rheum Dis 2004;63:703–8.
71. Silva LE, Valim V, Pessanha AP, et al. Hydrotherapy versus conventional land-based exercise for the management of patients with osteoarthritis of the knee: a randomized clinical trial. Phys Ther 2008;88(1):12–21.
72. Hurley M. Muscle dysfunction and effective rehabilitation of knee osteoarthritis: what we know and what we need to find out. Arthritis Care Res 2003;49:444–52.
73. Lynn SK, Costigan PA. Changes in the medial-lateral hamstring activation ratio with foot rotation during lower limb exercise. J Electromyogr Kinesiol 2008 March; [Epub].
74. Rogind H, Bibow-Nielsen B, Jensen B, et al. The effects of a physical training program on patients with osteoarthritis of the knees. Arch Phys Med Rehabil 1998; 79:1421–7.
75. Huang M, Lin Y, Yang R, et al. A comparison of various therapeutic exercises on the functional status of patients with knee osteoarthritis. Semin Arthritis Rheum 2003;32:398–406.
76. Suomi R, Collier D. Effects of arthritis exercise programs on functional fitness and perceived activities of daily living measures in older adults with arthritis. Arch Phys Med Rehabil 2003;84:1589–94.
77. Jan MH, Lin JJ, Liau JJ, et al. Investigation of clinical effects of high- and low-resistance training for patients with knee osteoarthritis: a randomized controlled trial. Phys Ther 2008 Jan [Epub].
78. Belza B, Topolski T, Kinne S, et al. Does adherence make a difference? Results from a community-based aquatic exercise program. Nurs Res 2002;51:285–91.
79. van Gool C, Penninx B, Kempen G, et al. Effects of exercise adherence on physical function among overweight older adults with knee osteoarthritis. Arthritis Rheum (Arthritis Care & Research) 2005;53(1):24–32.
80. Fielding R, Katula J, Miller M, et al. Activity adherence and physical function in older adults with functional limitations. Med Sci Sports Exerc 2007;39:1997–2004.
81. Campbell R, Evans M, Tucker M, et al. Why don't patients do their exercises? Understanding non-compliance with physiotherapy in patients with osteoarthritis of the knee. J Epidemiol Commun Health 2001;55:132–8.
82. Marks R, Allegrante J. Chronic osteoarthritis and adherence to exercise: a review of the literature. J Aging Phys Act 2005;13:434–60.
83. Castro C, King A, Brassington G. Telephone versus mail interventions for maintenance of physical activity in older adults. Health Psychol 2001;20:438–44.
84. Roddy E, Doherty M. Changing life-styles and osteoarthritis: what is the evidence? Best Pract Res Clin Rheumatol 2006;20:81–97.
85. King A, Taylor C, Haskell W, et al. Strategies for increasing early adherence to and long-term maintenance of home-based exercise training in healthy middle-aged men and women. Am J Cardiol 1988;61:628–32.

86. Noland M. The effects of self-monitoring and reinforcement on exercise adherence. Res Q Exerc Sport 1989;60:216–24.
87. Duncan K, Pozehl B. Effects of an exercise adherence intervention on outcomes in patients with heart failure. Rehabil Nurs 2003;28:117–22.
88. Litt M, Kleppinger A, Judge J. Initiation and maintenance of exercise behaviour in older women: predictors from the social learning model. J Behav Med 2002;25: 83–97.
89. Oka R, King A, Rohm Young D. Sources of social support as predictors of exercise adherence in women and men ages 50 to 65 years. Womens Health 1995;1: 161–75.

Knee Osteoarthritis: Primary Care Using Noninvasive Devices and Biomechanical Principles

K. Douglas Gross, PT, ScD[a],*, Howard Hillstrom, PhD[b]

KEYWORDS

- Osteoarthritis • Knee • Biomechanics • Devices • Braces
- Orthoses • Physical therapy

Osteoarthritis (OA) is an epidemic for which there is no known cure. In 1990, there were 21 million Americans who had physician-diagnosed OA.[1] By 2020, that number will have doubled,[2] due in large part to the rapid aging of our general population and its soaring rates of obesity. When OA becomes symptomatic in the knee, as it does in at least one out of every eight adults 60 years of age and older,[3,4] the impact can be debilitating. Mobility limitations account for 80% of all chronic disabilities among seniors[5] and knee OA is the single most prevalent cause.[6]

Despite increasing concern about the capacity of our current health care system to meet these demands, routine primary care for knee OA has changed little over several decades. Even today, a visit to the family doctor rarely results in much more than a prescription for palliative drugs and the promise of watchful waiting. Few attempts are made to identify interventions capable of supporting the structural integrity of an osteoarthritic knee so that it can bear weight, sustain loads, and perform the functions that allow continued participation in activities. Instead, this progressive disease is allowed to persist while narrowly focused treatments target short-term symptom reduction using palliative drugs. The two most widely prescribed drugs, the nonsteroidal anti-inflammatories (NSAIDs) and cyclo-oxygenase-2 (COX-2) inhibitors, have recently come under public scrutiny for their alarmingly high rate of adverse events[7,8] and their

A version of this article originally appeared in the 34:3 issue of the Rheumatic Disease Clinics of North America.
[a] MGH Institute of Health Professions, Graduate Programs in Physical Therapy, Charlestown Navy Yard, 36 First Avenue, Boston, MA 02129-4557, USA
[b] Hospital for Special Surgery, Leon Root, M.D., Motion Analysis Lab, The Dana Center, Ground Floor, 510 East 73rd Street, New York, NY 10021, USA
* Corresponding author.
E-mail address: kdgross@mghihp.edu (K.D. Gross).

grossly immoderate cost.[9] NSAIDs alone are responsible for an estimated 16,500 deaths and 103,000 hospitalizations each year in the United States.[10] Yet despite the risk, all NSAIDs have performed comparably in clinical trials, with subjects reporting a modest 30% reduction in short-term symptom intensity and only 15% improvement in functional activity.[11] Without physical protection from further damage, the knee with mild OA tends to worsen with time. Eventually a patient's activity limitations become severe enough to necessitate surgical joint replacement. If this pattern of medical practice continues, the number of primary total knee arthroplasties performed each year in the United States will increase 674% between 2005 and 2030, and the annual direct cost of knee and hip replacement will exceed $100 billion.[4]

With few conservative options available in the medical system, increasing numbers of seniors are turning to untested folk remedies and self-prescribed dietary supplements. There is enormous popular demand for nonpharmacologic and noninvasive therapies for OA, and there is a pressing need for primary care physicians to respond by updating their pattern of practice. This article introduces physicians to several of the most important noninvasive devices used in the conservative management of symptomatic knee OA. Each section of the article opens with a presentation of the device's anticipated biomechanical effects and then considers evidence of clinical efficacy. Where possible, we close each section with a summary of our own experience prescribing these devices, and the considerations that we believe are important for successful patient management.

TARGETING KNEE MECHANICS

The knee consists of three distinct joint compartments: the medial tibiofemoral (TF), lateral TF, and patellofemoral (PF). The shared goal of many noninvasive devices for knee OA is to alter lower limb biomechanics in such a way as to limit the exposure of one or more of these knee compartments to potentially damaging and provocative mechanical stresses. Optimal prescription of a device requires that physicians specify not only the knee compartments that require protection but also the types of mechanical stress that should be reduced. A basic understanding of lower limb biomechanics can valuably inform this determination.

CANES, WALKERS, AND GROUND REACTION FORCES

Nearly all patients with symptomatic knee OA report provocation with some type of weight-bearing activity. This finding indicates that sensitivity to mechanical load is a common feature of the most frequently symptomatic knee compartments. Physicians charged with caring for patients who have medial or lateral TF OA are familiar with the improvements that often occur when patients are provided with assistive walking devices that reduce compressive loading over TF joint surfaces.[12,13]

When body weight is borne on a limb during standing (**Fig. 1**) or walking (**Fig. 2**), the limb is subjected to an equal and opposite reaction force from the ground. The vertical component of this ground reaction force (GRF) exerts a compressive load on the weight-bearing surfaces of the TF joint. In bilateral standing, the GRF loads each limb with approximately 50% of body weight. By contrast, the stance phase of self-paced walking generates a peak GRF equal to 150% to 200% of body weight. For a knee with symptomatic TF OA, this amount of load can soon become excessive. Fortunately, when a cane, crutch, walker, or similar assistive walking device is used, a portion of this load can be shifted off of the symptomatic limb and onto the device. By shifting body weight off of the symptomatic limb and onto the cane, a patient enjoys a proportionate reduction of the GRF acting on that limb, and a consequent

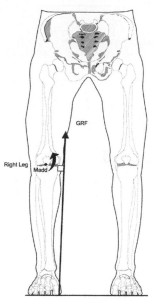

Fig. 1. Ground reaction force (GRF) through a normally aligned knee during standing. The perpendicular distance of the GRF from the knee's axis of rotation produces an adduction moment (M_{add}) that concentrates compressive load on the medial TF compartment.

lessening of the compressive load that is exerted on the symptomatic TF tissues.[14] It is by means of this reduction in the compressive load that canes and walkers are so often effective in improving tolerance for upright activities among patients who have TF OA. Shopping is an example of an upright activity for which cane use may be indicated. Shopping can involve long periods of uninterrupted standing and walking, and shopping is typically one of the first activity limitations reported by older women with TF OA.

There is a second means by which canes or walking sticks can be effective in reducing load over highly exposed portions of the TF joint. This second mechanism depends on the cane's placement relative to the knee's axis of frontal plane rotation (located near the center of the knee). To take full advantage of this second mechanism, a cane should always be held in the hand contralateral to the symptomatic joint, and made to contact the ground at some distance from the affected medial TF compartment.

During standing, the GRF normally passes a short distance medial to the knee and to its axis of frontal plane rotation (see **Fig. 1**). As a result of the short distance over which it is applied, the GRF generates a small torque, or adduction moment (M_{add}) that attempts to rotate the tibia around the knee's axis of frontal plane motion in the direction of knee adduction. The additional adduction stress serves to concentrate compressive load on the medial TF compartment. Although the medial TF loading may still be tolerable during quiet standing, the heightened stresses of walking can quickly overwhelm a knee with symptomatic medial TF OA. Not only is the GRF of a greater magnitude in walking than in standing, but its vector is also a greater distance medial of the knee (see **Fig. 2**). At its peak in the early stance phase of a normal

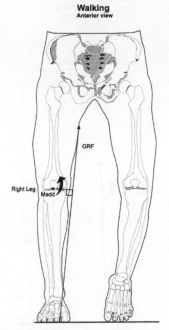

Walking
Anterior view

GRF

Right Leg
Madd

Fig. 2. Ground reaction force (GRF) through a normally aligned knee during walking. Although the magnitude of the GRF is only 50% of body weight during standing, it may be 150% to 200% of body weight during walking. The perpendicular distance of the GRF from the knee's axis of rotation produces an adduction moment (M_{add}) that concentrates compressive load on the medial TF compartment.

gait cycle, the resulting M_{add} forces the medial TF compartment to absorb at least 60% to 70% of the knee's total compressive load.[15] Given the magnitude of compressive load to which the medial TF compartment is repeatedly exposed during walking, it is advisable for many patients who have symptomatic medial TF OA to use a cane held in the contralateral hand whenever they are ambulating for long periods.

The downward force that a patient applies to the cane generates its own equal and opposite ground reaction force at the point where the cane contacts the ground. This ground reaction force (labeled GRF_{cane} in **Fig. 3**) acts through the contralateral hand and the trunk to generate a moment of force at the symptomatic knee (labelled M_{cane} in **Fig. 3**), which counteracts the usual M_{add} by attempting to rotate the femur in the direction of knee abduction. Allowing the cane to make ground contact at some distance contralateral to the symptomatic knee, the patient is able to take useful advantage of a long lever arm over which to apply this protective abductory moment of force. More importantly, by effectively resisting the forces that drive the knee into greater adduction, the patient succeeds in protecting the medial TF compartment against potentially damaging levels of compressive load.[14] To make use of a cane for this purpose, however, proper sizing and placement are critical.

To properly fit a cane to a patient, the cane should be aligned alongside the leg so that it contacts the ground just lateral of the lateral malleolus. The height of the cane is then adjusted until the handle is approximately level with the superior tip of the greater trochanter (**Fig. 4**). The user's arm should maintain 20 to 30 degrees of elbow flexion while holding the cane in this position. To successfully bolster against the effects of the

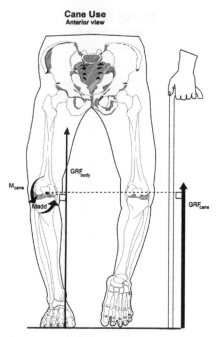

Cane Use
Anterior view

Fig. 3. Partial weight-bearing on a cane also generates a ground reaction force (GRF_{cane}). When the cane is held in the hand contralateral to the symptomatic knee, the GRF_{cane} is applied over a long lever arm to generate a moment of force (M_{cane}) that counteracts the usual adduction moment (M_{add}) at the knee. In so doing, contralateral cane use is effective in reducing load over the medial tibiofemoral compartment.

M_{add} at the time that it reaches its peak magnitude during walking, the patient must be able to initiate partial weight-bearing through the cane at the same instant that the opposite foot strikes the ground (ie, at the onset of stance phase). Directed rehearsal of the correct walking pattern is often necessary, especially for older patients.

The authors are not aware of any trials that have specifically evaluated the clinical efficacy of cane use. Both the American College of Rheumatology[16] and the European League Against Rheumatism[17] recommend cane prescription as an important component of primary medical care for knee and hip OA. A cane used in the contralateral hand has been shown to reduce intra-articular loading at the hip joint by 50% during self-paced walking,[18] and reductions in the knee M_{add} in excess of 10% have been reported in association with cane use by patients who have medial TF OA.[14] Because the PF compartment is not directly exposed to weight-bearing load during most upright standing or level-ground walking activities, cane use is not expected to serve any essential purpose for patients whose symptoms are of strictly PF origin.

TIBIOFEMORAL MALALIGNMENT AND THE UNLOADER BRACE

Although the GRF determines how much overall compressive load the TF joint routinely sustains, it is the relative alignment of the tibia and femur that determines the manner in which this load is distributed over the medial and lateral TF compartments. As little as 5 degrees of genu varum (bowlegged) malalignment results in an

Cane Sizing
Anterior view

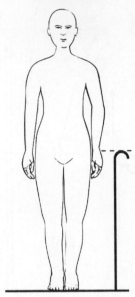

Fig. 4. To properly fit a cane to a patient, the cane should be aligned alongside the leg and contacting the ground just lateral of the lateral malleolus. The height of the cane is then adjusted until the handle is approximately level with the superior tip of the greater trochanter.

estimated 70% to 90% increase in compressive load over the medial TF compartment (**Fig. 5**).[19] Not surprisingly, this dramatic increase in compressive load corresponds to a fourfold increase in the odds of OA worsening in the medial TF compartment over 18 months.[20] Conversely genu valgum (knock-kneed) malalignment increases compressive load on the lateral TF compartment and elevates the odds of worsening lateral TF OA by fivefold over the same period.[20]

Relevant frontal plane malalignments are often identifiable during visual inspection of a patient's relaxed standing posture. Busy physicians should be reassured to know that simple clinical measurements of TF alignment correlate well (r=0.70, p<0.01) with more cumbersome measurements taken from long limb radiographs.[21] When genu varum malalignment is accompanied by knee instability, as is often the case with more severe OA, the bowlegged posture of the limb may become visibly exaggerated under the influence of the large M_{add} that occurs during walking. In such instances, observation of the patient's walking pattern reveals an abrupt thrust of the knee into an exaggerated varus (bowlegged) attitude with each successive footfall. Among knees with moderate genu varum malalignment in standing, the additional presence of an exaggerated varus thrust during walking has been found to elevate the odds of medial TF OA progression by threefold over an 18-month period.[22]

Improved frontal plane alignment and mediolateral stability are commonly cited reasons for prescribing either a valgus unloader brace to patients who have medial TF OA, or (less commonly) a varus unloader brace to patients who have lateral TF OA.[23] When a realigning force is applied to the knee using a valgus unloader brace (**Fig. 6**), the expectation is that slight improvements in tibiofemoral alignment and

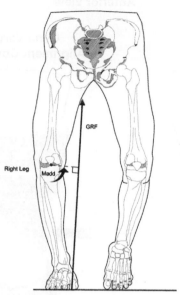

Genu Varum Malalignment
Anterior View in Walking

GRF

Right Leg

Madd

Fig. 5. Loading of the knee with genu varum, or bowlegged, malalignment. Genu varum increases the adduction moment (M_{add}) at the knee and the magnitude of compressive load on the medial TF compartment.

stability will result in meaningful reductions in the magnitude of the M_{add} and consequent improvement in the distribution of compressive load over TF joint surfaces. Using video fluoroscopy, Komistek and colleagues[24] confirmed that a custom-fitted unloader brace is capable of producing desirable changes in tibiofemoral alignment that are maintained during walking. Among 15 men and women who had unicompartmental OA in either the medial or lateral TF joint, only the 3 most obese subjects in the Komistek study failed to maintain the expected improvements in joint alignment at the time of heel contact during treadmill ambulation. The mean change in TF alignment was 2.2 degrees, which corresponded to a mean increase in joint space of 1.2 mm in the targeted TF compartment. These desirable changes help to explain the 10% to 13% reductions in the M_{add} that other investigators have reported in association with valgus unloader bracing.[25,26] As the knee assumes a more erect alignment, the distance between the knee and the GRF is reduced, causing the M_{add} to decrease and the compressive load to become more evenly distributed over the medial and lateral TF compartments.

Although the mechanical effects of a properly fitted unloader brace can be safely inferred from gait laboratory investigations, few high-quality clinical trials are available to help inform an assessment of the likely clinical effects of an unloader brace. A 2008 update of a 2005 Cochrane review[27] still succeeded in identifying only two trials that were of sufficient quality to satisfy all criteria for inclusion. In one, Kirkley and colleagues[28] compared the mean change in measured pain and function following 6 months of a prescribed valgus unloader brace (n = 41) to the effects of either no brace (n = 33) or a neoprene sleeve (n = 36). All subjects had medial TF OA with varus malalignment in standing. The prescribed valgus unloader brace was custom fitted and

Valgus Unloader Brace

Anterior view

**Genu Varum
Malalignment**

**Genu Varum
Alignment Corrected**

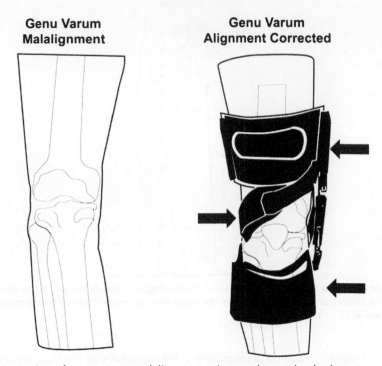

Fig. 6. Correction of genu varum malalignment using a valgus unloader brace.

consisted of lightweight calf and thigh shells connected on the medial side by an adjustable hinge (see **Fig. 6**). Tension in the brace was adjusted to apply as much as 4 degrees of valgus correction.

Results of the Kirkley and colleagues[28] trial indicated that the group receiving the valgus unloader brace achieved greater mean improvements in pain and function after 6 months than either of the two comparison groups. The mean change score for pain (lowest score possible, −500 mm) was −13.1 mm for the control group, 13.1 mm for the neoprene sleeve group, and 43.2 mm for the unloader brace group (P = .001). Even more impressively, the mean change score for physical function (lowest score possible. −1700 mm) was −6.5 mm for the control group, 68.9 mm for the neoprene sleeve group, and 157.2 mm for the unloader brace group (P = .004).

The second trial, a multicenter randomized controlled trial by Brouwer and colleagues,[29] enrolled 117 subjects who had unicompartmental OA in either the medial or lateral TF compartments. The prescribed unloader braces in this trial consisted of calf and thigh shells in four generic sizes that were connected by heavy metal hinges on the medial and lateral sides. The hinges allowed for adjustment of up to 12.5 degrees valgus correction for subjects who had medial TF OA and up to 10 degrees varus correction for subjects who had lateral TF OA. At 12 months, an intent-to-treat comparison of 60 subjects in the treatment group (including those who had either varus or valgus knee braces) and 57 subjects in the unbraced control group revealed only nonsignificant differences with respect to overall pain reduction. However, brace users also reported a mean increase in walking tolerance that was 1.8 km greater than the increase reported by controls ($P = .04$). A treatment effect of this magnitude is likely to be of substantial benefit to patients experiencing difficulty walking long distances because of unicompartmental TF OA.

Before recommending an unloader brace to a patient who has unicompartmental TF OA, it is important to note that of the 60 subjects originally assigned to intervention in the Brouwer[29] trial, more than one third (n = 24) stopped using the generically sized brace before completion of the assigned 12-month treatment period. The most commonly cited reasons for noncompliance were a lack of noticeable benefit (n = 20) and poor fit (n = 4). This report reinforces our own clinical experience. Obese patients have particular trouble with generically sized unloader braces, and older women commonly express frustration with the bulkiness and inconvenience of many metal-hinged braces. Younger and slimmer patients are easier to fit with an unloader brace, but some customization is often necessary to ensure that the desired mechanical effects are retained. There is increasing evidence that the mediolateral stability offered by a snugly fitting brace may be critical to ensuring that the desired reductions in mechanical stress are achieved.[23]

A challenge faced by prescribing physicians is how best to match a particular unloader brace with a particular patient's needs and preferences. Consultation with a knowledgeable physical therapist or orthotist may be helpful. In the interest of improving patient compliance, it is best to specify that the patient use the brace only during particular aggravating activities. Compliance is far more likely when the brace is used successfully to improve tolerance for shopping, walking, tennis, or some other weight-bearing pastime.

JOINT CONTACT AREA AND PATELLAR TAPING OR BRACING

It had long been assumed that knee OA was less common in the PF than in the TF compartments. It now appears that this assumption is incorrect.[30] Among subjects reporting knee symptoms in the Framingham Study, 40% had radiographic OA that remained isolated to one or both of the TF compartments, whereas 60% exhibited OA that was either isolated to (20%) or inclusive of (40%) the PF compartment.[31] PF joint involvement is even more common among women,[32] and because pathologic changes at the PF joint less frequently exhibit early osteophytosis, OA in the PF compartment probably goes undiagnosed more often than OA elsewhere in the knee.[33] When radiographic OA is finally identified in the PF compartment, the changes there generally provide a better explanation for the activity limitations that a person experiences than do osteoarthritic changes in either of the TF compartments.[32]

Because we now know that involvement of the PF compartment is common among older people who have knee pain, it is surprising that so few trials have yet been undertaken to evaluate the efficacy of patellar taping and bracing interventions for people who have PF OA. Instead, the great majority of what we currently know about PF devices has been abstracted from previous studies of their use among young adults who have PF pain syndrome. Studied application of these interventions to older patients with knee OA is long overdue. We still understand little about how the design of these devices might be modified to maximize their usefulness in older populations.

The knee typically flexes less than 15 degrees during the weight-bearing phase of level ground walking.[34] As a result, the patella rarely engages the femur during many upright activities. By contrast, the actions of climbing a stair and rising from a chair can require maximum joint angles of more than 90 degrees.[35,36] During these activities, with the GRF passing a substantial distance posterior of the knee's axis of sagittal plane rotation, the quadriceps muscle must contract powerfully to counteract a sizable external moment of force for knee flexion (**Fig. 7**). In fact, when ascending stairs, the peak external knee flexion moment increases to four times the magnitude of the peak M_{add} during the same effort.[37] The required quadriceps contraction exerts enormous compressive load on the PF joint. Load on PF joint is equivalent to three to four times body weight during unassisted stair climbing, and may be as much as seven to eight times body weight when rising from a low chair.[38]

Despite the enormous stress that is exerted on the PF joint during weight-bearing knee flexion, clinical experience tells us that knee flexion in a closed kinematic chain (foot planted on a stationary ground) is often far better tolerated than similarly resisted knee flexion in an open kinematic chain (foot free to move). This apparent inconsistency is explained by the retropatellar contact area being markedly increased during closed chain knee function.[39] The increased contact area means that the overall compressive load on the PF joint is distributed over a greater surface area. With a greater surface area over which to distribute the compressive load, focal pressure on the articular surfaces of the PF joint is reduced (**Fig. 8**).

PF taping and bracing interventions seek to reduce retropatellar pressure by maximizing PF contact area during weight-bearing activities that involve knee flexion. These treatments are believed to be ideal in cases where focal pressure on the lateral PF joint surfaces is made excessive by lateral patellar malalignment or lateral instability. Contrary to theory, however, the benefits of patellar taping and bracing may not be entirely specific to patients who have either of these clinical findings. Indeed, one

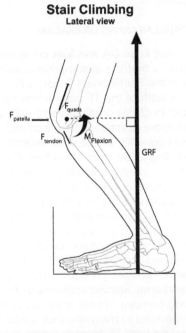

Stair Climbing
Lateral view

$F_{patella}$

F_{quads}

F_{tendon} $M_{Flexion}$

GRF

Fig. 7. In stair climbing, with the GRF passing a substantial distance posterior of the knee's axis of rotation, the quadriceps muscle must contract powerfully (F_{quads}) to counteract a sizable external moment of force for knee flexion ($M_{flexion}$). The contraction increases compressive load at the patellofemoral joint ($F_{patella}$).

Compressive Force

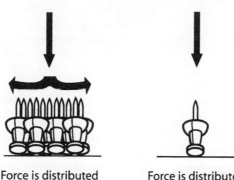

| Force is distributed over greater contact area = less pressure | Force is distributed over less contact area = more pressure |

Fig. 8. Focal compressive stress is measured as pressure. Because pressure is equal to the compressive force per unit of contact area, pressure declines when contact area is increased.

recently derived clinical prediction rule[40] suggests that the likelihood of a younger patient who has PF pain responding to medially-directed patellar taping (**Fig. 9**) actually increases when there is sufficient suppleness and flexibility in the lateral patellar soft tissues. This suggestion is contrary to the usual notion that tightness in the lateral soft tissues is a primary cause of the lateral patellar malalignment that indicates the need for realigning interventions. Moreover, there is little evidence supporting the claim that the usual methods of applying tape actually succeed in maintaining a measurable medial displacement of the patella once weight-bearing knee flexion activity has been initiated.[41,42] Instead, a far more consistent effect of taping and bracing is to increase contact area between the load-bearing facets of the patella and the articulating trochlea of the femur. For example, Powers and colleagues[43] used dynamic MRI to image PF contact at four different angles of weight-bearing knee flexion. Among the 15 symptomatic female participants, both of the patellar braces evaluated were effective in increasing mean PF contact area by 20% to 25% in comparison with the no-brace condition. This sizable increase in PF contact area was concurrent with a mean reduction in pain of 45% to 50%. Neither lateral patellar malalignment nor lateral patellar instability was prerequisite for participation in the study.

A recent systematic review and meta-analysis[44] synthesized current best evidence relating to the clinical effects of patellar taping and bracing for the treatment of chronic knee pain in both older and younger adults. Of the 16 studies that satisfied the criteria for inclusion, 13 investigated taping or bracing effects in nonspecific anterior knee pain, whereas only 3 studies evaluated the effects of patellar taping among subjects who had diagnosed knee OA. Of these 3, none required that study participants exhibit any radiographic or clinical confirmation of PF compartment involvement. Consequently, the results of these trials must be interpreted as possibly relevant to all patients who have knee OA, regardless of their specific compartmental diagnosis.

A pooling of the available data indicated that medially directed patellar taping was effective in decreasing chronic knee symptoms by 16.1 mm on a 100-mm pain scale (95% CI: 10.0 to 22.2 mm, $P<.01$) and 10.9 mm (95% CI: 3.4 to 18.4 mm, $P<.01$) in comparison with no tape and sham taping, respectively. When limiting the analyses

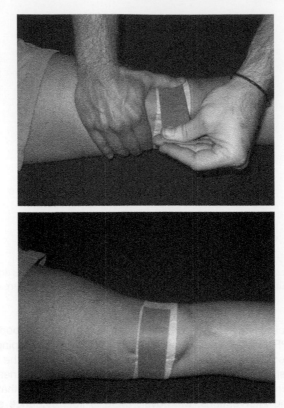

Fig. 9. Medially directed patellar taping serves the purpose of increasing patellofemoral contact area so that retropatellar pressure is reduced.

to only those three studies involving subjects who had diagnosed knee OA, the efficacy of patellar taping increased, resulting in pain decreases of 20.1 mm (95% CI: 14.3 to 26.0, *P*<.01) in comparison with no tape, and 13.3 mm (95% CI: 8.4 to 18.1 mm, *P*<.01) in comparison with sham taping. Although additional studies are needed to clarify the specific radiographic and physical findings that most strongly indicate its use, an examination of the current evidence suggests that patellar taping is effective in reducing chronic knee pain among patients who have knee OA. The cost of the intervention is minimal, and the most serious side effects reported are local irritation of the skin. Unfortunately, although many patients can be taught to apply patellar tape themselves, daily long-term use is unrealistic. If patients demonstrate a positive short-term response to taping, a comparable patellar brace should be sought for longer-term use.

Given the encouraging results about patellar taping, it is surprising that no trials have yet examined the effects of patellar bracing (**Fig. 10**) among subjects who have knee OA. We are hopeful that the results of our own ongoing crossover trial (Bracing in Patellofemoral Osteoarthritis: A Clinical Trial; DJ Hunter, principal investigator) will help to fill this obvious void. For now we are forced to infer the likely effects of patellar bracing on knee OA from studies of patients who have nonspecific anterior knee pain. Among such studies, three trials (n = 119) compared patellar bracing to no bracing, and two trials (n = 94) compared patellar bracing to sham bracing. Pooling of data from this limited set indicated that patellar bracing was successful in decreasing

Patellar Brace
Anterior view

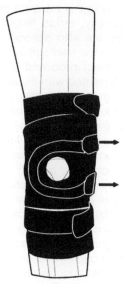

Fig. 10. Medially directed patellar bracing.

pain by 14.6 mm (95% CI: 3.8 to 25.5 mm, $P<.01$) in comparison with no bracing. Patellar bracing did not differ in its measured effects from sham bracing ($P = .76$). Again, it is unclear whether any of the observed effects of patellar bracing pertain to older patients who have knee OA.

In light of the evidence supporting the efficacy of patellar tape in reducing pain among patients who have knee OA, the clinician should feel confident introducing patellar taping as a safe and inexpensive, albeit impermanent, first line of therapy. Because there is currently no convincing evidence suggesting that patellar taping actually succeeds in markedly realigning the patella during weight-bearing function, or that the beneficial effects of patellar taping are limited to those patients whose OA remains confined to the lateral PF compartment, we recommend patellar taping as a treatment modality with potential application to lateral or medial PF OA or to mixed TF and PF OA diagnoses.

Given the absence of any published clinical trials of patellar bracing among patients who have knee OA, we feel less confident in offering firm guidelines for prescription of patellar braces. One method that we have found to be helpful in the clinic is to select an activity, such as stair climbing or standing from a low chair, that is typically provocative of a patient's knee pain. The patient is asked to pay close attention to the intensity of their knee symptoms while repeating the aggravating activity with and without a generically sized patellar brace. If the brace is successful in improving knee symptoms, our prescription is made on that basis.

TRANSIENT SHOCK AND VISCOELASTIC INSOLES

Each footfall during walking requires an abrupt deceleration of the limb at the moment that ground contact is made. Within milliseconds following initial contact, the GRF rises to a sharp peak and a shock wave is rapidly transmitted up the limb. Left unattenuated, the GRF, which at the moment of initial ground contact is referred to as the "heel strike transient," will pass jarringly up though the contacting heel and the tibia before eventually imparting a transient impulse to the tissues of the tibiofemoral joint. The magnitude and frequency of this transient impulse depends on several external factors, including gait velocity, stride length, and the compliance of the contacting ground surface. There are also several important internal mechanisms that serve to dampen and disperse the heel strike transient. The fat pad of the heel is one such mechanism. It has been proposed that the protective action of the cushioning fat pad may be supplemented with the addition of a viscoelastic insole.

As far back as the early 1970s, Simon and colleagues[45] and Radin and colleagues[46] proposed that repeated exposure to heel strike transient forces might increase the risk for TF OA. This hypothesis was later supported by findings from a series of animal studies that demonstrated that repetitive impulse loading, even at levels well below the threshold for gross tissue failure, could eventually trigger pathologic changes in the articular cartilage[47,48] and subchondral bone.[49] Radin and colleagues[50] followed up on these animal studies with a small cross-sectional study of 18 human subjects who had a history of recurrent knee pain (cases) and 14 age-matched subjects who had no history of knee pain (controls). Biomechanical analysis of the subjects' walking patterns indicated significant group differences in both the peak magnitude of the heel strike transient and the peak magnitude of measured tibial deceleration during the same brief period. There were no group differences in self-selected walking velocity, stride length, or other parameters that might serve to confound the observed association. Unfortunately, the presence of knee OA was not confirmed in any of the Radin study subjects, and when a similar case-control study was performed among 9 subjects who had radiographically confirmed TF OA, none of the previously observed differences were replicated.[51]

A causal link between the heel strike transient and TF OA still remains to be convincingly demonstrated. To date, there have been no high-quality trials evaluating the effects of viscoelastic insoles on pain and function outcomes among patients who have knee OA. Nevertheless, the possibility that viscoelastic insoles might help to relieve symptoms and reduce damaging impulse stresses at the knee should not be ruled out. Viscoelastic insoles made of silicone have been shown to markedly decrease the peak heel strike transient among healthy subjects.[52] In one randomized clinical trial involving 100 nursing students, these insoles also reduced weight-bearing–induced low back pain.

Given their low cost and negligible risk profile, we feel confident in recommending viscoelastic insoles as part of a more comprehensive prescription for TF OA that may include athletic shoes with thick foam midsoles. In addition, we advise patients whose symptoms are provoked primarily with walking to concentrate on slowing their gait speed and making gentle contact with the ground at heelstrike. The combination of interventions is often successful in improving tolerance for walking on noncompliant surfaces, such as asphalt or concrete.

LATERALLY WEDGED INSOLES

The apparent success of valgus realigning braces for the treatment of medial TF OA has invigorated efforts to develop less obtrusive interventions with similar realigning capabilities. Interventions intending to unload the medial TF compartment by way of laterally wedged shoe insoles that encourage a reduction of genu varum malalignment have so far not demonstrated comparable success in the few well-controlled clinical trials that have examined their effectiveness.[53]

Laboratory studies indicate that laterally wedged insoles probably do help to realign the genu varum limb, and reduce the M_{add} that is responsible for the concentration of load on the medial TF joint (**Fig. 11**).[54] The magnitude of these changes tends to be small, however. Kerrigan and colleagues[55] found that in comparison with no insole, 5 degrees of lateral wedging succeeded in reducing the peak M_{add} by only about 6%. Ten degrees of lateral wedging reduced the peak M_{add} by 8%. These findings are entirely consistent with those of Crenshaw and colleagues[56] who found that the M_{add} was reduced by 7% when walking with a 5-degree laterally wedged insole.

These small mechanical effects probably occur by way of slight alterations in the frontal plane alignment of the tibiofemoral joint.[57] Any resulting reductions in activity-related knee symptoms require a minimum of 5 to 10 hours of daily use, however,[58] and result in symptom improvements that are not much greater than the reductions achieved by placebo alone.[53,59] In one of only two randomized trials meeting the criteria for inclusion in a Cochrane-sponsored review,[27] Maillefert and colleagues[59] reported slightly reduced NSAID use (4 fewer days over 3 months) and somewhat greater compliance among a group of subjects who had medial TF OA who were assigned a 5-degree laterally wedged insole versus a comparison group that used

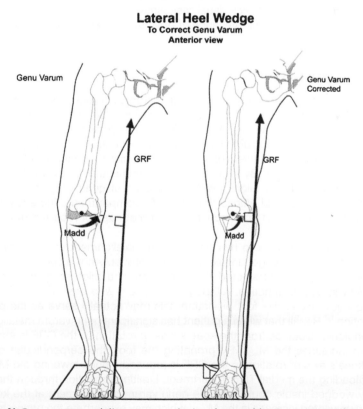

Lateral Heel Wedge
To Correct Genu Varum
Anterior view

Genu Varum

GRF

Madd

Genu Varum
Corrected

GRF

Madd

Fig. 11. (*Left*) Genu varum malalignment results in a large adduction moment (M_{add}), which concentrates compressive load on the medial TF compartment. (*Right*) The same limb with a laterally wedged insole has improved TF alignment and a commensurate reduction in the adduction moment (M_{add}).

a neutral insole. After 6 months, there were no differences in pain or function scores between the two groups. Similarly, Baker and colleagues,[60] in a well-conducted crossover study of 90 subjects who had medial TF OA, reported a mean difference in pain reduction over the 6-week treatment period (5-degree laterally wedged insole) versus the 6-week control period (neutral insole) equal to just 13.8 points on a 500-point pain scale (95% CI: −3.9 to 31.4). Comparably small and nonsignificant effects were reported for all of the secondary outcomes, including measured disability and several different physical performance tests.

Attempts to improve on the efficacy of laterally wedged insoles by increasing their inclination have met with only modest reductions in measured stress on the knee. The more pronounced effect of increasing the angle of inclination of the wedge is an increase in the number of new musculoskeletal complaints.[55] Any effort to significantly reduce painful compressive loading on tissues of the medial TF compartment by way of valgus realignment of the rearfoot also brings with it the unwanted risk for provoking problems related to excessive rearfoot pronation.[61] To the extent that excessive rearfoot pronation can adversely affect habitual loads on the knee, lateral heel wedges may in the long run lead to more harm than good among certain patients who have a pre-existing tendency to excessively pronate. We therefore recommend that before any serious consideration is given to the use of a laterally wedged insole in the treatment of medial TF OA, the patient is cleared for any significant history of pre-existing foot or ankle problems, and a quick visual assessment is made of the patient's habitual standing posture to rule out the presence of obviously excessive foot pronation (flat-footedness).

MEDIALLY WEDGED INSOLES

The application of conservative realignment therapies is both malalignment- and treatment strategy–dependent.[62–65] In the patient who has genu valgum malalignment and lateral TF OA, a medially wedged insole may provide benefit. If the patient demonstrates excessive foot pronation, then improvements to foot alignment and function may result from interventions, such as medially wedged insoles, that are designed to limit pronation. By improving foot alignment, it is hoped that the tibia will become more vertically aligned with a reduction of genu valgum. Improved tibiofemoral alignment should offload the lateral TF compartment. There is an apparent interaction between foot and knee alignment that has not received much formal study.

In the case of a patient who has genu varum malalignment and medial TF OA, application of medially wedged insole by itself is probably not a sensible approach. Kahler and colleagues[66] attempted this approach in a pilot study and found no improvement in pain or function. Although the patient who has medial TF OA may also demonstrate excessive foot pronation, this may actually serve as the patient's compensation.[67] Recall that when a patient has significant genu varum malalignment, the perpendicular distance from the knee's axis of rotation to the GRF is increased, which then increases the M_{add}. By pronating the foot, the perpendicular distance from the knee's axis of rotation to the GRF is reduced, hence lowering the M_{add} and slightly offloading the medial TF compartment. Limiting pronation through the use of a medially wedged insole could increase genu varum malalignment at the knee and result in an unwanted increase in the M_{add}, which may exacerbate the patient's medial TF symptoms.

An alternative approach was described in a pilot study[68] that treated 24 limbs in 15 patients who had medial TF OA using a combination of a valgus unloader knee brace and a medially wedged (ie, neutral) foot orthosis (**Fig. 12**). The patients were randomly assigned to one of two groups: (1) valgus unloader knee brace only, and (2) valgus unloader knee brace with custom-molded foot orthosis (medially wedged insole). Both groups demonstrated improved pain and function after 3 months, but the group with the combined prescription had significantly greater reductions in pain during upright activities than the group treated with the valgus unloader knee brace alone. Based on these findings and our own clinical experience, we believe that interventions that combine knee and foot orthoses hold great potential, especially for patients exhibiting both medial TF OA and excessive foot pronation.

A FINAL WORD OF CAUTION

Most conservative realignment therapies, including unloader knee braces and medially or laterally wedged insoles, are specifically designed to treat unicompartmental TF OA. Intuitively, if you increase the joint space in the medial TF compartment with the intention of unloading the medial joint, you can expect a reduction in joint space and an increase in loading in the lateral TF compartment. Such a strategy may be contraindicated for symptomatic bicompartmental disease.

The clinical term used to describe knee braces and shoe insoles is "orthoses." Over-the-counter orthoses are typically only available in discrete sizes (eg, small, medium, and large) and are often made of lighter duty, albeit less expensive, materials than their custom-molded counterparts. Some orthotic designs may be significantly more effective than others.[62,65] A full-length custom-molded foot orthosis is shown in **Fig. 13**. Notice the deep heel cup, medial longitudinal arch support, and forefoot cushioning material. The custom-molded foot orthosis is made by some form of a foot impression (eg, plaster slipper cast) and, in this case, a trilaminate

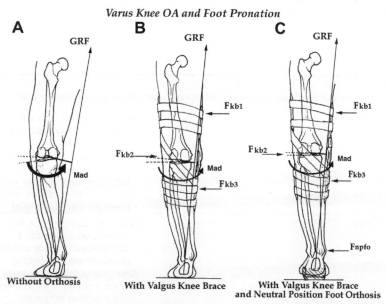

Varus Knee OA and Foot Pronation

A Without Orthosis

B With Valgus Knee Brace

C With Valgus Knee Brace and Neutral Position Foot Orthosis

Fig. 12. Posterior view of lower limb. (*A*) Genu varum malalignment with excessively pronated foot. (*B*) The same limb with a valgus unloader knee brace. (*C*) The same limb with a valgus unloader knee brace and a neutral foot orthosis (medially wedged insole).

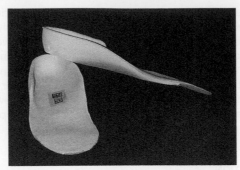

Fig. 13. Full-length custom-molded foot orthosis. Notice the deep heel cup, medial longitudinal arch support, and forefoot cushioning material. The custom-molded foot orthosis is made from some form of a foot impression (eg, plaster slipper cast) and, in this case, a trilaminate of materials supplying support, realignment, and shock absorption.

of materials supplying support, realignment, and shock absorption. These devices are most often "medially wedging" the foot. There is a lack of cost-benefit and efficacy data on which to base a decision about which specific orthosis will work for a given type of patient.

Based on the current literature and our own clinical experience, we recommend the approach summarized in **Table 1** for treating TF OA. It is our hope and our expectation that as more research is completed in this still understudied area we will be compelled to modify and amend these suggestions to integrate new evidence into clinical practice. We are confident that the revaluing of conservative care strategies that make frequent use of noninvasive devices is a justifiable imperative for the future medical management of knee OA.

Table 1	
Conservative realignment therapy considerations for managing tibiofemoral osteoarthritis	
Medial TF OA	When managing with a foot orthosis only, consider a laterally wedged insole When managing with a knee brace, consider a valgus unloader brace with or without a custom-molded foot orthosis (medially wedged insole)
Lateral TF OA	When managing with a foot orthosis only, consider a custom-molded foot orthosis (medially wedged insole) When managing with a knee brace, consider a varus unloader brace with or without a custom-molded foot orthosis (medially wedged insole)

REFERENCES

1. Lawrence R, Helmick C, Arnett F, et al. Estimates of the prevalence of arthritis and selected musculoskeletal disorders in the United States. Arthritis Rheum 1998; 41(5):778–99.
2. Centers for Disease Control and Prevention. Arthritis prevalence and activity limitations – United States, 1990. MMWR Morb Mortal Wkly Rep 1994;43(24):433–8.
3. Third National Health and Nutrition Examination Survey (NHANES III). In: Centers for Disease Control and Prevention. 1998–1994.
4. Burden of musculoskeletal diseases in the United States: prevalence, societal and economic cost. Rosemont (IL): American Academy of Orthopaedic Surgeons; 2008.
5. Health Canada. Arthritis in Canada: an ongoing challenge. Ottawa: Health Canada; 2003.
6. Guccione A, Felson D, Anderson J, et al. The effects of specific medical conditions on the functional limitations of elders in the Framingham Study. Am J Public Health 1994;84(3):351–8.
7. Ofman JJ, MacLean CH, Straus WL, et al. A metaanalysis of severe upper gastrointestinal complications of nonsteroidal antiinflammatory drugs. J Rheumatol 2002;29(4):804–12.
8. Ortiz E. Market withdrawal of Vioxx: is it time to rethink the use of COX-2 inhibitors? J Manag Care Pharm 2004;10(6):551–4.
9. Smalley WE, Griffin MR, Fought RL, et al. Excess costs from gastrointestinal disease associated with nonsteroidal anti-inflammatory drugs. J Gen Intern Med 1996;11(8):461–9.
10. Wolfe MM, Lichtenstein DR, Singh G. Gastrointestinal toxicity of nonsteroidal antiinflammatory drugs. N Engl J Med 1999;340(24):1888–99.
11. Todd PA, Clissold SP. Naproxen. A reappraisal of its pharmacology, and therapeutic use in rheumatic diseases and pain states. Drugs 1990;40(1):91–137.
12. Hochberg MC, Perlmutter DL, Hudson JI, et al. Preferences in the management of osteoarthritis of the hip and knee: results of a survey of community-based rheumatologists in the United States. Arthritis Care Res 1996;9(3):170–6.
13. Willson J, Torry MR, Decker MJ, et al. Effects of walking poles on lower extremity gait mechanics. Med Sci Sports Exerc 2001;33(1):142–7.
14. Kemp G, Crossley KM, Wrigley TV, et al. Reducing joint loading in medial knee osteoarthritis: shoes and canes. Arthritis Rheum 2008;59(5):609–14.
15. Andriacchi TP. Dynamics of knee malalignment. Orthop Clin North Am 1994; 25(3):395–403.
16. Recommendations for the medical management of osteoarthritis of the hip and knee: 2000 update. American College of Rheumatology Subcommittee on Osteoarthritis Guidelines. Arthritis Rheum 2000;43(9):1905–15.
17. Pendleton A, Arden N, Dougados M, et al. EULAR recommendations for the management of knee osteoarthritis: report of a task force of the Standing Committee for International Clinical Studies Including Therapeutic Trials (ESCISIT). Ann Rheum Dis 2000;59(12):936–44.
18. Neumann DA. Biomechanical analysis of selected principles of hip joint protection. Arthritis Care Res 1989;2(4):146–55.
19. Tetsworth K, Paley D. Malalignment and degenerative arthropathy. Orthop Clin North Am 1994;25(3):367–77.
20. Sharma L, Song J, Felson DT, et al. The role of knee alignment in disease progression and functional decline in knee osteoarthritis. JAMA 2001;286(2):188–95.

21. Kraus VB, Vail TP, Worrell T, et al. A comparative assessment of alignment angle of the knee by radiographic and physical examination methods. Arthritis Rheum 2005;52(6):1730–5.

22. Chang A, Hayes K, Dunlop D, et al. Thrust during ambulation and the progression of knee osteoarthritis. Arthritis Rheum 2004;50(12):3897–903.

23. Ramsey DK, Briem K, Axe MJ, et al. A mechanical theory for the effectiveness of bracing for medial compartment osteoarthritis of the knee. J Bone Joint Surg Am 2007;89(11):2398–407.

24. Komistek RD, Dennis DA, Northcut EJ, et al. An in vivo analysis of the effectiveness of the osteoarthritic knee brace during heel-strike of gait. J Arthroplasty 1999;14(6):738–42.

25. Lindenfeld TN, Hewett TE, Andriacchi TP. Joint loading with valgus bracing in patients with varus gonarthrosis. Clin Orthop Relat Res 1997;344:290–7.

26. Pollo FE, Otis JC, Backus SI, et al. Reduction of medial compartment loads with valgus bracing of the osteoarthritic knee. Am J Sports Med 2002;30(3):414–21.

27. Brouwer RW, Jakma TS, Verhagen AP, et al. Braces and orthoses for treating osteoarthritis of the knee. Cochrane Database Syst Rev 2005;(1):CD004020.

28. Kirkley A, Webster-Bogaert S, Litchfield R, et al. The effect of bracing on varus gonarthrosis. J Bone Joint Surg Am 1999;81(4):539–48.

29. Brouwer RW, van Raaij TM, Verhaar JA, et al. Brace treatment for osteoarthritis of the knee: a prospective randomized multi-centre trial. Osteoarthritis Cartilage 2006;14(8):777–83.

30. Hinman RS, Crossley KM. Patellofemoral joint osteoarthritis: an important subgroup of knee osteoarthritis. Rheumatology (Oxford) 2007;46(7):1057–62.

31. Zhang Y, Xu L, Nevitt MC, et al. Comparison of the prevalence of knee osteoarthritis between the elderly Chinese population in Beijing and Whites in the United States: the Beijing Osteoarthritis Study. Arthritis Rheum 2001;44(9):2065–71.

32. McAlindon TE, Snow S, Cooper C, et al. Radiographic patterns of osteoarthritis of the knee joint in the community: the importance of the patellofemoral joint. Ann Rheum Dis 1992;51(7):844–9.

33. Duncan RC, Hay EM, Saklatvala J, et al. Prevalence of radiographic osteoarthritis–it all depends on your point of view. Rheumatology (Oxford) 2006;45(6):757–60.

34. Perry J. Gait analysis: normal and pathological function. Thorofare (NJ): Slack, Inc.; 1992.

35. Walker CR, Myles C, Nutton R, et al. Movement of the knee in osteoarthritis. The use of electrogoniometry to assess function. J Bone Joint Surg Br 2001;83(2):195–8.

36. Rowe PJ, Myles CM, Walker C, et al. Knee joint kinematics in gait and other functional activities measured using flexible electrogoniometry: how much knee motion is sufficient for normal daily life? Gait Posture 2000;12(2):143–55.

37. Costigan PA, Deluzio KJ, Wyss UP. Knee and hip kinetics during normal stair climbing. Gait Posture 2002;16(1):31–7.

38. Grelsamer RP, Weinstein CH. Applied biomechanics of the patella. Clin Orthop Relat Res 2001;389:9–14.

39. Besier TF, Draper CE, Gold GE, et al. Patellofemoral joint contact area increases with knee flexion and weight-bearing. J Orthop Res 2005;23(2):345–50.

40. Lesher JD, Sutlive TG, Miller GA, et al. Development of a clinical prediction rule for classifying patients with patellofemoral pain syndrome who respond to patellar taping. J Orthop Sports Phys Ther 2006;36(11):854–66.

41. Gigante A, Pasquinelli FM, Paladini P, et al. The effects of patellar taping on pa-tellofemoral incongruence. A computed tomography study. Am J Sports Med 2001;29(1):88–92.
42. Powers CM, Heino JG, Rao S, et al. The influence of patellofemoral pain on lower limb loading during gait. Clin Biomech (Bristol, Avon) 1999;14(10):722–8.
43. Powers CM, Ward SR, Chan LD, et al. The effect of bracing on patella alignment and patellofemoral joint contact area. Med Sci Sports Exerc 2004;36(7):1226–32.
44. Warden SJ, Hinman RS, Watson MA Jr, et al. Patellar taping and bracing for the treatment of chronic knee pain: a systematic review and meta-analysis. Arthritis Rheum 2008;59(1):73–83.
45. Simon S, Radin EL, Paul IL, et al. The response of joints to impact loading. II. In vivo behavior of subchondral bone. J Biomech 1972;5(3):267–72.
46. Radin E, Parker HG, Pugh JW, et al. Response of joints to impact loading. 3. Relationship between trabecular microfractures and cartilage degeneration. J Biomech 1973;6(1):51–7.
47. Radin EL, Ehrlich MG, Chernack R, et al. Effect of repetitive impulsive loading on the knee joints of rabbits. Clin Orthop Relat Res 1978;131:288–93.
48. Radin EL, Orr RB, Kelman JL, et al. Effect of prolonged walking on concrete on the knees of sheep. J Biomech 1982;15(7):487–92.
49. Burr DB, Radin EL. Microfractures and microcracks in subchondral bone: are they relevant to osteoarthrosis? Rheum Dis Clin North Am 2003;29(4):675–85.
50. Radin EL, Yang KH, Riegger C, et al. Relationship between lower limb dynamics and knee joint pain. J Orthop Res 1991;9(3):398–405.
51. Henriksen M, Simonsen EB, Graven-Nielsen T, et al. Impulse-forces during walk-ing are not increased in patients with knee osteoarthritis. Acta Orthop 2006;77(4): 650–6.
52. Folman Y, Wosk J, Shabat S, et al. Attenuation of spinal transients at heel strike using viscoelastic heel insoles: an in vivo study. Prev Med 2004;39(2):351–4.
53. Pham T, Maillefert JF, Hudry C, et al. Laterally elevated wedged insoles in the treatment of medial knee osteoarthritis. A two-year prospective randomized con-trolled study. Osteoarthritis Cartilage 2004;12(1):46–55.
54. Ogata K, Yasunaga M, Nomiyama H. The effect of wedged insoles on the thrust of osteoarthritic knees. Int Orthop 1997;21(5):308–12.
55. Kerrigan DC, Lelas JL, Goggins J, et al. Effectiveness of a lateral-wedge insole on knee varus torque in patients with knee osteoarthritis. Arch Phys Med Rehabil 2002;83(7):889–93.
56. Crenshaw SJ, Pollo FE, Calton EF. Effects of lateral-wedged insoles on kinetics at the knee. Clin Orthop Relat Res 2000;375:185–92.
57. Toda Y, Tsukimura N. A 2-year follow-up of a study to compare the efficacy of lat-eral wedged insoles with subtalar strapping and in-shoe lateral wedged insoles in patients with varus deformity osteoarthritis of the knee. Osteoarthritis Cartilage 2006;14(3):231–7.
58. Toda Y, Tsukimura N, Segal N. An optimal duration of daily wear for an insole with subtalar strapping in patients with varus deformity osteoarthritis of the knee. Osteoarthritis Cartilage 2005;13(4):353–60.
59. Maillefert J, Hudry C, Baron G, et al. Laterally elevated wedged insoles in the treatment of medial knee osteoarthritis: a prospective randomized controlled study. Osteoarthritis Cartilage 2001;9(8):738–45.
60. Baker K, Goggins J, Xie H, et al. A randomized crossover trial of a wedged insole for treatment of knee osteoarthritis. Arthritis Rheum 2007;56(4):1198–203.

61. Friedlaender GE, Strong DM, Tomford WW, et al. Long-term follow-up of patients with osteochondral allografts. A correlation between immunologic responses and clinical outcome. Orthop Clin North Am 1999;30(4):583–8.
62. Hillstrom HW, Whitney K, McGuire J, et al. Evaluation and management of the foot and ankle. In: Clinical care in the rheumatic diseases. 2nd edition. Atlanta (GA): American College of Rheumatology; 2001. p. 203–11.
63. Hillstrom H, Whitney K, McGuire J, et al. Lower extremity conservative realignment therapies and ambulatory aids. In: Robins L, Hannan MT, Burkhardt C, editors. Clinical care in the rheumatic diseases. 2nd edition. Atlanta (GA): American College of Rheumatology; 2001. p. 213–20.
64. Hillstrom H, Brower DJ, Whitney K, et al. Lower extremity conservative realignment therapies for knee osteoarthritis. In: Brander VA, editor. Physical medicine and rehabilitation: state of the art reviews. Philadelphia: Hanley & Belfus, Inc; 2002. p. 507–20.
65. Hillstrom H, Whitney K, McGuire J, et al. Evaluation and management of the foot and ankle. In: Bartlett S, Bingham CO, Maricic MJ, editors. Clinical care in the rheumatic diseases. 3rd edition. Atlanta (GA): American College of Rheumatology; 2006. p. 267–70.
66. Kahler M, Hillstrom H, McGuire J, et al. Gait posture. Proceedings of the 3rd Annual Gait and Clinical Movement Anaylsis Meeting. San Diego, California, 1998.
67. Riegger-Krugh C, Keysor JJ. Skeletal malalignments of the lower quarter: correlated and compensatory motions and postures. J Orthop Sports Phys Ther 1996; 23(2):164–70.
68. Hillstrom H, Brower DJ, Bhimji S, et al. Assessment of conservative realignment therapies for the treatment of various knee osteoarthritis: biomechanics and pathophysiology. Gait and Posture 2000;11(2):170.

The Role of Analgesics and Intra-Articular Injections in Disease Management

William F. Harvey, MD[a],*, David J. Hunter, MBBS, MSc, PhD[b]

KEYWORDS

• Osteoarthritis • Pharmacology • Analgesics • NSAIDS
• Intra-articular • Hyaluronic acid

Osteoarthritis (OA) is the most prevalent form of arthritis and one of the leading causes of chronic disability among older individuals.[1] The health resource use imposed by OA is increasing due to the increasing prevalence of obesity and the aging of the community.[2] The largest increases will occur among older adults, for whom OA also has the greatest functional impact.

OA has been previously described as a "degenerative joint disease." Although OA is characterized by degradation of the cartilage, this moniker understates the significance of genetic, biologic, biochemical, nutritional, and mechanical factors that contribute to the process.[3,4] Successful management of the disease requires a comprehensive approach to address all of these factors. In light of the potential for adverse events from the use of pharmacologic agents, the authors endorse the use of nonpharmacologic treatments before, or in concert with, pharmacologic therapy.

The focus of pharmacologic treatment of OA includes targets from the cell and cytokine level to the larger joint components such as cartilage, bone, innervations, and vascular supply. The most important goals of therapy in patients with OA are pain management, improvement in function and disability, and, ultimately, disease modification. This review discusses the current pharmacologic regimen available to address these goals. Specific attention is paid to current trends and controversies related to pharmacologic management, including the use of oral, topical, and injectable agents.

A version of this article originally appeared in the 34:3 issue of the *Rheumatic Disease Clinics of North America*.
[a] Division of Rheumatology, Tufts Medical Center, 800 Washington Street, Box 406, Boston, MA 02111, USA
[b] Division of Research, New England Baptist Hospital, Boston, MA 02111, USA
* Corresponding author.
E-mail address: wharvey@bu.edu (W.F. Harvey).

ANALGESICS

Symptom management in OA can be achieved with analgesic medications. These agents include drugs with various routes of administration. Although symptom management does not alter the disease course, it can lead to improvements in functional status and disability. Because delaying disease progression in OA is so challenging, ultimately, an asymptomatic individual may be the only realistic goal until the science of disease modification in OA is more advanced. This approach also directly leads to delay of surgical intervention and potential reductions in the overall cost to patients and the health care system.

Acetaminophen (paracetamol) is the most commonly used analgesic for mild-to-moderate pain in OA.[5] Having no known disease-modifying properties, it represents a pure analgesic, in contrast to non-steroidal anti-inflammatory drugs (NSAIDs), which have analgesic and anti-inflammatory properties. The mechanism of action of acetaminophen is not well understood but likely involves some modification of the cyclo-oxygenase (COX) system without affecting the inflammatory cascade. The drug is notable for its rapid onset of action (less than 1 hour) and short duration of action (4–6 hours).[6] It is metabolized by the liver, and potentially toxic metabolites are excreted in the urine; therefore, it must be dosed with caution in patients with liver or kidney disease. Care should also be taken in patients who regularly consume even moderate amounts of alcohol because the liver toxicity of each can be synergistic. In standard doses, the drug is usually well tolerated, causing few gastrointestinal or hematologic side effects.[7]

The use of acetaminophen as the first-line drug in mild-to-moderate OA has been controversial within the medical community. Numerous studies have demonstrated its efficacy in reducing the pain of OA;[8,9] however, its status as a pure analgesic has made it arguably less favorable than the NSAID class of drugs. This controversy has become more apparent due to the balance between the increasing recognition of the inflammatory components (such as presence of synovitis and bone marrow lesions) of OA and the association of NSAIDs with significant toxicities (cardiovascular and others).[10,11] There are clearly large subsets of people for whom the relative safety of acetaminophen makes it a clear choice as the first-line agent for OA. Acetaminophen in doses greater than 2000 mg/d and 2600 mg/d, respectively, has also been associated with higher rates of gastrointestinal adverse events.[12,13] The role of acetaminophen in the treatment of OA requires a balance of potential toxicities, patient preference, and an understanding by patient and physician alike of the potential benefits.

Tramadol is a non-narcotic opioid analgesic that is useful in the treatment of moderate-to-severe pain in OA. Its mechanism of action is different from, and synergistic with, that of acetaminophen. The combination of this drug with acetaminophen allows a lower dosage of tramadol with the same analgesic benefit. Tramadol interacts with the serotonergic, GABAergic, and noradrenergic systems centrally to produce its effect. It is metabolized in the liver and excreted in the urine, requiring dosage adjustment in patients with renal and hepatic impairment.[14] It must be used with some caution in elderly patients owing to central nervous system depression and in patients with a seizure disorder or in combination with other medications that alter seizure threshold. Tramadol has been associated with an increased risk of serotonin syndrome when used in combination with monoamine oxidase inhibitor and selective serotonin reuptake inhibitor medications. The most common side effects are nausea, flushing, and drowsiness. Like acetaminophen, tramadol is a pure analgesic with no disease-modifying properties. Its efficacy has been demonstrated in subjects with OA, but the authors recommend its use only in subjects with contraindications to NSAIDs or when analgesic benefit is not fully achieved with other agents.[15]

Narcotic-containing medications of varying potencies are available. Their efficacy in treating acute and chronic pain conditions is well established;[16,17] however, because of the restricted prescribing, potential for central nervous system depression, addiction potential, and lack of disease-modifying effects, the authors do not recommend the routine use of these medications for pain control in OA. In patients with inadequate response or contraindications to other therapies, treatment with long-acting narcotic medications may be an option. When prescribing these medications, the use of a comprehensive institutional guideline (commonly called "narcotics contracts") is an inexpensive and effective way to minimize the potential for abuse and assist with regulatory oversight.[18]

NON-STEROIDAL ANTI-INFLAMMATORY DRUGS

NSAIDs are a large group of drugs with both analgesic and anti-inflammatory properties. Although OA has been thought of as a non-inflammatory disease, MRI studies have demonstrated the presence of inflammatory type lesions including synovitis and bone marrow lesions.[10,11] Because NSAIDs have both anti-inflammatory and analgesic properties, many clinicians consider these drugs the most important first-line agents in the treatment of OA; however, there is no clear evidence that these agents impact measures of inflammation in patients with OA.

NSAIDs inhibit the COX enzymes which convert arachadonic acid into prostaglandins, a major mediator of inflammation. The two well-known isoenzymes of the COX enzymes (COX-1 and COX-2) are inhibited by various NSAIDs to varying degrees. The COX-1 isoenzyme is of particular importance in mediating the gastric toxicities of the NSAID class, whereas the COX-2 isoenzyme has been implicated in mediating the cardiovascular toxicity of the enzyme. COX-2 is only expressed in cells activated by inflammatory cytokines and is thought to be most relevant to systemic anti-inflammatory effects.

There are six major classes of NSAID medications with a significant amount of individual variation in pharmacologic properties.[19] Although numerous preparations have been shown to be efficacious in treating OA, there is a large apparent variation in individual patient response to each drug. There are no clear clinical data regarding the relative potency of the various medications, although drugs such as indomethacin and diclofenac are anecdotally thought to be more effective. In clinical trials, all NSAIDs have performed similarly, with persons reporting approximately 30% reduction in pain and 15% improvement in function.[20] Additionally, there is no evidence that NSAIDs alter the natural history of the disease. Studies have controversially suggested that the reduction in pain that results in improvements in walking speed (and therefore increased joint-loading forces) may increase the risk of structural deterioration.[21,22]

Toxicity remains the most troublesome aspect of prescribing NSAIDs for the treatment of OA. The most common toxicity of NSAIDs is gastrointestinal.[23,24] Through inhibition of prostaglandin synthesis by COX-1 enzyme, NSAIDs cause increased rates of gastritis and ulceration. This risk is highest among patients with a prior history of ulcer or gastrointestinal tract bleeding, an age over 60 years, more than twice the normal dosage of NSAID, concurrent use of corticosteroids, and concurrent use of anticoagulants.[25] Evidence from clinical trials indicates that primary prevention of adverse gastrointestinal events can be accomplished with misoprostol and proton pump inhibitors.[26,27] H_2 blockers such as famotidine have not been shown to prevent gastric ulceration in persons on concomitant NSAIDs.[28] COX-2–selective NSAIDS showed a relative risk reduction of 0.49 in large trials as distinct from use of standard NSAIDs, but their use must be weighed against potential cardiovascular toxicity.[29] Proton pump inhibitors have the strongest evidence for healing and prevention of further ulceration.[30]

Nephrotoxicity is also a significant problem with the use of NSAIDs and is mediated by both prostaglandin inhibition at the afferent arteriole of the glomerulus and by interstitial nephritis through unclear mechanisms.[31,32] Both of these toxicities are usually self-limited and are associated more often with individuals with pre-existing renal disease.

Cardiovascular complications are increasingly being recognized as an adverse effect of NSAID use, particularly with the COX-2–selective medications. Inhibition of vasodilatory prostaglandins results in hypertension, and coadministration with aspirin reduces the antiplatelet effects of aspirin. Early studies showed a possible cardiovascular benefit of NSAIDs other than aspirin; however, a more recent long-term study of celecoxib and naproxen showed an increase in cardiovascular events.[33] The American Heart Association and the American College of Cardiology have each published guidelines recommending extreme caution when COX-2–selective NSAIDs are used in patients who have or are at risk for cardiovascular disease.[34] Numerous ongoing studies are being performed to further examine this relationship. Currently, the authors use COX-2–selective agents only in patients who have low cardiovascular risk and who have another indication such as documented gastrointestinal toxicity from nonselective NSAIDs or concomitant warfarin use.

Despite toxicities, NSAIDs have been and will continue to be an important component of pharmacologic management of OA. The authors' current practice is to prescribe nonselective NSAIDs, often nonacetylated salicylates, as a first choice. If patients do not tolerate this drug, switching to another NSAID of a different class may be an effective alternative before moving away from NSAIDs as a whole.

TOPICAL AGENTS

Topical agents are gaining in popularity because of the recognized toxicity of oral agents. Study of these medications has largely been restricted to small randomized trials of short duration; therefore, the medications have only been proven useful for short-term use of mild-to-moderate pain in OA.

Topical NSAIDs have been studied and are available. Topical diclofenac diethylamine gel has been shown to provide good short-term pain relief with less gastrointestinal and renal toxicity than oral diclofenac.[35,36] Topical NSAIDs are effective in relieving pain when compared with placebo for OA of the hand and knee.[36,37] Diclofenac sodium gel was recently approved for use in the United States on the basis of studies that have been published thus far only in abstract form.[38] There is no reason to suspect the sodium compound will be less effective, and because it is available now in the United States, this represents a potential alternative for use in patients when there is concern over systemic toxicity.

Topical salicylate-containing compounds work as rubefacients that presumably reduce pain through increasing local blood flow. Studies involving these agents also show only short-term benefit.[39] Examples include methyl salicylate, diethylamine salicylate, and hydroxyethylsalicylate, and several are available over the counter in the United States. These medications, like topical NSAIDs, provide an alternative to systemically absorbed compounds. The main side effects are local skin irritation and strong odor.

Capsaicin-containing products contain the oil extract from hot pepper plants. Application of capsaicin to the skin results in a burning sensation that can be severe. It is proposed that the neurologic stimulus caused by this local irritation depletes substance P in the sensory nerve fibers. Substance P is a powerful pain stimulus, and its depletion results in generalized pain sensitization in the local area. It has been shown to be effective for hand and knee OA when used three to four times daily.[40] Capsaicin in a concentration of 0.025% is better tolerated than 0.075%. It should be applied three to four times per day for at least 3 to 4 weeks for an adequate trial. A randomized controlled trial showed that capsaicin (0.075%) reduced pain and tenderness in patients with hand OA when compared with placebo over 4 weeks.[41] A similar study in patients with knee OA produced similar results, with 80% of capsaicin-treated patients (0.025%) experiencing pain relief after 2 weeks.[42] Skin irritation is the major side effect. Accidental application to any mucous membrane, including the eyes, nose, mouth, and genitals, should be avoided, and careful counseling of the patient is essential.

Topical lidocaine has been used to treat the pain in OA, particularly of the spine.[43] Lidocaine depolarizes the sensory nerve fibers, rendering them unable to transmit pain signals. Commercial patches are expensive, but gels and creams can be used effectively in some patients if applied under occlusive dressings.

INTRA-ARTICULAR CORTICOSTEROIDS

There is a long history of injection of steroids into joints for the purpose of pain relief and anti-inflammatory effects. Many studies show the efficacy of various preparations.[44] Although OA is not primarily an inflammatory disease, there are some inflammatory features, and there seems to be a response in OA patients to anti-inflammatory medications. Triamcinolone and methylprednisolone preparations are the most common, although there are others. In general, the authors believe the low-solubility compounds have a longer duration of action.[45] Nevertheless, clinical trials have not shown long-term benefits in OA patients treated with intra-articular steroids, and there is no evidence that injection of corticosteroids alters the natural history of the disease.[46] In fact, some evidence suggests that they may have deleterious consequences on structure.[47,48] How this relates to the frequency of use is unknown, although current armchair wisdom suggests that no single joint should be injected more than four times in the course of 1 year. Studies indicate that, when otherwise not contraindicated, intra-articular corticosteroids are of short-term benefit (1 week only) for pain and function.[45] Despite their widespread use to treat the pain associated with OA, patients should be counseled that the best evidence suggests minimal short-term benefit. Although clinical wisdom suggests that the presence of an effusion indicates likely therapeutic benefit, based on current data this wisdom is inaccurate.[49]

HYALURONIC ACID

Hyaluronic acid has been touted as a potentially disease-modifying drug for OA and has been investigated for OA of the hip, knee, ankle, and temporomandibular joint. In vitro and ex vivo studies have demonstrated growth of cartilage in a dose-related fashion and suppression of IL1β-induced metalloproteinases.[50,51] Indeed, two meta-analyses have been able to demonstrate statistically significant improvements in pain and function, although the degree of clinical response and duration of response were varied and most of the response was placebo related.[52,53] No study has been able to demonstrate a change in the rate of progression of disease. Furthermore, the meta-analysis by Lo and colleagues suggests that the molecular weight of the compound may have an important role, with high molecular weight compounds showing better effect. A more recent meta-analysis that looked specifically at high molecular weight hylan versus low molecular weight hyaluronic acid showed a trend toward benefit of the larger compounds but also showed large heterogeneity between trials and more local adverse reactions to hylan.[54] These findings were recently confirmed in a randomized controlled trial directly comparing these agents by the same group, supporting that there was little or no difference between high and low molecular weight compounds in their efficacy but greater potential for adverse effects with hylan.[55] As is true for glucosamine and chondroitin, there is a large amount of variation between studies, and the significant possibility of publication bias makes conclusions about intra-articular hyaluronic acid difficult. In light of the fact that these agents are essentially equivalent to placebo and considering the high rate of adverse events and cost, the authors do not currently recommend clinical use of these compounds.

GLUCOSAMINE AND CHONDROITIN

Glucosamine and chondroitin as treatments for OA have received a great deal of attention and controversy. These compounds are important components of cartilage and, theoretically, by increasing the level of these substrates could aid in cartilage repair or slow cartilage destruction. At present, most of the controversy lies in whether these agents have any proven efficacy for symptom or structure modification. A meta-analysis performed in 2005 indicated a modest benefit for glucosamine in reducing symptoms and slowing joint space narrowing of the knee on radiography.[56] Methodologic concerns have been raised about some of these studies. When only trials with adequate blinding are analyzed, no benefit is found. Furthermore, the most positive studies have been done using a proprietary glucosamine sulfate compound. Proponents of glucosamine use believe that this compound is more effective than glucosamine hydrochloride, whereas opponents have raised concerns about industry and publication bias.[57] Resolution of this matter will likely require a non–industry-sponsored study of glucosamine sulfate as opposed to the recent expensive National Institutes of Health investment on the GAIT trial.[58] That study found that glucosamine hydrochloride was no more effective than placebo but ultimately raised more questions than it answered because of concerns about the preparation used, the large placebo effect, and the multiple additional subset analyses performed. In the authors' opinion, glucosamine and chondroitin may be of potential benefit in treating the pain and function of OA, but widespread use of this expensive supplement should not be endorsed until more transparent large-scale studies are completed.

NUTRITIONAL SUPPLEMENTATION

A great deal of research has been performed on the nutritional aspects of OA. Numerous vitamin and mineral deficiencies have been linked with an increased risk of OA, and clinical trials are underway. Vitamin K has been linked with the risk of OA; however, a clinical trial of supplementation published in abstract form failed to show a benefit.[59,60] The trial included subjects with and without vitamin K deficiency and showed a trend toward significance in the group that was vitamin K deficient at baseline. Selenium has been demonstrated to be a risk factor for OA, but no clinical trial has been performed.[61] Vitamin D deficiency has been demonstrated to be a risk factor for OA, and two large ongoing clinical trials are investigating the effect of its replacement on the development and progression of disease. Other antioxidant nutrients have been studied and discussed, including beta carotene, vitamin E, and vitamin C, with some suggestion that they may slow the progression of disease but do not prevent its occurrence.[62] A more detailed review of nutritional risk factors for OA was published by McAlindon and Felson in 1997.[63]

EMERGING THERAPEUTIC TARGETS

A vast number of agents are currently under development for the treatment of OA. A comprehensive review of these targets has been performed by Dray and Read[64] and includes discussions of cytokines such as TNF-α and IL1β, receptors such as kinin, cannabinoid, and prostanoid receptors, and numerous ion channels. The large numbers of potential therapeutic targets bring hope that treatment will move away from analgesia and toward disease modification. A later section of this issue is dedicated to this new modality of therapeutic intervention in OA, namely, disease-modifying drugs.

SUMMARY

Management of OA is focused on relief of pain and improvement of function. These goals are achieved through a comprehensive treatment plan including pharmacologic and nonpharmacologic therapies. In addition to the recommendations in this article, several well-written guidelines are available that describe the management of OA based on evidence from trials and expert consensus.[65–67] Of these guidelines, the most recent and rigorously developed are those published by the Osteoarthritis Research Society.[68]

Pharmacologic management begins in most patients with analgesia through acetaminophen or NSAIDs, with careful attention to potential toxicities. In particular, the cardiovascular and gastrointestinal toxicities of NSAIDs must be monitored carefully. Tramadol and narcotic medications can be useful adjunctive therapies. Topical NSAIDs, salicylates, and capsaicin can be useful as adjuncts or in patients in whom systemic medications are problematic. Intra-articular glucocorticoids should be reserved for the short-term management of acute pain flares; however, a note of caution is needed given their short duration of effect and potential for long-term harm. Due to the continuing controversies and lack of clear beneficial evidence, glucosamine and chondroitin and intra-articular hyaluronic acid should be avoided.

The future of OA prevention and treatment may involve nutritional supplements such as vitamin D or selenium, but conclusive trials have not been completed. Likewise, numerous potential targets for therapy are under intense investigation. Regardless, the management of OA pain will continue to require a multifaceted approach and, in the absence of agents that can modify the disease, should be the preeminent focus of clinical management.

REFERENCES

1. Center for Disease Control. Arthritis prevalence and activity limitations—United States, 1990–1990. MMWR Morb Mortal Wkly Rep 1994;43(24):433–8.
2. Badley E, DesMeules M. Arthritis in Canada an ongoing challenge. Ottawa (Ontario): Health Canada; 2003.
3. Martin JA, Buckwalter JA. Roles of articular cartilage aging and chondrocyte senescence in the pathogenesis of osteoarthritis. Iowa Orthop J 2001;21:1–7.
4. Felson DT. An update on the pathogenesis and epidemiology of osteoarthritis. Radiol Clin North Am 2004;42(1):1–9, v.

5. Hochberg MC, Altman RD, Brandt KD, et al. Guidelines for the medical management of osteoarthritis. Part II. Osteoarthritis of the knee: American College of Rheumatology. Arthritis Rheum 1995;38(11):1541–6.
6. Clissold SP. Paracetamol and phenacetin. Drugs 1986;32(Suppl 4):46–59.
7. Graham GG, Scott KF, Day RO. Tolerability of paracetamol. Drug Saf 2005;28(3): 227–40.
8. Shen H, Sprott H, Aeschlimann A, et al. Analgesic action of acetaminophen in symptomatic osteoarthritis of the knee. Rheumatology (Oxford) 2006;45(6): 765–70.
9. Altman RD, Zinsenheim JR, Temple AR, et al. Three-month efficacy and safety of acetaminophen extended-release for osteoarthritis pain of the hip or knee: a randomized, double-blind, placebo-controlled study. Osteoarthritis Cartilage 2007; 15(4):454–61.
10. Hill CL, Hunter DJ, Niu J, et al. Synovitis detected on magnetic resonance imaging and its relation to pain and cartilage loss in knee osteoarthritis. Ann Rheum Dis 2007;66(12):1599–603.
11. Hunter DJ, Zhang Y, Niu J, et al. Increase in bone marrow lesions associated with cartilage loss: a longitudinal magnetic resonance imaging study of knee osteoarthritis. Arthritis Rheum 2006;54(5):1529–35.
12. Garcia Rodriguez LA, Hernandez-Diaz S, Garcia Rodriguez LA, et al. Relative risk of upper gastrointestinal complications among users of acetaminophen and nonsteroidal anti-inflammatory drugs [see comment]. Epidemiology 2001;12(5): 570–6.
13. Rahme E, Pettitt D, LeLorier J, et al. Determinants and sequelae associated with utilization of acetaminophen versus traditional nonsteroidal anti-inflammatory drugs in an elderly population [see comment]. Arthritis Rheum 2002;46(11): 3046–54.
14. Dayer P, Collart L, Desmeules J. The pharmacology of tramadol. Drugs 1994; 47(Suppl 1):3–7.
15. Cepeda MS, Camargo F, Zea C, et al. Tramadol for osteoarthritis: a systematic review and meta-analysis. J Rheumatol 2007;34(3):543–55.
16. Kalso E, Edwards JE, Moore RA, et al. Opioids in chronic non-cancer pain: systematic review of efficacy and safety. Pain 2004;112(3):372–80.
17. Markenson JA, Croft J, Zhang PG, et al. Treatment of persistent pain associated with osteoarthritis with controlled-release oxycodone tablets in a randomized controlled clinical trial. Clin J Pain 2005;21(6):524–35.
18. Weaver M, Schnoll S. Abuse liability in opioid therapy for pain treatment in patients with an addiction history. Clin J Pain 2002;18(4 Suppl):S61–9.
19. Tannenbaum H, Davis P, Russell AS, et al. An evidence-based approach to prescribing NSAIDs in musculoskeletal disease: a Canadian consensus. Canadian NSAID Consensus Participants. CMAJ 1996;155(1):77–88.
20. Todd PA, Clissold SP, Naproxen. A reappraisal of its pharmacology, and therapeutic use in rheumatic diseases and pain states. Drugs 1990;40(1):91–137.
21. Blin O, Pailhous J, Lafforgue P, et al. Quantitative analysis of walking in patients with knee osteoarthritis: a method of assessing the effectiveness of non-steroidal anti-inflammatory treatment. Ann Rheum Dis 1990;49(12):990–3.
22. Huskisson EC, Berry H, Gishen P, et al. Effects of anti-inflammatory drugs on the progression of osteoarthritis of the knee: LINK Study Group. Longitudinal Investigation of Nonsteroidal Anti-inflammatory Drugs in Knee Osteoarthritis. J Rheumatol 1995;22(10):1941–6.

23. Flower RJ. Studies on the mechanism of action of anti-inflammatory drugs: a paper in honour of John Vane. Thromb Res 2003;110(5–6):259–63.
24. Flower RJ. The development of COX-2 inhibitors. Nat Rev Drug Discov 2003;2(3): 179–91.
25. Lanza FL. A guideline for the treatment and prevention of NSAID-induced ulcers: members of the Ad Hoc Committee on Practice Parameters of the American College of Gastroenterology. Am J Gastroenterol 1998;93(11):2037–46.
26. Silverstein FE, Graham DY, Senior JR, et al. Misoprostol reduces serious gastrointestinal complications in patients with rheumatoid arthritis receiving nonsteroidal anti-inflammatory drugs: a randomized, double-blind, placebo-controlled trial. Ann Intern Med 1995;123(4):241–9.
27. Scheiman JM, Yeomans ND, Talley NJ, et al. Prevention of ulcers by esomeprazole in at-risk patients using non-selective NSAIDs and COX-2 inhibitors. Am J Gastroenterol 2006;101(4):701–10.
28. Taha AS, Hudson N, Hawkey CJ, et al. Famotidine for the prevention of gastric and duodenal ulcers caused by nonsteroidal anti-inflammatory drugs. N Engl J Med 1996;334(22):1435–9.
29. Silverstein FE, Faich G, Goldstein JL, et al. Gastrointestinal toxicity with celecoxib vs nonsteroidal anti-inflammatory drugs for osteoarthritis and rheumatoid arthritis: the CLASS study. A randomized controlled trial: Celecoxib Long-term Arthritis Safety Study. JAMA 2000;284(10):1247–55.
30. Lai KC, Chu KM, Hui WM, et al. Esomeprazole with aspirin versus clopidogrel for prevention of recurrent gastrointestinal ulcer complications. Clin Gastroenterol Hepatol 2006;4(7):860–5.
31. Huerta C, Castellsague J, Varas-Lorenzo C, et al. Nonsteroidal anti-inflammatory drugs and risk of ARF in the general population. Am J Kidney Dis 2005;45(3): 531–9.
32. Abraham P, Keane W. Glomerular and interstitial disease induced by nonsteroidal anti-inflammatory drugs. Am J Nephrol 1984;4(1):1–6.
33. Hippisley-Cox J, Coupland C. Risk of myocardial infarction in patients taking cyclo-oxygenase-2 inhibitors or conventional non-steroidal anti-inflammatory drugs: population based nested case-control analysis. BMJ 2005;330:1366–9.
34. Bennett JS, Daugherty A, Herrington D, et al. The use of nonsteroidal anti-inflammatory drugs (NSAIDs): a science advisory from the American Heart Association. Circulation 2005;111(13):1713–6.
35. Niethard FU, Gold MS, Solomon GS, et al. Efficacy of topical diclofenac diethylamine gel in osteoarthritis of the knee. J Rheumatol 2005;32(12):2384–92.
36. Lin J, Zhang W, Jones A, et al. Efficacy of topical non-steroidal anti-inflammatory drugs in the treatment of osteoarthritis: meta-analysis of randomised controlled trials. BMJ 2004;329(7461):324.
37. Bookman AA, Williams KS, Shainhouse JZ, et al. Effect of a topical diclofenac solution for relieving symptoms of primary osteoarthritis of the knee: a randomized controlled trial [see comment]. CMAJ 2004;171(4):333–8.
38. Altman RD, Longley S, Rachidi S. Topical diclofenac sodium gel for knee osteoarthritis [abstract]. Osteoarthritis Cartilage 2007;15(Suppl C):C225.
39. Mason L, Moore RA, Edwards JE, et al. Systematic review of efficacy of topical rubefacients containing salicylates for the treatment of acute and chronic pain. BMJ 2004;328(7446):995.
40. Mason L, Moore RA, Derry S, et al. Systematic review of topical capsaicin for the treatment of chronic pain. BMJ 2004;328(7446):991.

41. McCarthy GM, McCarty DJ. Effect of topical capsaicin in the therapy of painful osteoarthritis of the hands. J Rheumatol 1992;19(4):604–7.
42. Deal CL, Schnitzer TJ, Lipstein E, et al. Treatment of arthritis with topical capsaicin: a double-blind trial. Clin Ther 1991;13(3):383–95.
43. Burch F, Codding C, Patel N, et al. Lidocaine patch 5% improves pain, stiffness, and physical function in osteoarthritis pain patients: a prospective, multicenter, open-label effectiveness trial. Osteoarthritis Cartilage 2004;12(3):253–5.
44. Arroll B, Goodyear-Smith F. Corticosteroid injections for osteoarthritis of the knee: meta-analysis. BMJ 2004;328(7444):869.
45. Bellamy N, Campbell J, Robinson V, et al. Intra-articular corticosteroid for treatment of osteoarthritis of the knee. Cochrane Database Syst Rev 2006;(2): CD005328.
46. Raynauld JP, Buckland-Wright C, Ward R, et al. Safety and efficacy of long-term intra-articular steroid injections in osteoarthritis of the knee: a randomized, double-blind, placebo-controlled trial. Arthritis Rheum 2003;48(2):370–7.
47. Behrens F, Shepard N, Mitchell N, et al. Alterations of rabbit articular cartilage by intra-articular injections of glucocorticoids. J Bone Joint Surg Am 1975;57(1): 70–6.
48. Papacrhistou G, Anagnostou S, Katsorhis T, et al. The effect of intra-articular hydrocortisone injection on the articular cartilage of rabbits. Acta Orthop Scand Suppl 1997;275:132–4.
49. Jones A, Doherty M. Intra-articular corticosteroids are effective in osteoarthritis but there are no clinical predictors of response. Ann Rheum Dis 1996;55(11): 829–32.
50. Akmal M, Singh A, Anand A, et al. The effects of hyaluronic acid on articular chondrocytes. J Bone Joint Surg Br 2005;87(8):1143–9.
51. Waddell DD, Kolomytkin OV, Dunn S, et al. Hyaluronan suppresses IL-1beta-induced metalloproteinase activity from synovial tissue. Clin Orthop Relat Res 2007;465:241–8.
52. Arrich J, Piribauer F, Mad P, et al. Intra-articular hyaluronic acid for the treatment of osteoarthritis of the knee: systematic review and meta-analysis. CMAJ 2005; 172(8):1039–43.
53. Lo GH, LaValley M, McAlindon T, et al. Intra-articular hyaluronic acid in treatment of knee osteoarthritis: a meta-analysis. JAMA 2003;290(23):3115–21.
54. Reichenbach S, Blank S, Rutjes AW, et al. Hylan versus hyaluronic acid for osteoarthritis of the knee: a systematic review and meta-analysis. Arthritis Rheum 2007;57(8):1410–8.
55. Juni P, Reichenbach S, Trelle S, et al. Efficacy and safety of intra-articular hylan or hyaluronic acids for osteoarthritis of the knee: a randomized controlled trial. Arthritis Rheum 2007;56(11):3610–9.
56. Towheed TE, Maxwell L, Anastassiades TP, et al. Glucosamine therapy for treating osteoarthritis. Cochrane Database Syst Rev 2005;(2):CD002946.
57. Vlad SC, LaValley MP, McAlindon TE, et al. Glucosamine for pain in osteoarthritis: why do trial results differ? Arthritis Rheum 2007;56(7):2267–77.
58. Clegg DO, Reda DJ, Harris CL, et al. Glucosamine, chondroitin sulfate, and the two in combination for painful knee osteoarthritis [see comment]. N Engl J Med 2006;354(8):795–808.
59. Neogi T, Booth SL, Zhang YQ, et al. Low vitamin K status is associated with osteoarthritis in the hand and knee. Arthritis Rheum 2006;54(4):1255–61.

60. Neogi T, Felson DT, Sarno R, et al. Vitamin K in hand osteoarthritis: results from a randomized clinical trial [abstract]. Osteoarthritis Cartilage 2007;15(Suppl C): C228–9.
61. Jordan JM, Fang F, Schwartz TA, et al. Low selenium levels are associated with increased odds of radiographic hip osteoarthritis in African American and white women [abstract]. Osteoarthritis Cartilage 2008;15(Suppl C):C33.
62. McAlindon TE, Jacques P, Zhang Y, et al. Do antioxidant micronutrients protect against the development and progression of knee osteoarthritis? Arthritis Rheum 1996;39(4):648–56.
63. McAlindon T, Felson DT. Nutrition: risk factors for osteoarthritis. Ann Rheum Dis 1997;56(7):397–400.
64. Dray A, Read SJ. Arthritis and pain: future targets to control osteoarthritis pain. Arthritis Res Ther 2007;9(3):212.
65. Anonymous. Recommendations for the medical management of osteoarthritis of the hip and knee: 2000 update. American College of Rheumatology Subcommittee on Osteoarthritis Guidelines. Arthritis Rheum 2000;43(9):1905–15.
66. Jordan KM, Arden NK, Doherty M, et al. EULAR recommendations 2003: an evidence based approach to the management of knee osteoarthritis. Report of a task force of the Standing Committee for International Clinical Studies Including Therapeutic Trials (ESCISIT). Ann Rheum Dis 2003;62(12):1145–55.
67. Zhang W, Doherty M, Arden N, et al. EULAR evidence based recommendations for the management of hip osteoarthritis: report of a task force of the EULAR Standing Committee for International Clinical Studies Including Therapeutics (ESCISIT). Ann Rheum Dis 2005;64(5):669–81.
68. Zhang W, Moskovitz R, Nuki G, et al. OARSI recommendations for the management of hip and knee osteoarthritis. Part II: OARSI evidence-based, expert consensus guidelines. Osteoarthritis Cartilage 2008;16(2):137–62.

Surgery for Osteoarthritis of the Knee

John C. Richmond, MD

KEYWORDS

• Osteoarthritis knee • Surgery • Arthroscopy
• Osteotomy • Arthroplasty

Currently available surgical techniques for the treatment of osteoarthritis of the knee range from arthroscopy to total joint arthroplasty. These techniques include procedures regarded as less invasive than total joint arthroplasty, including osteotomies and joint-preserving spacers or unicompartmental replacements. Total joint arthroplasty of either the hip or knee has been demonstrated to be one of the most cost-effective medical interventions available (**Fig. 1**). A recent study from Europe has confirmed again that total knee arthroplasty is a more cost-effective medical intervention than coronary artery bypass surgery.[1] Total joint arthroplasty is one of the most studied treatments in osteoarthritis because of the very high volume of joint replacements performed. (More than 300,000 total knee replacements are performed each year in the United States in the Medicare population alone, and the number is increasing annually.) This high volume and the significant expense of the procedure have resulted in many well-done studies investigating the long-term survivorship and effectiveness of this intervention in treating osteoarthritis of the knee. Although total knee replacement remains an excellent procedure in the older population (>70 years of age), there are significant issues concerning the long-term durability of total knee arthroplasty in the younger population (<55 years of age). One long-term study of more than 10,000 total knees demonstrated the failure of total knee replacement at 10 years was approximately three times higher in the population under age 55 years than in the population over age 70 years (15% versus 6%).[2] With this significantly higher risk of failure, multiple other alternative treatments often are recommended in this younger age group. This article reviews the alternative treatments to total knee arthroplasty, including arthroscopy, osteotomy, metal spacers, and unicompartmental arthroplasty, and also reviews the perceived advances in total knee arthroplasty that have been introduced during the past decade.

A version of this article originally appeared in the 34:3 issue of the *Rheumatic Disease Clinics of North America*.

Department of Orthopedic Surgery, New England Baptist Hospital, 125 Parker Hill Avenue, Boston, MA 02120, USA
E-mail address: jrichmon@nebh.org

Med Clin N Am 93 (2009) 213–222
doi:10.1016/j.mcna.2008.09.012
0025-7125/08/$ – see front matter

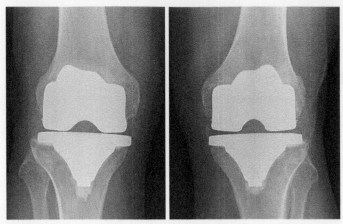

Fig.1. Bilateral total knee arthroplasties, an extremely cost-effective treatment for end-stage osteoarthritis of the knee. They are noted for high durability and excellent long-term survival.

ARTHROSCOPY

Arthroscopic treatment in osteoarthritis can range from lavage only to more complicated procedures that include removal of frayed articular cartilage (chondroplasty or debridement), removal of unstable meniscal tears and loose bodies, and synovectomy for hypertrophic synovium. For the first 25 years of arthroscopic surgery in the United States, debridement and/or lavage of the osteoarthritic knee was an accepted treatment, with little challenge as to its efficacy. In 2002, however, Moseley and colleagues[3] published a controlled trial of arthroscopic debridement/lavage versus sham surgery for osteoarthritis of the knee in *The New England Journal of Medicine*. This study, albeit imperfect, demonstrated that placebo surgery was as effective as lavage or debridement for the osteoarthritic knee. That paper provoked a protracted discussion concerning the potential role of arthroscopic surgery in osteoarthritis.[4,5] It has become clear through this discussion in the literature that lavage or lavage and debridement in prospective studies are no better than conservative care. A beneficial effect demonstrated by either of these treatments may be related to the cyclic nature of the symptoms or to the therapeutic benefit of placebo that occurs with osteoarthritis.[6,7]

There are, however, times when arthroscopic treatment of the osteoarthritic joint can be of benefit, particularly in that patient who has relatively mild to moderate osteoarthritis and a mechanically significant meniscal tear or loose body.[8,9] In these cases, the surgery is not performed for the osteoarthritis but rather to treat the mechanical derangement. More severe osteoarthritis does less well than mild or moderate osteoarthritis when treated arthroscopically. When preoperative weight-bearing views demonstrate bone-on-bone in an involved compartment, arthroscopy has little, if any, role. In that case the only indications for arthroscopy would be impinging osteophytes that prevent full extension or significant synovitis causing recurrent effusions.[10]

Although MRI scanning of an osteoarthritic knee has been of value in correlating the status of the meniscus with progression of the osteoarthritis, the author and colleagues find it of little value in identifying the patients who would benefit from arthroscopic surgery for osteoarthritis.[11–13] In fact, it is the author's personal experience that MRI scanning of the osteoarthritic joint can be counterproductive because of the high frequency of meniscal tears identified in this population. When the patient is made aware of a meniscal tear, he or she assumes that arthroscopic surgery will make the knee well by simple removal of the meniscal tear. This, in fact, is not the case, and significant effort is required to convince the patient that the underlying condition is osteoarthritis and that arthroscopic surgery has a very limited role in the treatment of osteoarthritis of the knee. Thus the widespread acquisition of MRI in osteoarthritis typically complicates rather than facilitates management.

This situation was confirmed again recently in another well-done level I study from Sweden. The authors randomly assigned patients who had mild osteoarthritis of the knee, an atraumatic medial meniscal tear demonstrated by MRI, and significant pain for 2 months or more to one of two treatments: arthroscopy and exercise or exercise alone.[7] In this series, arthroscopic partial medial meniscectomy and a subsequent supervised exercise program was not superior to supervised exercise alone when evaluating knee pain, knee function, or quality of life.

In summary, for osteoarthritis of the knee, the author recommends arthroscopic surgery be considered only in patients who have mild to moderate osteoarthritis as demonstrated radiographically on the Kellgren-Lawrence scale and symptoms suggestive of mechanical derangement. Secondary indications for arthroscopy in more advanced osteoarthritis (Kellgren-Lawrence stage 3) are the presence of anterior osteophytes in the intercondylar notch that block extension or significant synovitis leading to recurrent effusions. In these cases, resection of the osteophytes to regain extension and major synovectomy to reduce the recurrent effusions have proven beneficial and may delay more invasive surgery.

OSTEOTOMY

Unicompartmental osteoarthritis can exist in any of the three compartments (medial, lateral, or patellofemoral) of the joint. It is most common in the varus knee involving the medial compartment. The data as to efficacy and long-term outcomes following osteotomy are much better established for the medial compartment than for the lateral or patellofemoral compartments. Osteotomy to unload an overloaded compartment was described first in the 1960s for the medial compartment and in the 1970s for the patellofemoral compartment. Osteotomy for the treatment of lateral compartment tibiofemoral osteoarthritis is much less widely studied.

The Varus Knee with Medial Compartment Arthrosis

Osteotomy typically has been considered for a younger and more active population than joint replacement arthroplasty. It is recommended specifically for this group so that these patients can continue with high-impact, strenuous work or recreational activities. There is consensus that high-impact activities are deleterious after joint replacement arthroplasty and may lead to precocious failure of the implant through wear of the polyethylene and potential loosening of the prosthesis. It has been recommended that nothing more strenuous than cycling, low-impact aerobics, cross-country or light downhill skiing, or doubles tennis be performed following joint replacement arthroplasty.[14] Patients desirous of maintaining a more strenuous and active lifestyle, independent of age, can be considered for osteotomy when they have isolated unicompartmental disease. The Cochrane Review of valgus high tibial osteotomies concluded that these procedures improve function and reduce pain.[15] The reviewers concluded there was insufficient evidence to support osteotomy over unicompartmental arthroplasty. As noted previously, however, osteotomy should be preferred in the more vigorously active younger person desirous of strenuous work or athletic endeavors.

Identification of candidates for osteotomy requires long leg alignment views to determine the axis of weight bearing of the extremity as well as weight-bearing films of the knees done both in the anterior-posterior direction with the knee in full extension and in the posterior-anterior direction with the knee flexed ("Rosenberg views").[16] When the weight-bearing axis falls in the medial compartment, valgus high tibial osteotomy is an appropriate procedure. The goal of the procedure is to unload the damaged compartment and transfer weight bearing to the well-maintained lateral compartment. The combination of this mechanical overload of the noninvolved compartment and the degrative processes involved in osteoarthritis ultimately leads to progression of the osteoarthritis to involve the remainder of the joint, eventually necessitating total joint arthroplasty in the future.

There are multiple techniques for valgus-producing high tibial osteotomies as well as many different ways to fix these postoperatively. None has proved superior to the others. There are few direct comparative studies in the literature, and few meaningful differences have been demonstrated.[17,18] A closing wedge osteotomy, in which a wedge of bone is removed laterally from the tibia, with internal fixation using hardware, has the longest track record. There is detailed information about the durability of this osteotomy and the ease of revision to total joint arthroplasty when the osteotomy ultimately fails because of progression of the arthritis. Available data within the literature indicate there is approximately a 50% 10-year success rate for the osteotomy before revision.[19] Revisions of osteotomies performed with modern techniques of fixation to total knee arthroplasty when the osteoarthritis progresses have results comparable with those of primary total knee arthroplasties.[20]

Patellofemoral Arthrosis

Isolated osteoarthritis of the patellofemoral joint is not a common problem. Recognition of this condition is based on patellofemoral symptoms, with significant damage to the articular surface noted on plain radiographs, MRI scanning, or arthroscopy, with preservation of the tibiofemoral articulation. In the past treatment of this condition has included patellectomy. Patellectomy has fallen out of favor because of the potential loss of quadriceps strength and the need for a functioning patella to have optimal results with later total knee arthroplasty. Elevation of the tibial tubercle to decrease joint reactive forces across the patellofemoral joint was performed first in the 1960s and 1970s.[21] It has become a reliable alternative treatment when reasonable articular surface remains and the areas of most severe cartilage breakdown or exposed bone can be unloaded appropriately.[22] Because there is a spectrum from chondromalacia patella and patellar instability to patellofemoral arthrosis, there are no meaningful data in the literature to define accurately the indications or predictors for long-term success of procedures designed to unload the osteoarthritic patellofemoral joint by elevation of the tibial tubercle.

The Valgus Knee with Lateral Compartment Arthrosis

Significantly less information is available in the literature for treating the valgus knee with lateral compartment collapse via an osteotomy, in part because this condition is less common than the varus knee with medial degeneration. Also, patients who have lateral degeneration tend to be female, older, and more sedentary than patients who have varus medial compartment osteoarthritis. Because of the alignment of the knee and the relationship of the weight-bearing surface of the tibia to the floor, any realignment osteotomy for lateral compartment arthrosis usually needs be done on the distal femur. This procedure is more complicated, and fewer surgeons consider it as a treatment technique. From the few series in the literature, the success rates and durability of the procedure seem to be similar to those of proximal tibial osteotomy for varus malalignment and medial compartment arthrosis.[23] As in tibial osteotomies, there is no scientific evidence to support one technique over another.

INTERPOSITIONAL ARTHROPLASTY

Both biologic and metal interposition arthroplasty procedures currently are available for the treatment of unicompartmental osteoarthrosis. Information concerning the effectiveness and longevity of these procedures is sketchy at best. Current biologic interpositional arthroplasties use allograft meniscal transplantation. Data from meniscal transplantation series indicate that the presence of significant osteoarthritis within the involved compartment is a relative contraindication to performing the procedure. Although some authors believe there is a role for this procedure, the consensus is that meniscus transplantation in an isolated osteoarthritic compartment is not warranted.[24,25]

Metal interpositional arthroplasty procedures have a long history, dating back to the 1950s, and were virtually abandoned in the 1970s when modern techniques of joint replacement arthroplasty with methylmethacrylate fixation were introduced. The reason for this switch from interpositional implants to joint replacement was the dramatically greater success with joint replacement arthroplasty when compared with the metal interposition devices. When the US Congress added the Medical Device Amendment of 1976 to the Federal Food, Drug and Cosmetic Act, they created a category for exempting certain devices from premarket approval. This category, the 510(k) Exemption, required the device manufacturer only to demonstrate that the device to be marketed is substantially equivalent to a legally marketed device that was on the market in 1976. For devices on the market in 1976 that function well and are straightforward, such as bone screws and plates, this 510(k) Exemption has worked well. Some devices on the market in 1976, however, were not effective and have been replaced by much more effective techniques. This 510(k) Exemption has led to several devices being introduced for interpositional arthroplasty for which there was no evidence concerning safety or efficacy before their marketing. The first of these devices was the UniSpacer (Zimmer, Warsaw, Indiana). It was introduced in the United States in 2000 and was touted as restoring alignment of the knee by functioning the same way as an osteotomy might.[26] It is not known how many of these devices were implanted before independent surgeons published the results of a prospective trial in 2005.[27] That prospective trial indicated only one third of patients had good results, and more than 25% of patients required revision during the 2 years of the study. Subsequent to this publication, very few of these devices have been implanted.

A second interposition arthroplasty also has come recently on the market through the 510(k) Exemption: ConformMIS iForma (ConformiMIS Inc., Burlington, Massachusetts). This device is custom manufactured, using an MRI scan, to be fitted specifically for the individual patient (**Fig. 2**). To date, no studies as to its safety and efficacy have been published. Although the custom manufacturing process seems to hold promise that this device might alleviate pain caused by unicompartmental arthrosis of either the medial or lateral tibiofemoral compartment, well-done prospective studies are needed to determine if this technology will have a place in the treatment of unicompartmental osteoarthrosis of the knee joint.

UNICOMPARTMENTAL ARTHROPLASTY

Unicompartmental arthroplasty has been performed for many years. Current designs are considered superior to designs manufactured in the 1980s.[28,29] Success with these implants is definitely surgeon-specific, and many arthroplasty surgeons prefer

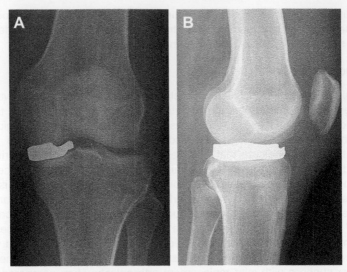

Fig. 2. (*A*) Anteroposterior and (*B*) lateral radiographs of a custom-manufactured spacer device. As yet, no studies have established the efficacy and durability of these new devices.

the reliability of total joint arthroplasty over unicompartmental replacement. A number of series, however, have noted that patient satisfaction is higher with unicompartmental arthroplasty than with total knee arthroplasty (**Fig. 3**). It is theorized this satisfaction is related to the preservation of two otherwise normal compartments within the joint. The problems with unicompartmental arthroplasty are related to the progression of the osteoarthritis in the remaining two compartments. This progression leads to a significantly higher revision rate over a 10- to 15-year time frame than seen with total joint

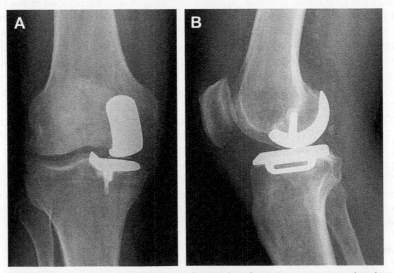

Fig. 3. (*A*) Anteroposterior and (*B*) lateral radiographs of a unicompartmental arthroplasty. These devices have the advantage of sparing normal parts of a joint with isolated compartmental degeneration, but they do not hold up as long as total joint replacements.

arthroplasty.[29] These data indicate the reason for failure is progression of the arthritis in the contralateral tibiofemoral compartment, not problems with the implant itself. The success rates for the revision of these unicompartmental replacements to total knee arthroplasty seem to be similar to the success rates for primary total knee arthroplasty. Interestingly, unicompartmental arthroplasty is touted as being best suited for the younger patient, in whom the preservation of normal tissues, with minimal bone resection, is a potential benefit when revision becomes necessary. It also is promoted for older patients who have isolated disease, whose osteoarthritis is not likely to progress to a degree that will affect the outcome of surgery before their demise.[30,31] For the younger, more active patient who has abnormal alignment, osteotomy seems to be a better choice than unicompartmental replacement. For the older, more sedentary patient, unicompartmental arthroplasty is supported by the literature as a more reliable operation.[32,33]

PATELLOFEMORAL REPLACEMENTS

Patellofemoral replacement has had a dubious long-term track record going back to the 1970s and 1980s. At that time, the implants were primitive, and the instrumentation to implant them was unreliable at best.[34] Current modifications of the implants and instrumentation have made the procedure more technically reproducible, but to date there are few long-term studies of the efficacy of these techniques.[35,36] As with the interpositional devices of tibiofemoral articulation, new custom-made implants have been designed. These implants show promising very early results, but to date patellofemoral replacement has little if any evidence base to support its use, particularly given the excellent long-term results related to total joint arthroplasty. Isolated patellofemoral replacement, like a unicompartmental arthroplasty, probably is done best by the surgeons most experienced in the technique.

EMERGING TECHNOLOGY FOR TOTAL KNEE REPLACEMENT

As noted in the introduction to this article, total knee arthroplasty is a very cost-effective, durable procedure for treatment of osteoarthritis of the knee joint. A recent review has indicated that the results are better, and the complications fewer, when the procedure is performed in specialty hospitals rather than general hospitals.[37] This difference probably is related to the volume in both the operating room and on the floors, with development of clinical pathways to improve clinical outcomes.

During the past 8 years a number of new technologies have been introduced into the realm of total joint arthroplasty, and a review of the most publicized and potentially important changes is warranted. These changes include minimally invasive total knee arthroplasty, computer-assisted or navigated total knee replacement, and gender-specific total knee replacement. Unfortunately, these three technologies have become marketing tools for surgeons, hospitals, and orthopedic implant manufacturers. In general, the length of the incision used for total knee replacement has become shorter. Many surgeons believe that total knee replacement through these mini-incisions is very demanding technically. Computer navigation can assist with joint replacement arthroplasty through these small incisions because bony anatomic landmarks can be identified precisely without extensile exposure. It allows the surgeon to obtain excellent alignment of the prosthesis (with higher reproducibility than traditional alignment guides). Computer navigation involves a significant learning curve as well as prolonged operative time and expense. The benefit of improved alignment may extrapolate to long-term durability of the prosthesis, although this benefit is yet to be demonstrated.[38] Although a number of surgeons have embraced the technology, many high-volume arthroplasty surgeons believe that the additional operative time, increased expense, and limited improvements in alignment do not warrant its adoption.

Several orthopedic implant manufacturers have introduced total knee prostheses that are marketed as gender specific. There are anatomic differences between men and woman, which previously had not been accounted for in implant manufacture. The gender-specific knee replacement for women has been promoted as being better because it reflects the anatomic variations between men and women recognized when the prosthesis was designed. To date, there is no evidence to support an advantage of these gender-specific devices for women; in fact, when the literature for traditional total knee arthroplasty is reviewed in detail for outcomes based on sex, the risk of failure is not greater in women than in men.[39]

SUMMARY

The surgical treatment in osteoarthritis of the knee continues to evolve. The indications for arthroscopy have narrowed. Orthopedic surgeons continue to explore options less invasive than total knee replacement for isolated unicompartmental arthritis of the knee joint. As in all therapeutic interventions, the practice of evidence-based medicine will drive surgeons to use only those surgical techniques that have been proven safe and efficacious by long-term prospective outcome studies.

REFERENCES

1. Räsänen P, Paavolainen P, Sintonen H, et al. Effectiveness of hip or knee replacement surgery in terms of quality-adjusted life years and costs. Acta Orthop 2007; 78(1):108–15.
2. Rand JA, Trousdale RT, Ilstrup DM, et al. Factors affecting the durability of primary total knee prostheses. J Bone Joint Surg Am 2003;85:259–65.
3. Moseley JB, O'Malley K, Petersen NJ, et al. A controlled trial of arthroscopic surgery for osteoarthritis of the knee. N Engl J Med 2002;347:81–8.
4. Felson DT, Buckwalter J. Débridement and lavage for osteoarthritis of the knee [correspondence]. N Engl J Med 2002;347:132–3.
5. Jackson RW, Ewing W, Ewing JW, et al. Arthroscopic surgery for osteoarthritis of the knee [correspondence]. N Engl J Med 2002;347:1717–9.
6. Siparsky P, Ryzewicz M, Peterson B, et al. Arthroscopic treatment of osteoarthritis of the knee: are there any evidence-based indications? Clin Orthop Relat Res 2007;455:107–12.
7. Herrlin S, Hållander M, Wange P, et al. Arthroscopic or conservative treatment of degenerative medial meniscal tears: a prospective randomised trial. Knee Surg Sports Traumatol Arthrosc 2007;15(4):393–401.
8. Dearing J, Nutton RW. Evidence based factors influencing outcome of arthroscopy in osteoarthritis of the knee. Knee 2008;14(3):159–63.
9. Aaron RK, Skolnick AH, Reinert SE, et al. Arthroscopic débridement for osteoarthritis of the knee. J Bone Joint Surg Am 2006;88:936–43.
10. Steadman JR, Ramappa AJ, Maxwell RB, et al. An arthroscopic treatment regimen for osteoarthritis of the knee. Arthroscopy 2007;23(9):948–55.
11. Bhattacharyya T, Gale D, Dewire P, et al. The clinical importance of meniscal tears demonstrated by magnetic resonance imaging in osteoarthritis of the knee. J Bone Joint Surg Am 2003;85:4–9.
12. Berthiaume MJ, Raynauld JP, Martel-Pelletier J, et al. Meniscal tear and extrusion are strongly associated with progression of symptomatic knee osteoarthritis as

assessed by quantitative magnetic resonance imaging. Ann Rheum Dis 2005; 64(4):556–63.

13. Hunter DJ, Zhang YQ, Niu JB, Tu X, et al. The association of meniscal pathologic changes with cartilage loss in symptomatic knee osteoarthritis. Arthritis Rheum 2006;54:795–801.

14. Healy WL, Iorio R, Lemos MJ. Athletic activity after joint replacement. Am J Sports Med 2001;29(3):377–88.

15. Brouwer RW, Raaij van TM, Bierma-Zeinstra SMA, et al. Osteotomy for treating knee osteoarthritis. Cochrane Database Syst Rev 2005,(1):CD004019.

16. Rosenberg TD, Paulos LE, Parker RD, et al. The forty-five-degree posteroanterior flexion weight-bearing radiograph of the knee. J Bone Joint Surg Am 1988; 70(10):1479–83.

17. Brouwer RW, Bierma-Zeinstra SMA, van Koeveringe AJ, et al. Patellar height and the inclination of the tibial plateau after high tibial osteotomy: the open versus the closed-wedge technique. J Bone Joint Surg Br 2005;87:1227–32.

18. Brouwer RW, Bierma-Zeinstra SMA, van Raaij TM, et al. Osteotomy for medial compartment arthritis of the knee using a closing wedge or an opening wedge controlled by a Puddu plate: a one-year randomised, controlled study. J Bone Joint Surg Br 2006;88:1454–9.

19. Billings A, Scott DF, Camargo MP, et al. High tibial osteotomy with a calibrated osteotomy guide, rigid internal fixation, and early motion. Long-term follow-up. J Bone Joint Surg Am 2000;82:70–9.

20. Meding JB, Keating EM, Ritter MA, et al. Total knee arthroplasty after high tibial osteotomy: a comparison study in patients who had bilateral total knee replacement. J Bone Joint Surg Am 2000;82:1252.

21. Maquet P. Advancement of the tibial tuberosity. Clin Orthop Relat Res 1976;(115): 225–30.

22. Farr J, Schepsis A, Cole B, et al. Anteromedialization: review and technique. J Knee Surg 2007;20(2):120–8.

23. Backstein D, Morag G, Hanna S, et al. Long-term follow-up of distal femoral varus osteotomy of the knee. J Arthroplasty 2007;22(4 Suppl 1):2–6.

24. Stone KR, Walgenbach AW, Turek TJ, et al. Meniscus allograft survival in patients with moderate to severe unicompartmental arthritis: a 2- to 7-year follow-up. Arthroscopy 2006;22(5):469–78.

25. Lubowitz JH, Verdonk PC, Reid JB III, et al. Meniscus allograft transplantation: a current concepts review. Knee Surg Sports Traumatol Arthrosc 2007;15(5):476–92.

26. Hallock RH, Fell BM. Unicompartmental tibial hemiarthroplasty: early results of the UniSpacer knee. Clin Orthop Relat Res 2003;(416):154–63.

27. Sisto DJ, Mitchell IL. UniSpacer arthroplasty of the knee. J Bone Joint Surg Am 2005;87(8):1706–11.

28. Emerson RH Jr, Higgins LL. Unicompartmental knee arthroplasty with the Oxford prosthesis in patients with medial compartment arthritis. J Bone Joint Surg Am 2008;90(1):118–22.

29. Borus T, Thornhill T. Unicompartmental knee arthroplasty. J Am Acad Orthop Surg 2008;16(1):9–18.

30. Soohoo NF, Sharifi H, Kominski G, et al. Cost-effectiveness analysis of unicompartmental knee arthroplasty as an alternative to total knee arthroplasty for unicompartmental osteoarthritis. J Bone Joint Surg Am 2006;88(9):1975–82.

31. Slover J, Espehaug B, Havelin LI, et al. Cost-effectiveness of unicompartmental and total knee arthroplasty in elderly low-demand patients. A Markov decision analysis. J Bone Joint Surg Am 2006;88(11):2348–55.

32. Naal FD, Fischer M, Preuss A, et al. Return to sports and recreational activity after unicompartmental knee arthroplasty. Am J Sports Med 2007;35:1688–95.
33. Stukenborg-Colsman C, Wirth CJ, Lazovic D, et al. High tibial osteotomy versus unicompartmental joint replacement in unicompartmental knee joint osteoarthritis: 7–10-year follow-up prospective randomised study. Knee 2001;8(3):187–94.
34. Grelsamer RP, Stein DA. Current concepts review: patellofemoral arthritis. J Bone Joint Surg Am 2006;88:1849–60.
35. Sisto DJ, Sarin VK. Custom patellofemoral arthroplasty of the knee. J Bone Joint Surg Am 2006;88:1475–80.
36. Ackroyd CE, Newman JH, Evans R, et al. The Avon patellofemoral arthroplasty: five-year survivorship and functional results. J Bone Joint Surg Br 2007;89:310–5.
37. Cram P, Vaughan-Sarrazin MS, Wolf B, et al. A comparison of total hip and knee replacement in specialty and general hospitals. J Bone Joint Surg Am 2007; 89(8):1675–84.
38. Bauwens K, Matthes G, Wich M, et al. Navigated total knee replacement. a meta-analysis. J Bone Joint Surg Am 2007;89:261–9.
39. Rankin EA, Bostrom M, Hozack W, et al. Gender-specific knee replacements: a technology overview. J Am Acad Orthop Surg 2008;16:63–7.

How Close are We to Having Structure-Modifying Drugs Available?

David J. Hunter, MBBS, MSc, PhD[a],*,
Marie-Pierre Hellio Le Graverand-Gastineau, MD, DSc, PhD[b]

KEYWORDS

• Structure modification • Osteoarthritis

Osteoarthritis (OA) is a clinical condition that manifests with joint pain and functional limitation. It was previously described as a cartilage-centric condition, and the hallmark of the disease was described as cartilage loss. Although cartilage loss is a prominent feature of OA, contemporary models recognize that important structural and pathologic changes also occur in other articular tissues.

More precisely, OA can be viewed as the clinical and pathologic outcome of a range of disorders that result in structural and functional failure of synovial joints with menis-cal degeneration, subchondral bone alterations, bone and cartilage overgrowth (osteophytes), loss of articular cartilage, and a synovial inflammatory response.[1] OA occurs when the dynamic equilibrium between the breakdown and repair of joint tissues becomes unbalanced.[2] This progressive joint failure may cause pain and dis-ability,[3] although many persons with structural changes consistent with OA are asymptomatic.[4] This last point is particularly salient for this review, because many would advocate that we need to alter the structural progression of this disease and can do so without regard to the symptomatic benefits. The development of agents to modify the structure of OA, that is, disease-modifying OA drugs (DMOADs), needs to be viewed in this light and the current regulatory stance that this is a symptomatic condition, and any improvement in structural outcome should be accompanied by a clinical benefit. Furthermore, the multitude of risk factors, the complex

A version of this article originally appeared in the 34:3 issue of the *Rheumatic Disease Clinics of North America*.

[a] Division of Research, New England Baptist Hospital, 125 Parker Hill Avenue, Boston, MA 02120, USA

[b] Pfizer Global Research and Development, 50 Pequot Avenue, MS6025-A3166, New London, CT 06320, USA

* Corresponding author. Division of Research, New England Baptist Hospital, 125 Parker Hill Avenue, Boston, MA 02120.

E-mail address: djhunter@caregroup.harvard.edu (D.J. Hunter).

etiopathogenesis, and the heterogeneity of clinical presentations create a complex environment for therapeutic development aimed at modifying structure.

This review describes what structure modification is, distinguishing between preventing, retarding, stopping, and reversing disease and what might be clinically meaningful. The authors also describe whether there is any evidence to suggest that one can modify disease, and whether the current tissue that is predominantly focused on, namely, cartilage, is an appropriate target. The methodologic approaches and other obstacles to demonstrating efficacy of these agents in clinical trials are considered. This discussion is a narrative review in a field that is rapidly evolving. It is hoped the reader appreciates the complexity of the field and the likely road ahead to DMOAD development.

WHAT IS A DISEASE-MODIFYING OSTEOARTHRITIS DRUG?

Primarily because OA has had such a cartilage-centric focus, the first substances that protected articular cartilage during the course of destructive joint disorders were termed *chondroprotective agents* because they focused their activity on the chondrocyte. When the chondroprotective effect became linked to a clinical benefit and appeared to alter the course of the disease, these agents were termed *disease-modifying osteoarthritis drugs*.[5]

Bearing in mind that the typical course of OA is one of slowly advancing structural progression, there are several potential goals of these agents. In principle, one outcome of a structure-modifying trial could be that the agent was ineffective or deleterious to structure and, if so, would be unlikely to be licensed for that purpose. An example of this from another field was the therapeutic investigation of fluoride for osteoporosis which actually increased fracture risk rather than reducing it.[6]

Other possible outcomes of the use of DMOADs would be retardation (slowing of the rate of progression), stopping progression, reversing progression (regeneration of the target tissue), or even preventing the development of the disease. Given these outcome options, what is likely to be clinically meaningful? Before that question can be answered, it must be determined what is meant by "clinically meaningful." For some, this means delaying or mitigating the need for surgical intervention such as joint replacement.[7] For others, it means making a meaningful impact on the quality of life of patients and in particular their physical function.[8] From a regulatory perspective, the major licensing authorities (US Food and Drug Administration [FDA] and the European Medicines Agency) have provided draft guidance documents for industry for clinical development programs for agents that modify OA structure, requiring that the agent slows joint space narrowing and results in clinical benefit (eg, improvement of patient symptoms or function). Details of the draft guidance can be found on the Internet at http://www.fda.gov/Cber/gdlns/osteo.htm.

With these thresholds for detecting clinically meaningful effects, no disease-modifying efficacy has been convincingly demonstrated for any of the existing pharmacologic agents. Some agents have slowed structural progression without symptomatic benefit, suggesting that simply slowing progression may not be sufficient to lead to symptom improvement.[9,10]

IS THE MARRIAGE OF SYMPTOMS AND STRUCTURE RATIONAL?

Many would argue that slowing the rate of structural progression is a noble intent in and of itself. They could also argue that many of the trials of DMOADs which were interpreted as not demonstrating a clinical benefit suffered limitations, including a majority of patients with little-to-no pain at baseline or the need for the use of concomitant standard of care medications, introducing noise in the results of the symptom assessment questionnaires. Given these limitations, the demonstration of structural improvement might plausibly be dissociated from clinical benefit in the same clinical trial. It could also be argued that DMOAD trials in which structure preservation was suggested but without affecting symptoms did not follow participants for long enough, and that the eventual clinical outcome could have been favorable.[9,10] Parallels may be drawn between the treatment of hypertension or osteoporosis, which typically has no short-term symptomatic benefit but reduces the risk of an unfavorable long-term outcome. This approach would require that a person take an agent presumably before the onset of OA for an uncertain period of time to prevent the development of the disease or to prevent the development of symptomatic disease in a person with pre-existing structural damage.

First, let us consider this scenario in its fullest extent. OA affects the majority of the population aged more than 65 years. Many believe that there is a long lead time for the development of OA, with some data suggesting this is programmed from developmental shape,[11] malalignment during adolescence,[12] or obesity during young adult life,[13,14] suggesting that the structural failure that is OA may begin developing decades before it becomes symptomatic. If we were to adequately treat this scenario with pharmacologic agents, we would need to treat the majority of the population for the large part of their adult life. Given the proclivity to toxicity of most agents and the burden of expense to the health care system, this treatment is not justifiable.

In an alternate scenario, a young adult may sustain a tear of the anterior cruciate ligament (ACL) or a meniscal injury that is not reparable. There is a high incidence of knee OA in the years following ACL[15,16] or meniscal injury,[15,17] and credible evidence suggests that current arthroscopic procedures, including ACL reconstruction and meniscectomy, are not sufficient to fully restore normal joint mechanics or neutralize the long-term risk of OA.[18,19] Given the great potential for the development of OA over a shorter time frame (7–10 years) in a more limited segment of the population, treatment of this alternate scenario may be possible within our health care system. Obviously, this scenario needs to be formally evaluated before the latter statement is supported by any evidence. Potentially, this latter approach could also be used if we had an algorithm that allowed the detection of those at greatest risk of disease based on some genetic predisposition or risk factor for incident disease, such as obesity.

Next, one can consider the alternate position in which treatment is limited to those who present with symptomatic disease—a much more limited segment of the population—for what presumably would be a more finite period of time. As for the stance taken previously, there are many fundamental limitations to this position as well. Much of the current focus on agents to modify the disease is directed at preserving hyaline articular cartilage. In the OA Initiative progression cohort, the majority of subjects with symptomatic radiographic disease appeared to have full-thickness cartilage loss over extensive areas in weight-bearing portions of the knee joint.[20] Retarding loss in these individuals would be more focused on preserving what they have left. This loss appears to occur in joints that are malaligned, creating a harsh mechanical environment for putative agents to work in.

Furthermore, the current FDA regulatory stance would have structural modification defined as imparting an effect on radiographic joint space narrowing, yet articular cartilage is both aneural and avascular. As such, cartilage is incapable of generating pain, inflammation, stiffness, or any of the symptoms that patients with knee OA typically describe. Given its relative unimportance to the symptomatic presentation of OA, it may appear ironic that articular cartilage has received so much attention while other common symptom sources in the knee are ignored.[21] Joint space width is composed not only of articular cartilage but also of meniscus.[22] In contrast to articular cartilage, the meniscal tissue is vascularized and innervated. In addition, although articular cartilage may not appear to drive symptoms directly, cartilage breakdown may lead to OA symptoms by generating synovial inflammation and promoting meniscal degeneration and subchondral bone changes in relation to changes in cartilage biomechanical properties. Interventions that focus exclusively on nourishing, replenishing, or replacing articular cartilage may be viewed as having little chance of providing long-term symptomatic relief unless they also simultaneously relieve strain on other innervated structures; however, it is unlikely that therapeutic agents will have an effect on articular cartilage only. The molecular pathways of tissue degeneration associated with OA in joint tissues other than cartilage are similar and may actually precede those occurring in the articular cartilage as suggested by several reports on degenerative changes in the meniscus in preclinical models of OA and in humans.[23–26]

Both approaches have fundamental limitations, and before either approach could be embarked upon, further research is needed to adequately understand the implications of such a decision.

IS THERE EVIDENCE THAT SUGGESTS WE CAN MODIFY DISEASE?

Some studies with varying levels of evidence suggest that glucosamine sulfate, chondroitin sulfate, sodium hyaluronan, doxycycline, matrix metalloprotease (MMP) inhibitors, bisphosphonates, calcitonin, diacerein, and avocado-soybean unsaponifiables can modify disease progression.[27]

A great degree of research effort has been geared toward identifying small molecule inhibitors of MMPs that act downstream in the pathophysiologic cascade. Thus far, these compounds have failed in the early clinical phase, mainly because of a painful joint stiffening tendonitis-like side effect named musculoskeletal syndrome which seems to be due to the relative broad-spectrum MMP inhibition of these compounds.[28] Nevertheless, some MMP inhibitors with more selective specificity profiles are in preclinical or early clinical development. Several of these candidates are specific for MMP-13, which is overexpressed by OA cartilage, and have minimal effects on MMP-1, which has been implicated in the development of adverse musculoskeletal events.[29]

Tetracyclines have been shown to reduce the severity of OA in animals, probably by inhibiting MMP activity, and have also been studied in early human trials with some suggestion of efficacy in slowing the progression of joint space narrowing.[9] Brandt and colleagues[9] reported that doxycycline slowed joint space narrowing in patients with OA of the medial tibiofemoral compartment. In this placebo-controlled trial, 431 obese women (aged 45–64 years) with radiographically visible unilateral knee OA were randomly assigned to receive 30 months of treatment with 100 mg of doxycycline or placebo twice daily. Doxycycline reduced the mean loss of joint space width in the OA knee by approximately 30% at 30 months; however, it did not prevent the development of progressive joint space narrowing in the contralateral knee, and it did not improve measures of pain or function when compared with placebo. Although it may have a beneficial effect on structure, the clinical meaningfulness of this effect remains questionable.

In a 3-year study, Dougados and colleagues[10] reported that diacerein slowed the radiographic progression of hip OA, defined by a joint space loss of at least 0.5 mm. The effects were modest (54% of the patients in the diacerein group had radiographic progression versus 62% in the placebo group) and were not associated with symptomatic improvement. A recent 1-year study of structural progression in knee OA failed to indicate that diacerein had a structure-modifying effect.[30]

The strong increase in bone remodeling in OA has prompted investigations of the disease-modifying potential of the bisphosphonates. Despite promising preclinical data and observational data implicating antiresorptives (alendronate and estrogen) in reducing the prevalence of bone marrow lesions in subchondral bone,[31] the clinical results have been disappointing. In a recently conducted placebo-controlled, randomized, phase III clinical study in patients with knee OA, risedronate did not show any structural or symptomatic efficacy despite having salient benefits on biochemical markers of cartilage degradation[32] and on the architecture of subchondral bone.[33] The fact that the main study result was negative may have as much to do with study design issues as therapeutic efficacy, in particular, identifying a population of persons who progressed during the finite period of the trial. This problem made separation of the placebo and active intervention arms problematic.

More promising in its potential role on bone remodeling in OA are the results of a recent preclinical investigation into the role of calcitonin. Further clinical trial results are eagerly anticipated.[34]

Two of the more controversial areas of OA management relate to the use of glucosamine and hyaluronans. Neither agent is currently approved for a DMOAD indication. Much of the symptomatic data on these agents suggests that there is little difference between active agent and placebo in well-designed trials.[35–38] Further controversy extends to whether they have any effect on structure. Claims have been made that hyaluronic acids slow the rate of disease progression; however, clinical results do not support this claim.[30,39] Two published randomized longitudinal studies indicate that glucosamine sulfate slows the rate of progression of knee OA;[40,41] however, joint space width was assessed using standing anteroposterior knee radiographs, which has led to criticism of the findings. A change in knee pain might potentially affect the ability to extend the knee and thereby alter apparent joint space width.[42] The results of the recently completed Glucosamine/Chondroitin Arthritis Intervention Trial (GAIT), which included an 18-month imaging outcome, have not yet been reported.[37]

Avocado-soybean unsaponifiables have been reported to repress chondrocyte catabolic activities and to increase the accumulation of proteoglycan by OA chondrocytes in culture. Based on current clinical evidence, their efficacy in modifying structure is questionable;[43] however, further trials are of merit given the preliminary nature of this evidence.

WHAT PROMISING TARGETS ARE BEING EXPLORED?

OA is a disease of the whole joint organ, and current drug development has seen widespread focus on several different tissue targets.[44] Synovitis is frequently present in OA and may predict other structural changes and correlate with pain and other clinical outcomes.[45] The synovium is densely innervated by small-diameter sensory nerve fibers.[46] Interleukin-1 beta (IL-1β) and tumor necrosis factor alpha (TNF-α) have the capacity to excite and sensitize nociceptors and contribute in vivo to behavioral signs of inflammatory hyperalgesia through nerve growth factor (NGF).[44,47] Moreover, cytokines enhance the release of prostaglandin E_2 (PGE$_2$), inducible nitric oxide synthase (iNOS), and histamine from chondrocytes, meniscal cells, and mast cells, which, in turn, can (indirectly) increase the sensitization of nociceptors.[48]

NO-dependent tissue injury has been implicated in OA.[49] The expression of iNOS by endotoxin, cytokines, or other pathophysiologic stresses generates high sustained concentrations of NO. The sustained excess production of NO and resulting NO-derived metabolites (eg, peroxynitrate) elicit cellular cytotoxicity and joint tissue damage through activation of MMPs, cytokines, and cyclooxygenase 2, producing alterations in normal physiologic function in the articular joint leading to OA changes. The widespread expression of iNOS in human OA tissues, including synovial, meniscal, osteophytes, and articular cartilage tissues,[25,49–51] as well as data from several animal models of arthritis[52,53] and pain[54] suggest that iNOS inhibitors may have potential utility in the treatment of OA.

Bradykinin is generated in inflamed synovium, as it is in all inflamed tissue, and is able to excite and sensitize sensory nerve fibers.[55] The clinical relevance of bradykinin has recently been demonstrated in a phase II study in which intra-articular injection of a specific bradykinin-B_2 receptor antagonist reduced OA knee pain more potently than placebo injection.[56] HOE140 is a specific and potent bradykinin-B_2 receptor antagonist that is a decapeptide and is administered via intra-articular injection. In the first placebo-controlled, proof-of-mechanism study in patients with knee OA, one dose of HOE140 provided greater pain relief than placebo injection.[57]

Another target of interest is NGF, which exerts its action through two types of receptors: high-affinity tyrosine kinase A receptor (trkA) and low-affinity p75 receptor. Both NGF and its receptors are expressed in synovial, meniscal, and articular cartilage tissues, suggesting that they could be involved in joint physiopathology and OA.[58,59] RN624, tanezumab, is a humanized monoclonal antibody against NGF. In two recently completed randomized, placebo-controlled, double-blind studies in patients with chronic OA pain, a single dose of tanezumab showed significant improvement in WOMAC scores when compared with placebo.[60]

Widespread use of TNF inhibitors and other biologics in the treatment of rheumatoid arthritis has led to unprecedented success in disease management. Intra-articular injection of specific IL-1 inhibitors or antagonists has been shown to slow disease progression in animal models of OA. In the first randomized, placebo-controlled trial of a IL-1β antagonist, a single intra-articular injection of 50 or 150 mg had no analgesic effect during 3 months of follow-up,[61] although 150 mg of IL-1 ra had an early analgesic effect. Anti–TNF-α therapy has also been tested in isolated cases of digital and knee OA, with little success in clinical trials to date. Given the fact that synovitis appears to have a role in symptoms but is a response to cartilage degradation rather than a risk factor predisposing to it, it is unlikely that TNF inhibitors will impact anything else other than symptoms.

Given the importance of bone remodeling in OA, further work has been initiated investigating the potential structure-modifying role of vitamin D. Another promising line of inquiry is investigation into the role of the bone morphogenetic protein family of protein-signaling molecules.[62] Another potential therapeutic target in OA may be the strong vascularization of areas of OA bone remodeling.[63] Evidence suggests that enhanced vascular pressure in subarticular bone regions (especially in the femur or tibia), venous engorgement, and the chemical and mechanical stimulation of sensory nerve endings in the vascular wall or ischemia may contribute to severe ischemia- and pressure-induced rest or night pain in patients with advanced hip or knee OA.[64] Preliminary investigation of the role of iloprost, a synthetic analogue of PGI_2, in this regard appears promising but warrants further rigorous evaluation.[65,66]

The rationale for leaving the discussion of agents that have activity in hyaline articular cartilage as a last topic is to recognize the importance of studying other tissues. One of the major players during breakdown of articular cartilage is the proinflammatory cytokine IL-1β.[44] Chondrocytes and synoviocytes produce and release IL-1β. Intracellularly, the pro-form of IL-1β is converted by interleukin-converting enzyme

(ICE) to the active form of IL-1β. The importance of this enzyme has been elucidated by both Pralnacasan, an ICE inhibitor that reduces joint damage in two murine models of OA,[67] and gene transfer of a biologic IL-1 receptor antagonist.[68] IL-1β activates proteases. These MMPs cleave collagen II (MMP-1, MMP-13) and convert pro-MMPs into collagenases and gelatinases (MMP-3).

Other agents of particular interest are the cathepsin K and aggrecanase inhibitors. Although characteristic to osteoclasts, the expression of cathepsin K has also been observed at other sites in the skeleton. Several recent observations have demonstrated up-regulation of cathepsin K in OA cartilage and inflamed synovial tissue.[69] Because cathepsin K is one of the few extracellular proteolytic enzymes capable of degrading native fibrillar collagen, it may have an important role in the progressive destruction of articular cartilage in OA and inflammatory arthritides.

A major component of the cartilage extracellular matrix is aggrecan, a proteoglycan that imparts compressive resistance to the tissue. Aggrecan is cleaved at a specific "aggrecanase" site in human OA cartilage by several members of the ADAMTS family of MMPs. ADAMTS5 is the primary aggrecanase responsible for aggrecan degradation in a murine model of OA,[70] and inhibition of this protease is now undergoing clinical investigation.

OBSTACLES TO DRUG DEVELOPMENT

Several well-known risk factors for the structural progression of OA are likely to be operational in the setting of investigation and use of DMOADs.[71] We need to pay greater attention to the pathogenesis of this complex disease in therapeutic trials. Recent studies have highlighted the importance of mechanical factors in the etiopathogenesis of this disease.[72] Knee alignment and the stance-phase adduction moment[73] are key determinants of the disproportionate medial transmission of load.[74] Mechanics of the joint environment have a pivotal role, and ignoring their importance will eliminate any chance of finding an effective product. Attempts to treat failing tissue in a grossly malaligned joint are equivalent to moving a mountain. If pharmacologic intervention as a single therapy is to be trialed effectively, selecting patients who have less advanced disease before the development of marked aberrant mechanics is a preferable solution. As Brandt and colleagues[21] have suggested, "if efforts to develop a DMOAD or biological treatment for osteoarthritis, which are almost always aimed at stimulating the osteoarthritic cartilage with growth factors or inhibiting matrix-degrading enzymes, do not concomitantly correct the mechanical disorder that is the proximate cause of the arthropathy, these treatments are unlikely to produce long-lasting benefit."

Current trials are wanting for more responsive outcome measures for symptoms and structure to identify change. Clinical research efforts are ongoing to develop and validate new pain and function questionnaires that may be more sensitive in detecting improvement in patient symptoms.[75,76] As is true in rheumatoid arthritis and osteoporosis, the advent of one therapy successful in modifying the disease will rapidly change the playing field. Persons in the OA community are readily looking forward to the dawn of a new age when this treatment breaks through, providing fertile ground for further therapeutic development.

The development of many agents is being stopped because of inefficacy in animal models, whereas the human model in which they may ultimately be tried is markedly different. Alternate preclinical methods that more closely mimic the human condition to assess efficacy in humans are highly desirable.

Therapeutic development should be tailored toward the clinical presentation. Typically, OA manifests with prominent symptoms in a limited number of weight-bearing joints or a few hand joints and lacks extra-articular manifestations. As such, it is well suited to local therapy administered by intra-articular injection. Although injection into joints is not without side effects, many products given systemically may have systemic side-effect profiles that would limit their chronic use in OA.

Similarly, it is important to change the current paradigm of focusing on hyaline articular cartilage at the expense of other joint tissues that have a more pivotal role in disease symptoms and etiopathogenesis, especially synovium, bone, fat, meniscus, and ligaments. We need to widen our perspective and study these other important structures and target them appropriately. Cartilage may reflect the underlying condition, but its contribution to symptoms and progression should not be considered in isolation. Obesity is the single most important risk factor for the development of severe OA of the knee and more so than other potentially damaging factors including heredity.[77] Important determinants of the local mechanical environment of the knee joint are the integrity and function of the periarticular muscles, meniscus, and ligaments.[78,79] Despite the prominent role obesity and these target tissues have in disease etiopathogenesis, they do not appear to have been sufficiently targeted through a biologic or pharmacologic approach for OA management. Their importance in disease would suggest that they would be a worthwhile therapeutic target.

SUMMARY

Improving our understanding of tissues in the joint other than hyaline cartilage (especially of bone, fat, meniscus, and synovium) and their role in OA pathophysiology will likely yield treatment breakthroughs. Therapeutic development needs to be viewed with the realization that, because we are treating a complex disease with a wide variety of clinical presentations, one single therapy is unlikely to be effective in treating this heterogeneous condition. We need to pay greater attention to the mechanics of the joint environment in developing therapies. Although promising therapies are being developed, these lessons and obstacles to development must be recognized if they are to be effective.

REFERENCES

1. Nuki G. Osteoarthritis: a problem of joint failure [review]. Z Rheumatol 1999;58(3): 142–7.
2. Eyre DR. Collagens and cartilage matrix homeostasis [review]. Clin Orthop Relat Res 2004;(427 Suppl):S118–22.
3. Guccione AA, Felson DT, Anderson JJ, et al. The effects of specific medical conditions on the functional limitations of elders in the Framingham study. Am J Public Health 1994;84(3):351–8.
4. Hannan MT, Felson DT, Pincus T. Analysis of the discordance between radiographic changes and knee pain in osteoarthritis of the knee. J Rheumatol 2000;27(6):1513–7.
5. Verbruggen G, Verbruggen G. Chondroprotective drugs in degenerative joint diseases. Rheumatology 2006;45(2):129–38 [review].
6. Haguenauer D, Welch V, Shea B, et al. Fluoride for the treatment of postmenopausal osteoporotic fractures: a meta-analysis [see comment]. Osteoporos Int 2000;11(9):727–38.

7. Gossec L, Hawker G, Davis AM, et al. OMERACT/OARSI initiative to define states of severity and indication for joint replacement in hip and knee osteoarthritis. J Rheumatol 2007;34(6):1432–5.

8. Pham T, van der Heijde D, Altman R, et al. OMERACT-OARSI Initiative: Osteoarthritis Research Society International set of responder criteria for osteoarthritis clinical trials revisited. Osteoarthritis & Cartilage 2004;12(5):389–99.

9. Brandt KD, Mazzuca SA, Katz BP, et al. Effects of doxycycline on progression of osteoarthritis: results of a randomized, placebo-controlled, double-blind trial [see comment]. Arthritis Rheum 2005;52(7):2015–25.

10. Dougados M, Nguyen M, Berdah L, et al. Evaluation of the structure-modifying effects of diacerein in hip osteoarthritis: ECHODIAH, a three-year, placebo-controlled trial. Evaluation of the chondromodulating effect of diacerein in OA of the hip [see comment]. Arthritis Rheum 2001;44(11):2539–47.

11. Jacobsen S, Sonne-Holm S, Jacobsen S, et al. Hip dysplasia: a significant risk factor for the development of hip osteoarthritis. A cross-sectional survey. Rheumatology 2005;44(2):211–8.

12. Utting MR, Davies G, Newman JH. Is anterior knee pain a predisposing factor to patellofemoral osteoarthritis? Knee 2005;12(5):362–5.

13. Karlson EW, Mandl LA, Aweh GN, et al. Total hip replacement due to osteoarthritis: the importance of age, obesity, and other modifiable risk factors [see comment]. Am J Med 2003;114(2):93–8.

14. Flugsrud GB, Nordsletten L, Espehaug B, et al. The impact of body mass index on later total hip arthroplasty for primary osteoarthritis: a cohort study in 1.2 million persons. Arthritis Rheum 2006;54(3):802–7.

15. Roos H, Adalberth T, Dahlberg L, et al. Osteoarthritis of the knee after injury to the anterior cruciate ligament or meniscus: the influence of time and age. Osteoarthritis Cartilage 1995;3(4):261–7.

16. Lohmander LS, Ostenberg A, Englund M, et al. High prevalence of knee osteoarthritis, pain, and functional limitations in female soccer players twelve years after anterior cruciate ligament injury. Arthritis Rheum 2004;50(10):3145–52.

17. Englund M, Roos EM, Lohmander LS. Impact of type of meniscal tear on radiographic and symptomatic knee osteoarthritis: a sixteen-year follow-up of meniscectomy with matched controls. Arthritis Rheum 2003;48(8):2178–87.

18. Englund M, Lohmander LS. Risk factors for symptomatic knee osteoarthritis fifteen to twenty-two years after meniscectomy. Arthritis Rheum 2004;50(9):2811–9.

19. Andriacchi TP, Briant PL, Bevill SL, et al. Rotational changes at the knee after ACL injury cause cartilage thinning. Clin Orthop Relat Res 2006;442:39–44.

20. Hunter DJ, Niu J, Zhang Y, et al. Change in cartilage morphometry: a sample of the progression cohort of the Osteoarthritis Initiative. Ann Rheum Dis, in press.

21. Brandt KD, Radin EL, Dieppe PA, et al. Yet more evidence that osteoarthritis is not a cartilage disease [comment]. Ann Rheum Dis 2006;65(10):1261–4.

22. Hunter DJ, Zhang YQ, Tu X, et al. Change in joint space width: hyaline articular cartilage loss or alteration in meniscus? Arthritis Rheum 2006;54(8):2488–95.

23. Hellio Le Graverand MP, Sciore P, Eggerer J, et al. Formation and phenotype of cell clusters in osteoarthritic meniscus. Arthritis Rheum 2001;44(8):1808–18.

24. Hellio Le Graverand MP, Vignon E, Otterness IG, et al. Early changes in lapine menisci during osteoarthritis development. Part I. Cellular and matrix alterations. Osteoarthritis Cartilage 2001;9(1):56–64.

25. Hellio Le Graverand MP, Vignon E, Otterness IG, et al. Early changes in lapine menisci during osteoarthritis development. Part II. Molecular alterations. Osteoarthritis Cartilage 2001;9(1):65–72.

26. Englund M, Roos EM, Roos HP, et al. Patient-relevant outcomes fourteen years after meniscectomy: influence of type of meniscal tear and size of resection. Rheumatology 2001;40(6):631–9.
27. Abramson SB, Attur M, Yazici Y. Prospects for disease modification in osteoarthritis [review]. Nat Clin Pract Rheumatol 2006;2(6):304–12.
28. Hutchinson JW, Tierney GM, Parsons SL, et al. Dupuytren's disease and frozen shoulder induced by treatment with a matrix metalloproteinase inhibitor. J Bone Joint Surg Br 1998;80(5):907–8.
29. Johnson AR, Pavlovsky AG, Ortwine DF, et al. Discovery and characterization of a novel inhibitor of matrix metalloprotease-13 that reduces cartilage damage in vivo without joint fibroplasia side effects. J Biol Chem 2007;282(38):27781–91.
30. Pham T, Le Henanff A, Ravaud P, et al. Evaluation of the symptomatic and structural efficacy of a new hyaluronic acid compound, NRD101, in comparison with diacerein and placebo in a 1 year randomised controlled study in symptomatic knee osteoarthritis. Ann Rheum Dis 2004;63(12):1611–7.
31. Carbone LD, Nevitt MC, Wildy K, et al. The relationship of antiresorptive drug use to structural findings and symptoms of knee osteoarthritis. Arthritis Rheum 2004; 50(11):3516–25.
32. Bingham CO III, Buckland-Wright JC, Garnero P, et al. Risedronate decreases biochemical markers of cartilage degradation but does not decrease symptoms or slow radiographic progression in patients with medial compartment osteoarthritis of the knee: results of the two-year multinational knee osteoarthritis structural arthritis study [see comment]. Arthritis Rheum 2006;54(11):3494–507.
33. Buckland-Wright JC, Messent EA, Bingham CO III, et al. A 2 yr longitudinal radiographic study examining the effect of a bisphosphonate (risedronate) upon subchondral bone loss in osteoarthritic knee patients. Rheumatology 2007;46(2):257–64.
34. Papaioannou NA, Triantafillopoulos IK, Khaldi L, et al. Effect of calcitonin in early and late stages of experimentally induced osteoarthritis: a histomorphometric study. Osteoarthritis Cartilage 2007;15(4):386–95.
35. McAlindon T, Formica M, LaValley M, et al. Effectiveness of glucosamine for symptoms of knee osteoarthritis: results from an Internet-based randomized double-blind controlled trial. Am J Med 2004;117(9):643–9.
36. Towheed TE, Maxwell L, Anastassiades TP, et al. Glucosamine therapy for treating osteoarthritis. Cochrane Database Sys Rev 2005;(2) [review] [update of Cochrane Database Syst Rev 2001;(1):CD002946; PMID:11279782]:CD002946.
37. Clegg DO, Reda DJ, Harris CL, et al. Glucosamine, chondroitin sulfate, and the two in combination for painful knee osteoarthritis [see comment]. N Engl J Med 2006;354(8):795–808.
38. Lo GH, LaValley M, McAlindon T, et al. Intra-articular hyaluronic acid in treatment of knee osteoarthritis: a meta-analysis [see comment]. JAMA 2003;290(23): 3115–21.
39. Jubb RW, Piva S, Beinat L, et al. A one-year, randomised, placebo (saline) controlled clinical trial of 500-730 kDa sodium hyaluronate (Hyalgan) on the radiological change in osteoarthritis of the knee. Int J Clin Pract 2003;57(6):467–74.
40. Reginster JY, Deroisy R, Rovati LC, et al. Long-term effects of glucosamine sulphate on osteoarthritis progression: a randomised, placebo-controlled clinical trial [see comments]. Lancet 2001;357(9252):251–6.
41. Pavelka K, Gatterova J, Olejarova M, et al. Glucosamine sulfate use and delay of progression of knee osteoarthritis: a 3-year, randomized, placebo-controlled, double-blind study. Arch Intern Med 2002;162(18):2113–23.

42. Mazzuca SA, Brandt KD, Lane KA, et al. Knee pain reduces joint space width in conventional standing anteroposterior radiographs of osteoarthritic knees. Arthritis Rheum 2002;46(5):1223–7.
43. Lequesne M, Maheu E, Cadet C, et al. Structural effect of avocado/soybean unsaponifiables on joint space loss in osteoarthritis of the hip. Arthritis Rheum 2002;47(1):50–8.
44. Wieland HA, Michaelis M, Kirschbaum BJ, et al. Osteoarthritis: an untreatable disease? [review]. Nat Rev Drug Discov 2005;4(4):331–44.
45. Hill CL, Gale DG, Chaisson CE, et al. Knee effusions, popliteal cysts, and synovial thickening: association with knee pain in osteoarthritis. J Rheumatol 2001;28(6): 1330–7.
46. Mapp PI, Mapp PI. Innervation of the synovium [review]. Ann Rheum Dis 1995; 54(5):398–403.
47. Safieh-Garabedian B, Poole S, Allchorne A, et al. Contribution of interleukin-1 beta to the inflammation-induced increase in nerve growth factor levels and inflammatory hyperalgesia. Br J Pharmacol 1995;115(7):1265–75.
48. Chen X, Tanner K, Levine JD, et al. Mechanical sensitization of cutaneous C-fiber nociceptors by prostaglandin E_2 in the rat. Neurosci Lett 1999;267(2):105–8.
49. Abramson SB, Amin AR, Clancy RM, et al. The role of nitric oxide in tissue destruction [review]. Best Pract Res Clin Rheumatol 2001;15(5):831–45.
50. McInnes IB, Leung BP, Field M, et al. Production of nitric oxide in the synovial membrane of rheumatoid and osteoarthritis patients. J Exp Med 1996;184(4): 1519–24.
51. Nishida K, Doi T, Matsuo M, et al. Involvement of nitric oxide in chondrocyte cell death in chondro-osteophyte formation. Osteoarthritis Cartilage 2001;9(3):232–7.
52. Pelletier JP, Jovanovic D, Fernandes JC, et al. Reduced progression of experimental osteoarthritis in vivo by selective inhibition of inducible nitric oxide synthase. Arthritis Rheum 1998;41(7):1275–86.
53. Salvemini D, Wang ZQ, Wyatt PS, et al. Nitric oxide: a key mediator in the early and late phase of carrageenan-induced rat paw inflammation. Br J Pharmacol 1996;118(4):829–38.
54. Levy D, Kubes P, Zochodne DW. Delayed peripheral nerve degeneration, regeneration, and pain in mice lacking inducible nitric oxide synthase. J Neuropathol Exp Neurol 2001;60(5):411–21.
55. Manning DC, Raja SN, Meyer RA, et al. Pain and hyperalgesia after intradermal injection of bradykinin in humans. Clin Pharmacol Ther 1991;50(6):721–9.
56. Flechtenmacher J, Talke M, Veith D, et al. Bradykinin receptor inhibition: a therapeutic option in osteoarthritis? [abstract]. Osteoarthritis Cartilage 2004;12(Suppl 1002).
57. Walsh DA, Walsh DA. Angiogenesis in osteoarthritis and spondylosis: successful repair with undesirable outcomes [review]. Curr Opin Rheumatol 2004;16(5): 609–15.
58. Gigante A, Bevilacqua C, Pagnotta A, et al. Expression of NGF, Trka and p75 in human cartilage. Eur J Histochem 2003;47(4):339–44.
59. Manni L, Lundeberg T, Fiorito S, et al. Nerve growth factor release by human synovial fibroblasts prior to and following exposure to tumor necrosis factor-alpha, interleukin-1 beta and cholecystokinin-8: the possible role of NGF in the inflammatory response. Clin Exp Rheumatol 2003;21(5):617–24.
60. Lane N, Webster L, Lu S, et al. RN624 (anti-NGF) improves pain and function in subjects with moderate knee osteoarthritis: a phase I study [abstract]. Osteoarthritis & Cartilage 2005;1206:S461.

61. Chevalier X, Mugnier B, Bouvenot G, et al. Targeted anti-cytokine therapies for osteoarthritis [review] [French]. Bull Acad Natl Med 1475;190(7):1411–20.
62. Sandell LJ. Anabolic factors in degenerative joint disease [review]. Curr Drug Targets 2007;8(2):359–65.
63. Bonnet CS, Walsh DA. Osteoarthritis, angiogenesis and inflammation [review]. Rheumatology 2005;44(1):7–16.
64. Simkin PA. Bone pain and pressure in osteoarthritic joints [review]. Novartis Foundation Symposium 2004;260:179–86.
65. Meizer R, Radda C, Stolz G, et al. MRI-controlled analysis of 104 patients with painful bone marrow edema in different joint localizations treated with the prostacyclin analogue iloprost. Wien Klin Wochenschr 2005;117(7–8):278–86.
66. Mayerhoefer ME, Kramer J, Breitenseher MJ, et al. Short-term outcome of painful bone marrow oedema of the knee following oral treatment with iloprost or tramadol: results of an exploratory phase II study of 41 patients. Rheumatology 2007; 46(9):1460–5.
67. Rudolphi K, Gerwin N, Verzijl N, et al. Pralnacasan, an inhibitor of interleukin-1 beta converting enzyme, reduces joint damage in two murine models of osteoarthritis. Osteoarthritis Cartilage 2003;11(10):738–46.
68. Zhang X, Mao Z, Yu C, et al. Suppression of early experimental osteoarthritis by gene transfer of interleukin-1 receptor antagonist and interleukin-10. J Orthop Res 2004;22(4):742–50.
69. Salminen-Mankonen HJ, Morko J, Vuorio E, et al. Role of cathepsin K in normal joints and in the development of arthritis [review]. Curr Drug Targets 2007;8(2): 315–23.
70. Glasson SS, Askew R, Sheppard B, et al. Deletion of active ADAMTS5 prevents cartilage degradation in a murine model of osteoarthritis. Nature 2005;434(7033): 644–8.
71. Hunter D. In the clinic: osteoarthritis [review]. Ann Intern Med 2007;147(3):ITC8.
72. Sharma L, Song J, Felson DT, et al. The role of knee alignment in disease progression and functional decline in knee osteoarthritis [erratum appears in JAMA 2001;286(7):792]. JAMA 2001;286(2):188–95.
73. Andriacchi TP. Dynamics of knee malalignment [review]. Orthop Clin North Am 1994;25(3):395–403.
74. Schipplein OD, Andriacchi TP. Interaction between active and passive knee stabilizers during level walking. J Orthop Res 1991;9(1):113–9.
75. Hawker GA, Davis AM, French M, et al. Development and preliminary psychometric testing of a new OA pain measure: an OARSI/OMERACT initiative. Osteoarthritis Cartilage 2008;16(4):409–14.
76. Davis A, Perruccio A, Canizares M, et al. The development of a short measure of physical function for hip OA: HOOS-Physical Function Shortform (HOOS-PS). An OARSI/OMERACT initiative. Osteoarthritis Cartilage 2008;16(5):551–9.
77. Coggon D, Reading I, Croft P, et al. Knee osteoarthritis and obesity. Int J Obes Relat Metab Disord 2001;25(5):622–7.
78. Seedhom BB, Dowson D, Wright V. Proceedings: functions of the menisci. A preliminary study. Ann Rheum Dis 1974;33(1):111.
79. Verstraete KL, Verdonk R, Lootens T, et al. Current status and imaging of allograft meniscal transplantation [review]. Eur J Radiol 1997;26(1):16–22.

Index

Note: Page numbers of article titles are in **boldface** type.

A

Acetaminophen, 133, 200
ADAM12, 52
Aggrecanase inhibitors, 227
Alendronate, 225
Alpha1 antiproteinase antitrypsin, 52
American College of Rheumatology, diagnostic criteria of, 127
Analgesics, 199–201
Ankle osteoarthritis, 108
Antioxidants, 204
Arthritis, Diet, and Activity Program Trial, 149
Arthroplasty, knee
    interpositional, 215
    unicompartmental, 215–217
Arthroscopy, knee, 212–213
Asporin, 52
Association studies, genetic, 51–56
Avocado-soybean unsaponifiables, 225

B

Balance, loss of, 144
Bisphosphonates, 225
Bone
    changes in, **25–35**
        adaptive, 25–28
        cysts, 30–31
        in meniscal lesions, **37–42**
        marrow edema, 30–31
        osteophytes, 31–32
        patterns of, 28–29
        structural, 25–28
        subchondral, 29–30
        tidemark advancement in, 30
        trabecular, 29–30
    pain originating in, 14–16
Bone marrow lesions, 30–31, 86
    nuclear medicine studies of, 104
    pain originating in, 15–16

Med Clin N Am 93 (2009) 235–243
doi:10.1016/S0025-7125(08)00172-7
0025-7125/08/$ – see front matter © 2008 Elsevier Inc. All rights reserved.

medical.theclinics.com

Moving?

Make sure your subscription moves with you!

To notify us of your new address, find your **Clinics Account Number** (located on your mailing label above your name), and contact customer service at:

E-mail: elspcs@elsevier.com

800-654-2452 (subscribers in the U.S. & Canada)
314-453-7041 (subscribers outside of the U.S. & Canada)

Fax number: 314-523-5170

Elsevier Periodicals Customer Service
11830 Westline Industrial Drive
St. Louis, MO 63146

*To ensure uninterrupted delivery of your subscription, please notify us at least 4 weeks in advance of move.

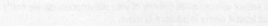